FROM ABSTRACT INTO ACTION

JEROME P. LYSAUGHT, Ed.D.
Director

*The National Commission for the Study of
Nursing and Nursing Education*

FROM ABSTRACT INTO ACTION

A nursing classic
.94

"Landmark Study"
SH 2/07

McGRAW-HILL BOOK COMPANY

A Blakiston Publication

*New York St. Louis San Francisco Dusseldorf Johannesburg
Kuala Lumpur London Mexico Montreal New Delhi Panama
Rio de Janeiro Singapore Sydney Toronto*

FROM ABSTRACT INTO ACTION

Library of Congress Cataloging in Publication Data

National Commission for the Study of Nursing and Nursing Education.
From abstract into action.

"A Blackiston publication."
1. Nurses and Nursing--Study and teaching--United States. I. Lysaught, Jerome P., ed. II. Title. [DNLM: 1. Education, Nursing--U. S. 2. Nursing--U. S. WY18 N273f 1973]
RT81.U6N26 1973 610.73'0973 73-10106
ISBN 0-07-045840-5 (pbk.)
ISBN 0-07-045841-3

1234567890 MAMB 79376543

This book was set in Press Roman by Creative Book Services, division of McGregor & Werner, Inc. The editor was Cathy Dilworth; the designer was Creative Book Services; and the production supervisor was Judi Frey. The printer and binder was The Maple Press Company.

This implementation effort
was supported by the W. K. Kellogg Foundation,
the American Nurses' Association,
the National League for Nursing,
and private individuals.

Contents

COMMISSIONERS

President of the Commission

LEROY E. BURNEY, M.D.

President
Milbank Memorial Fund
New York, New York

Vice President of the Commission

BOISFEUILLET JONES, LL.B.

President
Emily and Ernest Woodruff Foundation
Atlanta, Georgia

Secretary of the Commission

ELEANOR LAMBERTSEN, Ed.D.*

Dean, School of Nursing
Cornell University—New York Hospital
New York, New York

*Indicates members of Commission during study phase.

Members of the Commission

MARGARET B. DOLAN *
Head, Department of Public Health Nursing
School of Public Health
University of North Carolina
Chapel Hill, North Carolina

JOAN GUY
Executive Director
Michigan State Nurses' Association
East Lansing, Michigan

JOSEPH HAMBURG, M.D.
Dean
College of Allied Health Professions
University of Kentucky
Lexington, Kentucky

JAMES G. HAUGHTON, M.D.
Executive Director
Cook County Hospitals Governing Commission
Chicago, Illinois

C. A. HOFFMAN, M.D.
President
American Medical Association
Huntington, West Virginia

WILLIAM N. HUBBARD, Jr., M.D.
Vice President and General Manager
Pharmaceutical Division
The Upjohn Company
Kalamazoo, Michigan

LOIS TURNER JONES
Director
Playhouse Academy
Omaha, Nebraska

ANNE K. KIBRICK, Ed.D.
Chairman, Department of Nursing
Graduate School of Arts and Sciences
Boston College
Chestnut Hill, Massachusetts

*Indicates members of Commission during study phase.

MARY JANE McCARTHY*
Chief, Nursing Service
Veterans Administration Hospital
Dallas, Texas

LEONARD F. McCOLLUM*
Former Chairman of the Board
Continental Oil Company
Houston, Texas

STUART J. MARYLANDER
Executive Director
Cedars-Sinai Medical Center
Los Angeles, California

CHARLES S. PAXSON, Jr.
Executive Vice President
Hahnemann Medical College and Hospital
Philadelphia, Pennsylvania

JOHN D. PORTERFIELD, M.D.
Director
Joint Commission on Accreditation of Hospitals
Chicago, Illinois

BARBARA A. RESNIK
Associate Clinical Professor
Community Health Nursing
Division of Ambulatory and Community Medicine
School of Medicine
University of California
San Francisco, California

RALPH W. TYLER, Ph.D.*
Former Director
Center for Advanced Study in Behavioral Sciences, Palo Alto
Chicago, Illinois

HAROLD B. WISE, M.D.
Former Project Director
Martin Luther King, Jr., Health Center
New York, New York

*Indicates members of Commission during study phase.

NATIONAL ADVISORY COUNCIL*

RAY EVERETT BROWN
Executive Vice President
Northwestern University Medical Center
Chicago, Illinois

LOWELL T. COGGESHALL, M.D.
Former Assistant to the Secretary of Health, Education, and Welfare
Foley, Alabama

DOROTHY A. CORNELIUS
Executive Director
Ohio Nurses' Association
Columbus, Ohio

MARION B. FOLSOM
Former Secretary of Health, Education, and Welfare
Rochester, New York

WALTER E. HOADLEY, Ph.D.
Executive Vice President
Bank of America
National Trust and Savings Association
San Francisco, California

HERBERT E. LONGENECKER, Ph.D.
President
Tulane University
New Orleans, Louisiana

ROBERT K. MERTON, Ph.D.
Giddings Professor of Sociology
Department of Sociology
Columbia University
New York, New York

W. ALLEN WALLIS
Chancellor
University of Rochester
Rochester, New York

*All members of the Council previously had served as members of the Commission.

NATIONAL STAFF

DR. JEROME P. LYSAUGHT
Director

MS. SYDNEY A. SUTHERLAND
Assistant to the Director

MS. MARYANN E. PIERLEONI*
Staff Associate

DR. NATALIE S. PAVLOVICH
Staff Associate

MS. GILDA M. ORIOLI
Secretary

MS. ANN C. MURPHY
Secretary

Regional Associates

MYRTLE AYDELOTTE
Director, Department of Nursing Service
The University of Iowa
Iowa City, Iowa

*1070-72

VIRGINIA Z. BARHAM
Nursing Consultant
The Permanente Medical Groupe
Oakland, California

LUTHER CHRISTMAN
Dean, Rush College of Nursing and Allied Health Sciences
Rush-Presbyterian-St. Luke's Medical Center
Chicago, Illinois

GRACE L. DELOUGHERY
Dean, Inter-Collegiate Center of Nursing Education
Spokane, Washington

CHARLES H. RUSSELL
Dean of Instruction
Mattatuck Community College
Waterbury, Connecticut

MARYANN E. PIERLEONI**
Nurse Practitioner
Overland Park, Kansas

Preface

This volume is the report on the implementation efforts of the National Commission for the Study of Nursing and Nursing Education. It is a commentary on three years of effort to effect change in the health care system of the United States, particularly in the areas of nursing roles and functions, nursing education, and nursing careers.

Over the course of this work, progress has been made in many vital areas and disappointments have been experienced as well. This report attempts to discuss candidly and frankly what has been done, what have been the outcomes, and what remains as the unfinished agenda for others to take up.

It is essential that we express our gratitude to the W. K. Kellogg Foundation, to the American Nurses' Association, and to the National League for Nursing for their financial support and for their organizational aid throughout the course of these months. To the officers and directors, to the leaders and staffs of ANA and NLN, we express our appreciation for their initial organization of the Commission and for their subsequent involvement in the implementation phase. In particular, we thank Eileen Jacobi and Margaret Walsh for their help and interest.

The Commission has been unusual in its willingness to persevere and to seek implementation of its report long after many groups might have turned to other pursuits. It is entirely in keeping with its long-term commitment to an enhanced profession of nursing that it has planned a longitudinal follow-up in 1976 to consider the impact of its recommendations on the health care system of that day. The protocols for that assessment are provided in Appendix D to this volume.

To the Commissioners, present and former, I would like to express the appreciation of the staff and the advisory groups who have worked throughout the implementation effort. Your individual and collective wisdom, aid, and encouragement, bolstered by unerring composure, have made this work enjoyable as well as productive. While we know your greatest satisfactions will stem from the outcomes of processes still underway, we trust that our advances to date have been some reward for your time and effort.

Finally, our thanks must go to the McGraw-Hill Book Company, which has made remarkable efforts to ensure that the publication of this report is accomplished by the fall of 1973. Joseph Brehm, Cathy Dilworth, and Mary Murray have worked heroically, both on the earlier volumes and on this, to ensure that maximum currency and impact are provided. The Commission and staff are very grateful.

Jerome P. Lysaught

June 6, 1973

Acknowledgments

It is literally impossible to name, let alone fully acknowledge, the individuals who have contributed to the implementation phase of the Commission's work. We know of the graduate student in Indiana who personally took responsibility for contacting each area of the state to inform district nurses' groups about *An Abstract for Action.* We know of the nurse educator in Florida who broke all tradition with her announcement that a community college would offer a program in distributive nursing practice. We know of the practitioner in California who resigned from her position with a group of nursing homes after reviewing the Commission's writings on professional commitment and reflecting on the care being provided in the institutions she served. We know of the former nurse in Arkansas who provided a professional clipping service to our staff throughout the implementation period so that we might follow events in health care concerns over that state. These we know.

We know, too, the contributions of the Commissioners. The physicians who represented the viewpoint of joint practice with sometimes doubtful, sometimes hostile, colleagues. The hospital administrators who represented the concept of altered educational patterns to disapproving contemporaries. The consumer representatives and educators who represented enhanced career perspectives to the uninvolved, unconcerned public. The nurses who, in season and out, had to represent the Commission and staff in every real and imaginary circumstance to their 1,400,000 fellows. These, too, we know

We know the contributions of our regional associates and advisors and speakers' bureau. They have helped to carry the Commission's message to every state and to every organization that has called upon us. They have helped establish the enduring apparatus that will continue to effect change over the months and years ahead. These we know very well.

We know the contributions of staff people from state and national nursing organizations. We know the help afforded us by staff from medical societies and hospital associations, as well, at state and national levels. We know the support of individuals who served on committees, commissions, task forces, and all the other organizational paraphenalia that are involved in the planning, carrying out, and following up that are part and parcel to the perpetuation of our health care system.

We know the assistance of public officials and civil servants at all levels of government. We know their concerns and their dedication to improved health care in our society, and we know that our efforts have been magnified through their help.

In a very personal way, I know better than anyone the contributions of staff members. I know what Maryann Pierleoni and, later, Natalie Pavlovich did in working with our target states and on a host of other assignments. I know what Sydney Sutherland did in constructing the National Joint Practice Commission and in serving every aspect of our effort. I know that Jill Orioli, Bernie Trombetta, and Ann Murphy did in making our work efficient and effective.

What we will never know are the names of all those across the country who, at this time of critical need, made their own personal, professional commitment and contribution to change. Their actions, their prayers, and their support have sustained us throughout. To the unsung nurse and student, this work is truly dedicated. May yours be that unambiguous profession for which we have all striven.

Jerome P. Lysaught

June 25, 1973

ONE

PURPOSES, PRIORITIES, AND INITIAL ORGANIZATION FOR IMPLEMENTATION

In June of 1970, the National Commission for the Study of Nursing and Nursing Education culminated three years of study and analysis by publishing its report, *An Abstract for Action.*[1] This volume, together with a supplementary collection of *Appendices,*[2] described the findings, reported the conclusions, and proposed a series of recommendations intended to "improve the delivery of health care to the American people, particularly through the analysis and improvement of nursing and nursing education."

Six months earlier, the Commission had unanimously arrived at a decision to seek support and funding for an intensive period of implementation effort to follow the investigation and reporting phase. In communicating this decision to Emory W. Morris, then president and general director of the W. K. Kellogg Foundation, the president of the National Commission, W. Allen Wallis, said:

> Over the past several decades, beginning with the Goldmark study in 1923, continuing through the Brown report in 1948, and reinforced by the many state and regional studies recently completed or currently in progress, there has been widespread agreement concerning the advisability of enacting certain changes in nursing and nursing education. It is a distressing fact that lack of evidence of implementation has necessitated periodic repetition of such recommendations over nearly a half century.[3]

On cogitating the outcomes of prior studies—and their impact on the health care delivery system—the Commission determined that something different should be attempted *this time.* As the Wallis letter continued:

> A major intent of this Commission has always been that its report might include the mechanisms that could facilitate enactment of its recommendations—in the hope that 1990 will not see the funding of yet another study of nursing urging the profession and the public to look once again at these proposals for change.[4]

As one example of the consistent thread that has connected the long series of nursing studies, we need look no farther than the basic educational pattern for preparatory competence. In 1923, Josephine Goldmark[5] urged that nursing education move toward a collegiate system of education. Because of the controversial nature of that suggestion, and because of the economic impact of the great depression, little enough was done that in 1948 two other nursing studies, that of Brown[6] and of Ginzberg[7], again recommended this change—with increased urgency. Five years later, Bridgman[8] still found it necessary to return to the same theme and urge the ultimate merger of preparatory nursing education in the collegiate system. In the light of these recommendations, it is somewhat disconcerting to find that the National Commission in its 1970 report is again required to reiterate, "We feel that nursing education should be structured within the overall pattern of higher education, that is, within the collegiate institutions. . . ."[9]

For the better part of fifty years, then, there has been consistent agreement from independent and competent observers about this one particular aspect of nursing education. Yet, over that period of time, insufficient progress had been made in terms of change to permit the current Commission to pass on totally to other concerns. And this, of course, is illustrative of proposals in nursing education, practice, and career perspectives.

Not all of the recommendations of the National Commission had been anticipated by these earlier studies. It is significant to note, however, that much of the difference in emphasis, from one report to another, could better be attributed to those things that had happened in the general social and economic environment of the nation than to specific changes recorded as responses to prior proposals. Thus, differences in specific suggestions for nursing education reflected more surely the increasing acceptance of fourteen years of general education as the norm of public schooling, the phenomenal growth of the community and junior colleges after the Second World War, and the general upswing in the economy over the fifties and sixties rather than the reconstruction of patterns for nursing education per se.

Also, in fairness, it must be emphasized that social change can only occur when needs and proposals are seen in a positive relationship—and at a time favorable to "unfreezing" the status quo to facilitate movement toward a new configuration. If Goldmark, Brown, and others did not always succeed in their efforts to institute change, they nevertheless fostered an understanding among nurses, other health professionals, and the lay public concerning the need to solve some of these continuing problems. These prior investigators were never "voices crying in the wilderness," but they surely were those "who went before to prepare the way."

As the National Commission assessed the situation in early December of 1969,

> . . . [Our conferences with representatives of] nursing, medicine, health administration, health resource planning, educators and economists, and . . . individuals who are either providers or recipients of health care, have been a major resource in the formulation of the proposals and recommendations included in the report. Our contacts with these many representatives convince us that compromise and change are possible at this vital point in time. It is apparent in all these discussions, however, that widespread implementation will depend upon the existence of a definite, planned course of action to follow termination of the research work of the present Commission.[10]

The Commission then proposed to the W. K. Kellogg Foundation that support be given to the continuation of the body's life beyond the investigation phase, and that a three-year implementation effort be mounted. While such a period of time could hardly be expected to afford the opportunity to install each of the almost sixty specific recommendations in the final report, it would provide an opportunity to develop widespread understanding and participation among the affected publics, plan specific activities for overcoming initial inertia, and make substantial progress in the desired directions. Through such means, some success should be realized and an example established for succeeding implementation efforts.

OBJECTIVES OF THE IMPLEMENTATION EFFORT

In a broad sense, the overall objective of the implementation phase was to secure the enactment of each and all of the Commission's recommendations proposed in *An Abstract for Action.* Common sense and a recognition of the need to build relationships indicated, however, that more limited objectives established with a clear order of priorities had to be our principal approach. The primary thrust of the implementation phase could be derived from the areas of emphasis contained in the Commission report: These include:

1. The development and expansion of nursing practice together with a reexamination of role relationships among the health professions;
2. The repatterning of educational systems in nursing to meet current exigencies and provide a foundation for innovation; and
3. The emergence of an unambiguous profession that would, in fact, be

> a full partner in shaping health policy and in serving the needs of our people.[11]

There was, however, an even more fundamental task of education, better stated perhaps as reeducation, that had to precede a direct attack upon these concerns. This was the internalized reaction of many people to the familiar phrase, "manpower needs and supply." Since the Second World War, we have been so conditioned by the man- or woman-power needs in nursing that we have developed a conditioned verbal reflex. Just as we couple *day* with *night, right* with *wrong*, and *boy* with *girl*, most Americans will react to the word *nurse* with the label *shortage.*

The pervasive aspect of this perception is so encompassing that it played a significant part in the very establishment of the National Commission. In its 1963 report, *Toward Quality in Nursing,*[12] the Surgeon General's Consultant Group on Nursing recommended a national investigation to examine nursing education and high quality patient care, with concern for the numbers and kinds of individuals required. This group to some extent mirrored a host of commissions, committees, and task forces, working at federal, state, and local levels, most of which saw the "problems" of nursing as centering on a lack of personnel. This, in turn, channeled most solutions into concerns for increasing the supply—by recruitment, enlargement of programs, increased numbers of schools, etc.

Out of the Commission's study of nursing and nursing education, however, it was determined that the "shortage" of nurses is not nearly so simple and straightforward as is commonly considered. For example, over the twenty-year period from 1951 to 1971 the number of nurses in practice grew from 375,000 to 723,000, an increase of 93 percent. Over the same period of time, the nurse-to-population ratio climbed from 249 to 353 per 100,000.[13] Thus, the supply of nursing manpower not only grew significantly, but increased faster than our population, as indicated by the companion curves of Figure 1-1.

As a comparison, the profession of medicine over the same period of time was making valiant efforts to increase the number of its practitioners. Millions of dollars were laid out for new schools, improved teaching facilities, larger student classes, and faculty support. Yet over this twenty-year span, the number of active physicians climbed from 208,997 to 311,203, an increase of only 49 per cent. (Incidentally, the figure for 1971 includes more than 48,000 foreign medical graduates who were actively providing patient care; therefore, our internal growth rate was really only 26 percent.) The ratio of practicing physicians to population grew from 141 to 149 per 100,000, a figure which should be increased slightly to account for osteopathic physicians not included in the data thus presented.

The point, however, is not to make a judgment about these two professions' growth rates so much as to emphasize that nursing has done a remarkable job of responding to the public's demand for more health practitioners. In twenty years, it has almost doubled its numbers, and has increased the nurse-to-population ratio by 42 percent. Thus, by any standard of measurement, we have seen significant

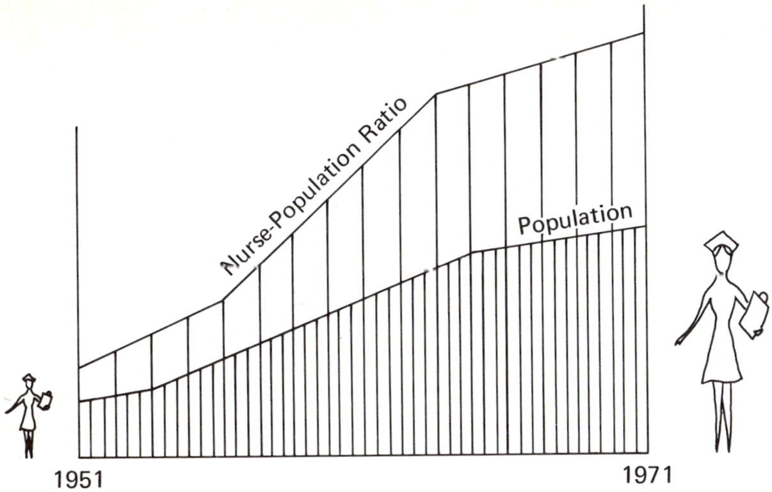

Figure 1-1. Relative growth of population and nurse-population ratios. The two-decade period from 1951 to 1971 provides a clear demarcation and a frequently used comparison period. Updated figures indicate that trends and analyses are continuing without deflection. At the end of 1972, there were 748,000 nurses in practice, a ratio of 361 per 100,000 population.

growth. A summary review of the relationship between actual manpower figures and previous estimates of need reveals the pattern displayed by Table 1-1. In short, over the period considered, most national estimates for nursing manpower needs have been equalled or exceeded. And, by straight line projection through 1975, or perhaps even 1980, it would appear that all but the most extreme forecasts of nurse

TABLE 1-1 COMPARISON OF FORECAST REQUIREMENTS FOR NURSING MANPOWER WITH ACTUAL SUPPLY

Estimating Agency	Forecast Need	Year	Actual Supply
U.S. Department of Labor	620,000	1966	621,000
U.S. Public Health Service	600,000	1966	621,000
Surgeon General's Consultant Group on Nursing	637,000	1968	659,000
Surgeon General's Consultant Group on Nursing	680,000	1970	700,000

Source: National Commission for the Study of Nursing and Nursing Education. *An Abstract for Action.*, Jerome P. Lysaught, Director. New York: McGraw-Hill Book Co., 1970, pp 50-52.

manpower requirements will continue to be met through the natural annual growth of the profession.

Why then is there so much concern over the matter of nurse manpower? In part, it is a lack of understanding of nursing's positive response to personnel quotas and goals. And, additionally, it includes related phenomena that are often confused with a national manpower shortage. There is, for example, a considerable maldistribution of nurses across the United States—just as there is a maldistribution of physicians, surgeons, and other health practitioners. Table 1-2 reflects the patterns to be observed among the states. Obviously, some states and regions are wealthy and some are poor in their relative nurse resources. These figures, however, are closely related to general population movements, and we find within states that there are areas, such as the urban ghetto or the rural community, which vary as considerably as does one state from another. The point to be made is that manpower maldistribution is different from manpower shortage per se, and must be attacked differently.

Of even greater significance, however, is the matter of retention in nursing. So long as we have concentrated on manpower shortage to the exclusion of other concerns, we have been emphasizing the supply curve without regard for the demand side of the picture. Economists and statisticians would find this peculiar in any event, but particularly so in the light of data on retention within the profession. As indicated in Figure 1-2, there is an extremely high withdrawal rate from nursing that materially affects our balance of manpower needs and supply.

Any enthusiasm we may have garnered over the growth rate in American nursing is rapidly chastened when we examine the withdrawal rate from the profession. While we have most certainly increased the numbers, and the nurse-

TABLE 1-2 COMPARISON OF NURSE-POPULATION RATIOS IN SELECTED STATES (1966)

State	Nurse-Population Ratio (per 100,000 persons)
Connecticut	536
District of Columbia	454
Colorado	425
National average	*313*
Utah	233
Mississippi	157
Arkansas	133

Source: *Facts About Nursing, 1970-71 Edition.* New York: American Nurses' Association, 1972.

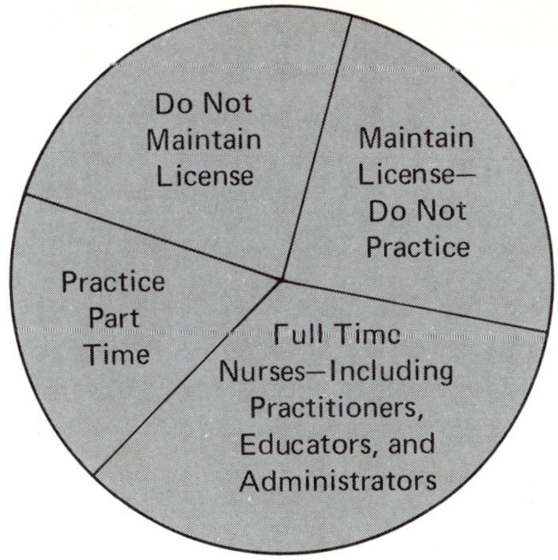

Figure 1-2. Professional activity level among American nurses.

client ratio, in practice, we have suffered sobering losses from the potential numbers we might have attained. In Figure 1-2, we have a graphic commentary on the "staying power" of nurses in professional practice. Of more than 1,400,000 registered nurses, almost one out of every four is totally inactive. Another 25 percent is active only to the extent of maintaining a license. Of the remaining 50 percent, almost one out of every three is a part-time nurse. Thus, our manpower "pool" has shrunk to approximately 525,000 full-time nurses, and this figure, of course, includes nurse educators, administrators, supervisors, and all manner of practitioners.

In the highest of all recorded estimates for future nursing personnel, the National Planning Association called for a total of 1,091,000 by 1975.[14] This figure, which seems so extreme, could be achieved by now were it not for the withdrawal of nurses from the profession—or, more accurately, our failure to retain them in active practice.

The entire sweep of the National Commission's recommendations—and their implementation—has been designed to provide a long-term solution to these vexing problems of maldistribution and retention. In terms of our more specific objectives, however, we found it necessary to reiterate time and time again that the "shortage" of nurses is a much more complicated thing than can be solved by merely urging recruitment, enlarged classes, and increased numbers of schools. These approaches which have been so often exercised and urged in the past are, in effect, only treating the symptoms of the problem. We need to address the underlying causes. And the causes are to be found in the difficulties which nurses encounter in practice roles and functions, education, and career perspectives. Solution of these difficulties will, in turn, obviate the concerns we have so long experienced in terms of manpower needs and shortages.

Nursing Roles and Functions

In its investigation of American nursing, the National Commission pointed out a paradox of the first dimension. While the overwhelming majority of nursing students select the program because of their wish to "help people" and to render care,[15] our utilization patterns tend inexorably to draw them away from direct patient involvement. The pyramidal structure of most health care facilities encourages the nurse to gravitate upward on the organizational chart to a point where contact with the patient, or client, is lost and the nurse, at best, may be one or two levels removed from where care is being dispensed.[16]

Related to this problem is the concurrent desire on the part of many nurses to expand their role in professional practice at the same time that physicians are reexamining their functions in an effort to make optimum use of their own time and skills. In the past, we have too often taken a cavalier attitude toward changing assigned roles and functions. Unilateral decisions have been announced, whole new occupations have emerged, and yet few are satisfied that we have significantly improved health care.

In order to meet the public need, and to encourage the interdisciplinary and interprofessional planning that is necessary to accomplish rational change, the Commission proposed that a first step in expanding nursing roles and functions would be to establish a joint committee between medicine and nursing to explore their mutual concerns and their congruent roles in a time of changing health care patterns and demands.[17]

Still another facet of the Commission's findings in the area of roles and functions is that there is serious need for redevelopment of nursing resources in terms of the articulated demands of our society. Most of the emphasis in nursing care–like that of other health professions–has been placed on episodic practice, that is, the provision of needed intervention to the acutely unwell person generally in the confines of an in-patient facility. Important as this care is, it has been estimated that perhaps fewer than 15 percent of actual health care problems are those related to cure, while more than 85 percent of the difficulties people encounter are really ones of a different dimension–health education, periodic examination, dietary advice, immunization, and nonacute regimens. To distinguish these kinds of care from episodic practice, the National Commission termed them *distributive*–care that is generally continuous in nature, seldom acute, taking place in community or emergent institutional settings and essentially aimed at health maintenance and disease prevention.[18]

In all, the National Commission recommended seventeen proposals in the area of nursing roles and functions that would get at the root problems of practice. In terms of specific priorities, however, a more modest agenda was established. The Commission and its staff proposed for the period of implementation to:

1. Secure the establishment of a National Joint Practice Commission between medicine and nursing to study and make proposals concerning new roles and functions for both professions.

2. Encourage the development of state counterpart committees of nurses and physicians to consider more specific and immediate needs and to interact with the national group in planning and obtaining change.

3. Stimulate nursing, the other health professions, and the consumer public to the possibilities of enlarged emphasis on distributive care, to the need for more health practitioners for that area, and the concomitant demands on facilities and personnel to change traditional patterns of operation.

4. Advocate the reexamination of traditional utilization patterns in nursing service so as to increase involvement of nurses in direct patient care and divest them of non-nursing functions—both to enhance patient care and improve the retention of nurse practitioners within the profession.

These, then, were the primary objectives of the implementation phase in the area of nursing roles and functions. In attacking them, the National Commission sought to accomplish indirectly many of the other specific recommendations—or at least to facilitate their later accomplishment through the amelioration afforded by the initial goals.

Nursing Education

One of the deep-rooted problems that has long beset nursing, and in turn the retention of its individual practitioners, is that of educational patterning. Like medicine, law, and education, nursing began with an apprentice-type approach to preparatory training. Unlike the other three professions, nursing is today still characterized by a bifurcated educational system. Slightly more than half of the preparatory programs for nursing education now reside in collegiate institutions; slightly less than half are housed in the hospital schools of nursing outside the common pattern of American higher education. While this may seem to be a matter of mere curiosity, it has tremendous import for hundreds of thousands of students who find their recognition, career mobility, and personal opportunity seriously affected. Nationwide, there has been a strong movement toward the development of a collegiate system of nursing education. From state to state, however, the pace of change has varied acutely. In the light of this somewhat confusing picture, the National Commission urged that nursing education be positioned within the mainstream of American collegiate education—and that master planning committees be erected in each state to establish guidelines and deadlines for the repatterning of the educational system.[19]

One of the major trends that has occurred in nursing education is the emergence of the two-year community or junior college as a primary agency in the preparation of beginning practitioners. As the hospital schools have declined in number, the greatest growth has taken place in these comparatively new institutions—colleges that have developed, for the most part, in the last twenty years. Unfortunately, the fact that two-year colleges have replaced noncollegiate institutions as preparatory programs has not, of itself, eliminated the problems of student mobility and curricular articulation. There are instances in which the psychological distance between the two- and four-year colleges is every bit as wide as that between a baccalaureate program and a hospital school. Absolutely unwilling to substitute one form of frustration for another, the National Commission urged the joint planning of articulated programs between and among the institutions for nursing education and proposed a concerted approach on statewide and regional bases to ensure the maximum freedom of movement along an educational career ladder.[20]

Because of the intense emphasis on the "manpower shortage" assumed to exist in nursing, the Commission became convinced that preparatory programs in nursing had received proportionately more attention than other necessary aspects of a total educational plan for professional development. Continuing and in-service education are extremely necessary, but seldom given the priority or support that they deserve. Graduate education in nursing, particularly in areas of expanded practice, faces many problems in terms of faculty availability, institutional support, and economic efficiency. At the same time, however, there has been a rapid expansion in some states of both preparatory and advanced programs in nursing that bespeaks a lack of interinstitutional planning and farsightedness. For all these reasons, the National Commission proposed that the master planning committees in each state look to the postpreparatory programs as well and seek regional and statewide approaches to handling the thorny problems of resources and allocations.[21]

Finally, there is the matter of ensuring that changing roles and functions in practice are anticipated and constructively advanced by the educational institutions. The vast majority of preparatory programs in nursing are primarily aimed at producing beginning practitioners for episodic care. The student nurse is prepared to give care to acutely ill patients in an institutional setting within a range of practices generally referred to as interventions. This educational approach is so pervasive that it is often referred to as "general nursing." In reality, as measured against health care needs of society, it is a very specialized form of nursing practice. Our Commission feels that we should identify more clearly than ever before what truly constitutes a general core in nursing preparation and then provide opportunities for elective concentrations in *both* episodic and distributive care so that we produce the practitioners needed in the evolving health care system that is already becoming discernible.[22]

To approach these and related concerns, the National Commission proposed twenty-two specific recommendations in the area of nursing education. In total, these were designed to eliminate most of the frustrations and impediments encountered by nurses wishing to expand their career opportunities. At the same time, the recommendations were intended to provide advanced and continuing education for improved practice in substantially better fashion than is found today. And, in both preparatory and graduate programs, the recommendations would provide for the inclusion of a broad range of clinical electives that adequately reflect the health care needs of all our people. Again, specific priorities for emphasis were established in the belief that advances made on some issues would help in the general implementation of other recommendations. The Commission and staff intended to:

1. Seek the establishment of statewide master planning committees to take nursing education under their purview for the purpose of determining and recommending needed changes, guidelines, and timetables for improvement of the institutional patterns and use of resources.
2. Encourage the development of articulated programs and curricula between two- and four-year programs so that an educational ladder might surely be established in nursing education.
3. Advocate the construction of electives, alternatives, and clinical concentrations in preparation for both episodic and distributive nursing practice within all collegiate programs.
4. Support increased attention to the needs for advanced and continuing education in nursing so that practitioners would maintain excellence in practice and resultant care might be enhanced.

By essentially increasing the range of choice afforded both students and institutions, the National Commission felt that sufficient leverage could be exerted to dislodge the status quo. Beyond this, the institutions themselves, supported by the state master planning committees and encouraged by the evolution in nursing roles and functions, could develop a new configuration of knowledge, understandings, and skills for the emergent nurse practitioner.

Career Perspectives in Nursing

In distinguishing between problems of "recruitment" and "retention" in nursing, the National Commission pointed out that most utilization patterns in our traditional health care facilities lead away from direct patient involvement. This tendency, of course, is reflected in the economic reward system developed to compensate nursing careers. Thus, we find higher salaries, as well as acclaim, being attached to positions in which the individual nurses find few of the intrinsic satisfactions that initially induced them to enter the profession. Such a double-bind system of approach-avoidance undoubtedly affects the attractiveness—and the actuality—of pursuing a career in this field.

Beyond this, however, there are a number of other basic problems throughout the entire system of recognition and reward presently offered American nursing. Most people simply assume that there is a positive relationship between the importance of a job to society and the amount of salary that is attached to the work. While economists could readily find general support for such a statement, they have long recognized significant exceptions. In our society, for example, those tasks "mainly directed at serving a person and his situation . . . are low status . . ." and consequently undervalued and underpaid.[23] Unfortunately, this generalization is quite widespread in America, and its boundary lines are diffuse. In terms of economic classification, nursing has often been grouped with such occupations as maid service, waitressing, and laundering simply because all of these occupations have elements of personal service rendered on demand. This is a long-existing perceptual problem that admits of no easy solution. It does explain, however, the relative depression of most nursing salaries as compared with equivalent positions in other fields requiring relative preparation and exacting similar responsibility and commitment.

The fact that 99 percent of our practicing nurses are women has undoubtedly affected the overall view of the profession and the urgency with which we have addressed problems of compensation and reward. To many men—and most individuals holding positions of ultimate authority in health management are men—such a preponderance of women constitutes ipso facto proof that nursing is high in maternal considerations, low in scientific content, and likely to be engaged in as an avocation, or as a job activity en route to marriage. Life being as it is, women must recognize that such a proposition does contain more than a germ of self-fulfillment. Much of the socialization process engaged in by parents, teachers, counselors, and friends tends to influence those entering nursing to recognize, and even accept, these considerations. Given these preconditions, it is true that most observers feel the level of commitment "among those who aspire to nursing would appear to be relatively low as measured by both women and men in college teaching, medicine, law, engineering, and the ministry."[24] There is comparative evidence of the validity of this feeling in the general finding that men who have entered nursing commonly gravitate into positions of influence and authority out of all proportion to their numbers. The irony, of course, is that we justify our inadequate compensation for nurses on the very propositions that we foster—without examining or seeking to alter them.

A further complication exists in the fact that two out of every three full-time nurses are presently employed in a hospital. These institutions, in turn, grew out of an eleemosynary and religious heritage that attached tremendous importance to the altruism and dedication of those engaged in caring for people. Nurses have long been underpaid, but so too have been aides, orderlies, technicians, interns, and residents. The prevalence of this practice is such that the entire health care system has long been subsidized by those working within it in terms of salaries unreceived and benefits unobtained. For those in medicine, there is the promise of eventual private practice outside, or alongside, the eleemosynary institution. For nurses and many others, however, there is less possibility for opportunity—and far greater probability of constraint. In addition to the "charity consciousness" of the hospital system, there also is a large ingredient of economic monopsony engendered by the understandings reached among hospital associations and area councils in the realm of salaries.[25] This means simply that demand is controlled while supply is encouraged and the hospital would "welcome additional employees at the going wage" which is set by inter-institutional agreement. A variety of factors has combined to challenge this traditional approach to economic rewards—collective bargaining, unionization, institutional competition—but much more thought is required to develop sounder career reward systems in nursing.

In the face of these cultural and economic restraints, it is surprising that nursing has been successful at all in marshalling the numbers of qualified practitioners we now have working within the health care system. Nor is there any wonder that in the struggle to overcome economic deprivation, male domination, and societal unconcern, nursing has sometimes evidenced suspicion, mistrust, and borderline paranoia. Unable to attack directly many of its problems, American nursing has frequently evidenced classic behavior patterns of projection and displacement. If you cannot assault administrators, or physicians, or society, then you can assault other nurses, their organizations, and their programs. The result has been fractionalization, loss of professional identity, and a high degree of isolation.

Of the more than 700,000 full- or part-time practitioners in nursing, approximately 160,000 belong to the largest professional organization, the American Nurses' Association, down from an all-time high of 200,000. The National League for Nursing has more than 1,800 agency members, but an individual membership of only 14,000 nurses. Approximately fifteen specialty practice groups in nursing enroll some additional thousands of American nurses, but when we make allowance for dual membership, we come to the sober recognition that less than 250,000 nurses belong to *any* organization dedicated to the long-term development of the profession. Moreover, there is considerable dispersion among this variety of organizations and associations, together with some history of rivalry, factionalism, and disagreement.[26]

In the general area of nursing careers, the National Commission advanced nineteen recommendations designed to solve the basic problems of reward systems, professional perspectives, and individual growth. To initiate activities in this regard, four specific priorities were established:

1. Disseminate information to health management administrators and other decision makers on the effects of depressed salaries in nursing and the probable consequences of altered career reward systems;
2. Encourage nursing organizations to cooperate in interpreting the characteristics of nursing to the public and to vital agencies throughout the country and to establish some continuing inter-organizational approach to consensus and unity;
3. Advocate that each individual nurse take personal responsibility for assuming an active role in professional development through organizational participation; and
4. Recommend that professional nursing organizations address continuing career concerns like those of licensure and certification while placing a moratorium on localized or ad hoc activities that could interfere with more generalized or articulated approaches.

While all of these approaches are considerably less tangible than most priority activities in both nursing roles and education, it was the belief of the Commission that the climate in which nursing exists had to be revealed and examined. Only through greater unity in nursing, and the supportive actions of other health professions and the public, could we begin to solve some of these basic problems which affect all other areas and concerns. Thus, the staff was charged with developing an educational program that could highlight aspects of concern and promise in the building of an unambiguous profession of nursing.

FUNDING OF THE IMPLEMENTATION PHASE

The investigation phase of the National Commission's work had been supported by grants from the W. K. Kellogg Foundation, the Avalon Foundation (now known as the Andrew W. Mellon Fund), and a generous gift from a private benefactor. In early 1971, the Commission contacted both foundations to explore their possible interest in financing an implementation effort. The Mellon Fund indicated immediately that its practice was not to continue support of a project beyond the stipulated period of the initial grant. The W. K. Kellogg Foundation, on the other hand, expressed considerable interest in the conduct of an implementation phase—providing that the nursing organizations of the country indicated their support and participation in the effort.

Based on this assurance, the National Commission next approached the two nursing organizations that had been instrumental in the preparation of the original proposal for the study—the National League for Nursing and the American Nurses' Association. On April 28, 1970, the Executive Committee of the NLN Board of Directors pledged $25,000 for support of the implementation project, and in May of that year, the House of Delegates of the ANA voted its endorsement and financial support of the implementation phase—without specifying an amount. Later, on October 27, 1971, the ANA Board of Directors took action to approve a grant in the amount of $25,000 for the third year of National Commission operations.

Meanwhile, the W. K. Kellogg Foundation, encouraged by the action of the NLN and the assurance of the ANA that assistance would be forthcoming, agreed to underwrite the entire project for two years and to share with nursing the support of the third and final year. To this end, the Foundation pledged a total of $361,000 over the three-year period, subject of course to annual review and analysis.

Figure 1-3 displays a comparison of sources from which financial aid was received over the two phases of the National Commission's existence. The total support for the investigation phase was $500,000 plus earned income accumulated over the first years of the project. Total requested support for the implementation phase was $411,000. This latter figure, however, was supplemented throughout the three years by generated income in the form of interest, royalties, small donations, and payments for publications—a total of approximately $35,000. Moreover, in 1972 the W. K. Kellogg Foundation appropriated $125,000 to the Commission for the purpose of assisting in the work of implementation within a selected number of states. While these funds were separately treated and accounted for, their availability materially aided the general program of activities.

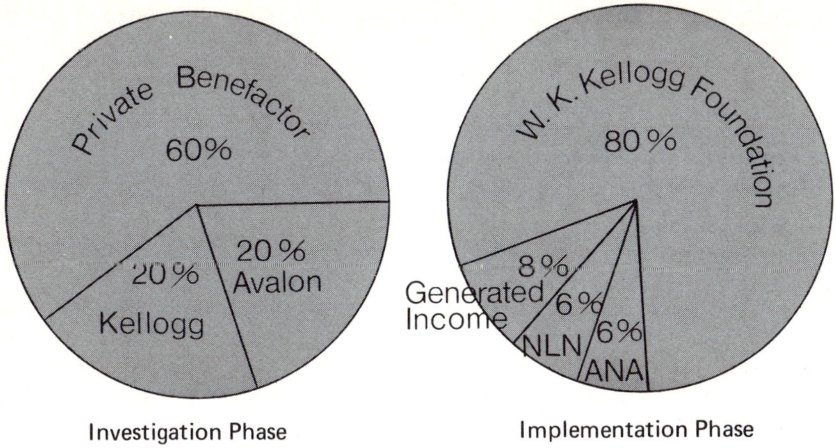

Figure 1-3. Comparative sources of support income for activities of the National Commission.

In addition to simple, factual recording of the sources of income received by the Commission, these figures may serve two particular purposes. First, it is significant that more money was directed toward the total effort involved in the implementation phase than to the investigatory period. Second, it is important to note that professional nursing did, indeed, participate in the total support of the implementation program–not only by means of the direct contributions of the large associations, but also through the category of "general income." At the same time, nursing's financial support was never determinative of Commission programming–nor was there ever an attempt to direct that function.

With the conclusion of negotiations for financial support, the implementation phase was assured and the National Commission could now set about the task of organizing for the second phase of its activities.

RECOMPOSITION OF THE NATIONAL COMMISSION

In moving from research processes to the functioning of a change agent, it was clear that some adjustments had to be made in the composition of the Commission. The original body had fully discharged its assigned responsibilities with the presentation of its report. All members had served longer than their original understanding would have led them to expect because of delays in the organization and funding of the investigation phase. Each commissioner had participated actively in the succeeding phases of the work, most particularly in the detailed discussion of the specific recommendations adopted by the group. Finally, the commissioners had taken part in the regional report meetings across the country and had individually met with groups and associations to discuss the findings and proposals.

Combined with the other demands on the commissioners' time, including that of their own employment, it was almost impossible for some members to continue at the same level of involvement, but no one wanted to see the matter end without full provision for intensive implementation.

Two basic agreements were reached in the spring of 1970. First, it was arranged that all those commissioners who had to restrict their activities would continue as members of a National Advisory Council. This would not only permit them to assist as needed on an occasional basis, but would underscore the solidarity and unanimity of the Commission's decisions. Second, it was accepted that the body should be enlarged and diversified to deal with the variety of concerns sure to be encountered. Upon consideration, six of the original commissioners asked to move to the advisory council; the other six, including all three nurses, expressed a willingness to continue their service on the governing board.

Chancellor W. Allen Wallis of the University of Rochester, who had served as president of the Commission throughout the first phase of the work, was one who asked to be relieved from the board. In June of 1970, the commissioners agreed to ask Dr. Leroy E. Burney, president of the Milbank Memorial Fund and former Surgeon General of the United States Public Health Service, to assume leadership of a reconstituted board for the implementation phase. With his acceptance, invitations were quickly extended and accepted by thirteen other individuals and a board of twenty commissioners, including the fourteen new members, was convened. This enlarged board included:

Leroy E. Burney, M.D., President, Milbank Memorial Fund.

Dorothy A. Cornelius, R.N., Executive Director, Ohio Nurses' Association, and former President of the American Nurses' Association.

Margaret B. Dolan, R.N., Head, Department of Public Health Nursing, School of Public Health, University of North Carolina, and former President of the American Nurses' Association.

Marion B. Folsom, former Secretary of Health, Education, and Welfare.

Joseph Hamburg, M.D., Dean, College of Allied Health Professions, University of Kentucky.

James G. Haughton, M.D., Executive Director, Cook County Hospitals Governing Commission.

Charles A. Hoffman, M.D., Medical Practitioner, now President, American Medical Association.

William N. Hubbard, Jr., M.D., Vice President and General Manager, Pharmaceutical Division, The Upjohn Company.

Boisfeuillet Jones, President, Emily and Ernest Woodruff Foundation.

Lois Turner Jones, R.N., Director, Playhouse Academy of Omaha.

Anne K. Kibrick, R.N., Ed.D., Chairman, Department of Nursing, Graduate School of Arts and Sciences, Boston College, and now President of the National League for Nursing.

Eleanor C. Lambertsen, R.N., Ed.D., Dean, School of Nursing, Cornell University-New York Hospital.

Mary Jane McCarthy, R.N., Chief, Nursing Service, Veterans Administration Hospital of Dallas.

Leonard F. McCollum, Chairman of the Board, Continental Oil Company.

Stuart J. Marylander, Executive Director, Cedars-Sinai Medical Center of Los Angeles.

Charles S. Paxson, Jr., Executive Vice President, Hahnemann Medical College and Hospital of Philadelphia.

John D. Porterfield, M.D., Director, Joint Commission on Accreditation of Hospitals.

Barbara A. Resnik, R.N., Division of Ambulatory and Community Medicine, School of Medicine, University of California at San Francisco.

Ralph W. Tyler, Ph.D., National Academy of Education, Office of the President, Chicago.

Harold B. Wise, M.D. .Medical Practitioner, Former Project Director, The Martin Luther King, Jr. Health Center.

Commissioners Dolan, Folsom, Lambertsen, McCarthy, McCollum and Tyler continued their service begun during the investigatory stage. All others were appointed at the beginning of the implementation period.

In addition to their services as commissioners, Dr. Burney served as president, Mr. Jones as vice president, and Dr. Lambertsen as secretary. The treasurer and assistant treasurer, LaRoy B. Thompson and Kenneth E. Wood, discharged the responsibilities of these offices, but were not members of the Commission and did not take part in its deliberations.

Designation of Advisory Council

One of the first acts of the new Commission was to implement the concept of the National Advisory Council. Appointed to this consultative body were:

Ray Everett Brown, Executive Vice President, Northwestern University McGaw Medical Center.

Lowell T. Coggeshall, M.D., former Assistant to the Secretary of Health, Education, and Welfare.

Walter E. Hoadley, Ph.D., Executive Vice President, Bank of America National Trust and Savings Association.

Herbert E. Longenecker, Ph.D., President, Tulane University.

Robert K. Merton, Ph.D. .Giddings Professor of Sociology, Columbia University.

W. Allen Wallis, Chancellor, The University of Rochester.

Over the period of the implementation phase, these individuals continued to receive all materials and documents distributed to the Commission, as well as invitations to attend Commission meetings and other functions. Several of the council members participated in specific activities related to implementation, and each of them responded in the case of specific requests for advice and assistance.

Changes in Membership

Over the entire course of the implementation phase, only three changes took place in the composition of the Commission and Advisory Council. On November 17, 1971, Dorothy A. Cornelius wrote to President Burney that her increased activities with the Ohio State Nurses' Association and the International Council of Nurses would seriously hamper her contribution to the National Commission. In January of 1972, the Commission appointed Miss Cornelius to the National Advisory Council and unanimously invited Joan S. Guy, R.N., Executive Director, Michigan Nurses' Association, to join the board.

In February of 1973, Marion B. Folsom, one of the original commissioners, asked to be shifted from the Commission to the Advisory Council and this was done in accordance with his wish. Thus the final membership of the two bodies stood at nineteen commissioners and eight advisors, each of whom had participated for some time as a member of the National Commission.

Reappointment of Staff

Coincident with the recomposition of the Commission and the installation of the National Advisory Council, Dr. Jerome P. Lysaught was reappointed director of the staff to plan and conduct the activities of the implementation phase. Ms. Sydney A. Sutherland was asked to continue to serve as assistant to the director, and a small staff was planned to carry out the objectives specified by the Commission.* The operational headquarters of the Commission were continued in Rochester, New York through the cooperation and support of the University of Rochester.

It was agreed between the Commission and its staff that wide use would have to be made of advisory groups, volunteers, and agencies throughout the country because it would be economically and administratively impossible to staff a national office that would have capacity to handle all the details of implementation. The Commission delegated broad latitude to the staff for determining the specific groups and bodies that should be asked to participate in implementation efforts while reserving final approval of these projects and their objectives.

Timetable for the Implementation

The primary purpose of the investigation phase was completed with the publication of *An Abstract for Action* in June of 1970. The period from June through September of 1970 represented a planning and assessment stage during which the manuscript for the volume of *Appendices* was completed, the objectives fixed for initial implementation efforts, and the Commission reconstituted. On October 1, 1970 the three year implementation began officially, and all activities related to the investigation ceased. The protocols for the implementation specified

*A listing and acknowledgement of the contributions of individuals on the staff is provided in the *Foreword* to this volume.

that the work would be planned over a thirty-six month period with emphasis on the priority items discussed earlier under the headings of: nursing roles and functions, nursing education, and nursing careers.

In very broad terms, the implementation phase was divided into three stages coinciding roughly with the three one-year time periods. In the first year of implementation, there was emphasis on educational and informational activities aimed at nursing, related health occupations, key decision-making agencies, and the general public. Over the course of the second year, emphasis was laid on the development of a National Joint Practice Commission between medicine and nursing together with counterpart state committees. And, in the third year, the thrust was aimed toward generation of statewide master planning committees and changes in patterns of education and practice.

These general objectives, however, must be viewed in a relative fashion because the informational priorities led clearly into both joint practice and state planning. Moreover, we became involved very early in working with a limited number of states interested in planning so that we could have that experience long before the third year of the implementation phase. Thus, some activities were undertaken in all three areas of the recommendations each year, but the proportion of time and effort was shifted rather significantly. As indicated in the sections on the separate recommendation areas, there was also a high degree of pragmatism involved. When obstacles appeared in terms of one priority, we shifted focus quickly in order to capitalize on those items in which more rapid accomplishment might be attained. In this way, we attempted to maximize progress while continuing to attack the residual, major problems encountered.

SUMMARY

Six months prior to the publication of its final report, *An Abstract for Action*, the National Commission for the Study of Nursing and Nursing Education initiated steps to ensure that there would be some form of systematic follow-up and implementation of its recommendations. It did so after considering the series of national studies of nursing, extending back to 1923, the consistency of their findings, and the discouraging fact that little effective change had resulted.

The Commission made overtures to the foundations which had supported the investigation phase of its work and proposed that a three year effort be mounted to attain priority objectives in each of three areas: nursing roles and functions, nursing education, and nursing careers. The purpose of this endeavor would be to foster progress over a variety of key recommendations, initiate change processes that could be followed up independently by other groups over time, and to engineer the development of new agencies or bodies that could ensure continuing attention to long-term recommendations of the Commission.

Through the support of the W. K. Kellogg Foundation, the National League for Nursing, and the American Nurses' Association, the implementation phase was undertaken. To direct this work, the National Commission was recomposed to broaden its representation and expertise while retaining all of the former commissioners either on the new board or on an advisory council to the board. Staff was organized, priorities and timetables were established in a general fashion to allow for tactical decision making, and in September of 1970 the Commission formally moved from investigation to implementation.

Three broad stages were planned to coincide roughly with the three years of the project. Stage one was to be an informational and educational effort directed at nursing, other health occupations, and the general public. Its primary purpose would be to explain the findings and recommendations of the Commission and, particularly, to cut through the confusions about a "manpower shortage" in nursing and expose the underlying problems which have long been obscured by our overemphasis on matters of personnel supply. In the second stage, the Commission and staff would address the establishment of a National Joint Practice Commission between medicine and nursing so that this body, in turn, could foster basic reexamination of the practice roles in an evolving health care delivery system calculated to better meet the needs of our society. The third stage would emphasize planning and change processes within the states and regions of the country aimed at reconstructing the patterns of education and practice in nursing.

Obviously no single group of commissioners, however talented, could adequately plan and cope with the full range of forces currently operating in the health scene. It was therefore agreed that advisory committees should be established, as needed, to ensure the consideration of alternatives and to provide for continuing commentary, criticism, and evaluation. In addition, the staff was charged with exploring ways of extending the reach of Commission efforts through securing assistance from individuals and groups in attaining the priority objectives.

FOOTNOTES

1. The National Commission for the Study of Nursing and Nursing Education. *An Abstract for Action.* Jerome P. Lysaught, Director. New York: McGraw-Hill Book Co., 1970.
2. The National Commission for the Study of Nursing and Nursing Education. *An Abstract for Action: Appendices.* Jerome P. Lysaught, Director. New York: McGraw-Hill Book Co., 1971.
3. Personal communication from W. Allen Wallis, President, The National Commission for the Study of Nursing and Nursing Education, to Emory W. Morris, President and General Director, The W. K. Kellogg Foundation, dated December 15, 1969, p. 1.
4. ibid., p. 2.
5. Goldmark, Josephine. *Nursing and Nursing Education in the United States.* New York: The Macmillan Co., 1923.
6. Brown, Esther L. *Nursing for the Future.* New York: Russell Sage Foundation, 1948.
7. Committee on the Function of Nursing. *A Program for the Nursing Profession.* Eli Ginzberg, Chairman. New York: The Macmillan Co., 1948.
8. Bridgman, Margaret. *Collegiate Education for Nursing.* New York: Russell Sage Foundation, 1953.
9. *An Abstract for Action.,* op. cit., p. 157.
10. Wallis, W. Allen, op. cit., p. 2.
11. Lysaught, Jerome P. "Progress Report from the National Commission on Nursing and Nursing Education: From Abstract into Action." *Nursing Outlook.,* 20:3:173-179 (March) 1972. p.173.

12. *Toward Quality in Nursing.* Report of the Surgeon General's Consultant Group on Nursing. Washington, D.C.: U.S. Department of Health, Education, and Welfare, Public Health Service, PHS Publication No. 992, 1963, p.55.
13. All data in this section are derived from: *Facts About Nursing, 1970-71 Edition.* New York: American Nurses' Association, 1971 and *Health Resources Statistics*, 1972. Washington, D.C.: U.S. Department of Health, Education, and Welfare, Public Health Service, DHEW Publication No. (HSM) 72-1509, 1972.
14. Lecht, Leonard A. *Manpower Needs for National Goals in the 1970's.* New York: Frederick A. Praeger, 1969. p.147.
15. Hughes, Everett et al. *Twenty Thousand Nurses Tell Their Story.* Philadelphia: J. B. Lippincott Co., 1958.
16. Lysaught, Jerome P. "The House Reunited: It Must Not Fall." *American Journal of Public Health.* 62:7:957-961 (July) 1972.
17. *An Abstract for Action.*, op. cit., pp.87-90.
18. "Distributive Nursing Practice: Development and Fusion of the Roles." Rochester, N.Y.: The National Commission for the Study of Nursing and Nursing Education, 1972 (pamphlet). See also, "Episodic Nursing Practice: Refinement and Expansion of the Roles." Rochester, N.Y.: The National Commission for the Study of Nursing and Nursing Education, 1972 (pamphlet).
19. "A Guide for Establishing Statewide Master Planning Committees." Rochester, N.Y.: The National Commission for the Study of Nursing and Nursing Education, 1970 (pamphlet).
20. *An Abstract for Action.*, op cit., pp.103-113.
21. "Continuing Education in Nursing: Necessity and Opportunity." Rochester, N.Y.: The National Commission for the Study of Nursing and Nursing Education, 1971 (pamphlet).
22. "Individualization, Articulation, Concentration: Emergent forces in Nursing Education." Rochester, N.Y.: The National Commission for the Study of Nursing and Nursing Education, 1972 (pamphlet).
23. Anderson, Odin W. *Toward an Unambiguous Profession? A Review of Nursing.* Chicago: University of Chicago Center for Health Administration. Pamphlet No. A6, 1968, p.3.
24. ibid., p.11.
25. Altman, Stuart H. *Present & Future Supply of Registered Nurses.* Washington, D.C.: U.S. Department of Health, Education, and Welfare, DHEW Publication No. NIH 72-134, 1971, pp.9-38.
26. Lysaught, Jerome P. "An Epistle to the New Corinthians." Paper presented at the National Nurses' Congress, Western White House, San Clemente, California, January 25, 1973.

TWO THE ENVIRONMENT OF CHANGE

In true perspective, any effort to effect change in nursing should be viewed as an attempt to alter a subsystem of health care which is, in turn, a major subsystem of our entire society. The sheer enormity of this complex relationship clearly means that one cannot defer change attempts until the time is *right*—for such a determination, in itself, is an impossibility. The best that can be done is to attempt a limited assessment of major related trends, analyze their likely impact upon one's own designs, and, then, strive to optimize the outcomes as much as possible.

In the course of its investigatory phase, the National Commission and its staff reviewed four general areas that seemed intimately related to the future of American nursing. These were:

1. Developing trends in American health care and its systems for delivery.
2. Related social and cultural changes both among consumers and practitioners of health care.
3. Advances in health sciences and research with concomitant changes in public expectations.
4. Changed economics for health care financing and insurance.[1]

The combined impact of these forces suggested that an entirely new configuration of health care was needed to ensure that quantitative and qualitative increases in service could be proffered to the American people. Some form of universal health care has to be provided in our society if our pledge of "access for all" is to have any substantive meaning. For these reasons, the NCSNNE staff attempted an on-going analysis of proposals for national health insurance and/or related schemes for widened care provision.

A second "trend of the times" emerged with the growing emphasis on feminine rights and liberation. If only for the fact that 99 percent of all nurse practitioners are women, the "women's lib" movement would have been important. As the program of several of the women's groups took form, however, there was a profound emphasis on health concerns—on the treatment accorded the female consumer as well as the opportunities for women to succeed as health professionals.

Still a third major trend, shaped in part by the interplay of the first two, appeared in the form of a reexamination of professional relationships between American medicine and nursing. If some major reconstruction is to occur in the health care delivery system, and if, coincidentally, we accept the better utilization of American women in health practice, then, there must be a reapportionment of roles and functions between the two largest groups of clinical providers.

Obviously, the exhaustive examination of any one of these three trends is beyond the concerns of this Commission. Our analysis of their development, configuration, and probable directions was limited strictly to the relationship this bore to the implementation of *An Abstract for Action*, and to the desired directions for change in American nursing. From this particularized perspective, however, it may be helpful to comment on all three developments, for they remain continuing elements in any formulation of change in nursing.

NATIONAL HEALTH INSURANCE

In a clear, concise analysis of American health care in transition, Somers points out a series of paradoxes between the promise and the reality of our present "system" for meeting societal needs.[2] She describes crucial changes in the outlook of both the practitioner and the consumer, finds related changes in the institutions and finances of health care, and concludes that ". . . there is now stronger and more widespread support for some form of national health insurance than at any time in the past."[3]

Certainly in terms of the number of legislative proposals, and the variety of their backers, there is corroboration of generalized public support. Such seemingly unlikely groups as the American Medical Association and the American Hospital Association have actually participated in the development of major bills pertaining to national health insurance; special-interest action committees have been formed to marshal opinion in favor of the different propositions.

Organized nursing has long been identified as a general advocate of some form of comprehensive system for national health care, although it has attempted to enumerate the qualities that such a plan should contain rather than draft its own legislative proposal. The House of Delegates of the American Nurses' Association, for example, voted at its 1970 convention to support a national health insurance program that would include "a restructuring of our present system . . . into a rational cohesive base for meeting the health needs of society." When a number of bills were introduced by Congressmen in 1971, the Executive Director of the ANA, Dr. Eileen Jacobi, elaborated on what was meant by a rational, cohesive base:

> If an optimal or near optimal state of health is to be reached the national health care program must be comprehensive and include preventive, health maintenance, diagnostic and treatment, restorative and protective services. A piecemeal approach to meeting health care needs will in the long run be more costly, will not meet the public's expectations, and will result in frustration of both the providers of services and their clients.
>
> We are opposed . . . to proposals for national health insurance that address themselves merely to providing more public funding to meet the costs of care . . . Such protection should be part of the comprehensive health care program.[4]

In a related statement prepared by the ANA Commission on Nursing Services, thirteen essential elements of a national health care system were tendered. Among these were two key points in relation to nursing's contribution to the delivery of care:

> 10. There should be joint planning by all health professions for recruitment, preparation, utilization, and compensation for health manpower.
>
> 13. There should be provisions within a health care system for the nursing profession to fulfill its function according to established nursing standards; and to collaborate with other professions in evaluating health care practices.[5]

These proposals for collaborative approaches to the preparation and utilization of professional practitioners and to the evaluation of their services defined the way that nursing viewed its involvement in any program of national health care—as a full and participating partner.

What had appeared in the spring of 1971 to be an early certainty—the passage of a national health insurance bill—grew less sure over the course of lengthy hearings before the House Committee on Ways and Means and the Senate Committee on Finance. The very multiplicity of proposed measures, as well as the variety of differences found among them, militated against an early decision.

The Ninety-second Congress adjourned in November 1972 with a national insurance program no closer to being realized than it was in early 1971. Political commentators predicted that it would be a central issue in the presidential and congressional races during the 1972 campaign since both parties had included health planks in their political platforms. In the course of the campaign itself, however, health insurance never surfaced as a viable point of controversy.

During the first five months of the Ninety-third Congress, a number of bills were introduced and referred to House and Senate committees. By May of 1973, two major bills were reported being drafted: one by Senator Edward Kennedy, Chairman of the Senate Committee on Health and Wilbur Mills, Chairman of the House Committee on Ways and Means; the other by Senator Russell Long, Chairman of the Senate Committee on Finance and Senator Abraham Ribicoff, member of the Senate Committee on Finance. It was indicated that Senator Long intended to schedule hearings on national health insurance late in 1973 regardless of actions by the House Committee on Ways and Means—a strict departure from tradition—to emphasize the need for definitive action by Congress in the near future.

Aside from the rumors and conjectures, however, there are presently no less than four significant proposals for national health insurance placed before the Congress. These include the bills for:

1. *Health Security*. (S. 3) (H.R. 22-23) introduced by Senator Edward Kennedy and Representative Martha Griffiths, and supported by the Committee of 100, the AFL-CIO, Teamsters, and United Auto Workers.
2. *Health Care* introduced by Senator Thomas J. McIntyre and Representative Omar Burleson, and supported by the Health Insurance Association of America.
3. *Medicredit* (S. 444) (H.R. 2222) introduced by Senator Clifford Hansen, Representative Joel Broyhill, and Representative Richard Fulton, and supported by the American Medical Association.
4. *Health Care Services* (H.R. 1) introduced by Representative Al Ullman, and supported by the American Hospital Association.

As indicated in Table 2-1, there are considerable differences among these bills in terms of benefits, administration, financing, and probable effects. They vary from relatively mild extensions of present concepts to the comprehensive overhaul and restructuring of the entire health care system. Health Security would provide for the greatest amount of public intrusion into the structuring and administration of the health care system. Health Care, on the other hand, would represent basically a widening of present private group insurance with federal subsidization for those individuals and families who are either economically deprived or suffer from conditions that would preclude coverage under normal circumstances. The Medicredit plan retains much of the voluntary system, but vastly enlarges the emphasis on preventive care and maintenance of health. The Health Care Services proposal would be nearly as comprehensive as the Health Security measure, but with greater emphasis on voluntary nonprofit agencies working along as partners with public agencies.

In addition to the major differences in purpose and arrangement, each of these proposals has its own emphasis on the role of nursing in the provision of health care in a reorganized approach to delivery systems. The specific mention of nursing in these four bills is presented in Table 2-2.

TABLE 2-1 SUMMARY COMPARISON OF FOUR PROPOSED PLANS FOR NATIONAL HEALTH INSURANCE

Category	Health Security	Health Care	Medicredit	Health Care Services
General Purpose	Comprehensive health insurance for all Americans.	Tax incentives for group coverage. Paid insurance for poor and uninsurables.	Voluntary income tax and tax credit plan.	Comprehensive health care insurance for all Americans.
Benefits	Complete health service including health maintenance, disease prevention, and treatment.	Phased benefits subject to deductions and co-insurance regulations.	Comprehensive coverage of both ordinary and catastrophic illness.	Comprehensive coverage of ordinary and catastrophic illness.
Administration	Publicly administered program through HEW.	Combination of public health and private insurers.	Coverage paid by government through private and prepaid group insurance.	Publicly administered through federal Department of Health.
Probable Effects	Restructure of health care system with emphasis on health maintenance organizations.	Few changes other than increased insurance coverage.	Few changes other than increased coverage and greater emphasis on preventive care.	Restructure of health care system with emphasis on voluntary health care corporations.

Source: Washington Office, the American Nurses' Association, June 1, 1973.

TABLE 2-2 SPECIFIC PROVISIONS FOR NURSING CARE IN FOUR PROPOSALS FOR HEALTH INSURANCE

Program	Specific Provisions Related to Nursing Care
Health Security	In general hospitals—provides 24-hour nursing service rendered by or supervised by a registered professional nurse. Licensed practical or registered nurses to be on duty at all times. In skilled nursing homes—provides 24-hour nursing service sufficient to meet needs in accordance with policies developed by professional personnel (one or more physicians and one or more registered nurses); professional staff responsible for executing policies; and at least one professional nurse employed full time.
Health Care	Provides funds for student loans for preparatory training. Provides grants for health professionals in areas of critical needs. Covers charges made by a licensed physician for professional services rendered by the physician or, at his direction, by his staff of nurses.
Medicredit	Covers home health services, including part-time or intermittent nursing care provided by or under the supervision of a registered professional nurse. In general hospitals—provides coverage for all nursing services. In skilled nursing homes—provides coverage for all nursing services.
Health Care Services	Covers home health services, including part-time or intermittent nursing care provided by or under the supervision of a registered professional nurse. In general hospitals—provides coverage of such nursing services as are ordinarily furnished by the hospital.

Source: Washington Office, the American Nurses' Association, June 1, 1973.

At best, these provisions for nursing care and intervention are quite traditional and contain little hint of the expanding role of the nurse clinician in both episodic and distributive practice. It is significant, in light of these proposals, that the NLN Council of Baccalaureate and Higher Degree Programs, through its legislative committee, distributed a set of "recommendations for inclusion in a position paper on national health insurance," at the biennial convention of the National League for Nursing on May 8, 1973. Among the ten items included on their priority list were these:

> 3. Recognition of the nurse in primary care delivery and in the nurse practice and patient advocate roles must be clearly identified.
>
> Professional nurses' services should be clearly recognized for reimbursement.
>
> Advanced clinical preparation beyond the basic professional level should be certified through the professional association.[6]

Unmistakeable in these recommendations is an enlarged view of nursing practice well beyond the confines of the traditionalist perspective of current national health insurance proposals. Organized nursing sees itself clearly as an equal member of the health care team, filling an extended role in primary and specialized service, and determined to receive recognition and compensation based on that contribution.

At present, the fate of current proposals for national health insurance is uncertain. The administration has yet to submit its own bill, and there is currently no indication of when it might be announced.[7] With the added likelihood that two additional bills will be introduced in the near future, it is even more probable that no single piece of legislation in its present form will move toward adoption. Rather, there will be continuing debate, modifications and amendments, and, quite possibly, a major confrontation between Congress and the administration before some compromise solution is reached.

Health Maintenance Organizations

If the future is uncertain in national health insurance, there is considerably more action to consider in terms of the development of health maintenance organizations which are an integral aspect of both the Health Security and Health Care Services proposals—although there are differences in concept and control in their individual formulations.

Two major bills were introduced in the Ninety-third Congress to provide for the development of health maintenance organizations designed to prevent catastrophic illness through early detection, regularly scheduled examinations, and prompt treatment of minor illness. The Senate bill (S. 14) was sent to the floor of the Senate on May 14, 1973 and, after considerable debate and the acceptance of a substitute amendment on fiscal authorization, was passed by a vote of sixty-nine to twenty-five on May 15.

In contrast to the somewhat traditional approaches delimited by the current health insurance proposals, the health maintenance organization bill states:

> It is hoped by the Committee that physicians, osteopaths, dentists, psychologists, and other health workers, podiatrists, optometrists, nurses, physiotherapists, nurse practitioners, health educators, physicians assistants, nutritionists, medical social workers, occupational therapists, and other health professionals will develop a team approach in the delivery of health care services so as to expand and increase the efficiencies of all these disciplines.[8]

Specifically, the bill provides for the development and expansion of prepaid group health insurance plans, for the development of innovation in care and in delivery, and for the establishment of a Commission on Quality Health Care Assurance to oversee and to energize the establishment of health maintenance as a primary priority in the national health system.

The related House bill (H.R. 51) had not been reported out of committee at the time the Senate bill was passed so that no prediction of its fate can be made. The major difference between the two bills lies in the amount of the financial authorization with the Senate version originally calling for $805 million over three years and the House bill authorizing $260 million over the same period. Since the substitute amendment substantially reduced the Senate authorization, it may be possible that the bill which emerges from conference, if it indeed does, will be modelled after the House version. Beyond that, it appears that the administration which strongly supported health maintenance legislation four years ago may have become very cool to the concept—particularly in the amounts authorized by even the House proposal.

Public Health Act Extensions

In the absence of an administration proposal on health, there was considerable concern over the June 30, 1973 expiration date for a series of amendments to the Public Health Service Act. The expiring legislation includes the migrant health program, the regional medical programs, community mental health centers, the Hill-Burton legislation on Hospital support, health care delivery research and development, and family planning. The administration had already indicated its desire to see much of the "special purpose" legislation expire, and make provisions to continue other programs under different categories or authorizations. In the present state of tension, Congress has more and more vigorously asserted its right and responsibility for determining which programs should be continued and the manner of their authorization. At a series of public hearings in the spring of 1973, it became evident that Congress intended to vote to extend the public service act provisions for at least one year in order to provide an opportunity for evaluation and decision making about each of the individual programs.

On Thursday, May 31, 1973, the House of Representatives took emphatic action to approve three bills by such overwhelming margins that presidential vetoes seemed futile. The *Washington Post* characterized the voting as "the session's greatest show of House resistance to administration wishes."[9] By a vote of 372 to 1, the House approved a bill to extend all twelve health programs for one year, despite the fact that the administration indicated that five of them should be completely eliminated and others changed drastically. By a vote of 361 to 5, the House authorized $208 million a year for two years for biomedical research and training; by a margin of 261 to 96, it authorized $145 million over three years for emergency health services. The one-year extension of all twelve public health act amendments was defended by Congressional advocates on the basis that study was required to properly determine which, if any, of the programs should be ended or otherwise redirected.

The Senate had already passed a related bill extending the programs; the two measures will now proceed to conference committee to resolve the differences in authorized amounts—an added Senate provision which seeks to forestall administration impoundment of any authorized and appropriated funds must also be debated.

Social Security Amendments of 1972

One of the most controversial provisions of all recent health legislation was included in the 1972 Social Security Amendments, and calls for the establishment of Professional Standards Review Organizations. The law requires that, by July of 1976, PSROs be established across the United States for the purpose of monitoring health care, particularly medical care as provided to Medicare and Medicaid recipients.

Essentially, the federal legislation mandates that doctors of medicine and osteopathy develop and maintain a system of peer review with the primary enforcement mechanism being bound up in economics—poor practice can be punished through lack of reimbursement for services rendered. While there have been vigorous dissents expressed by many physicians over the provisions of the law, there are movements now afoot to establish the required bodies. In contrast to the concern voiced by medicine and osteopathy, nursing has expressed interest in its voluntary inclusion in the legislation. The Legislative Committee of the NLN Council of Baccalaureate and higher Degree Programs, for example, has recommended that:

> 10. Quality control for the professional practitioner should allow for peer review.[10]

To what extent this nursing action is a professionally positive thrust, or to what extent it is a reaction to the possibility that the present legislation might place medicine and osteopathy in an unrivalled position to review all health care practice by themselves, is a moot point. Whatever the reason, professional nursing has indicated more than passing interest in legislated peer review.

A more controversial aspect of PSRO operations from the viewpoint of nursing is the employment of nurse coordinators to collect data and make judgments concerning patient care. Some in nursing see this as inappropriate and a continuation of the subservient role nurses have played for years. Some, however, see the real possibility that the nurse coordinators are a logical first step toward achieving the inclusion of nurses in peer review within the PSRO concept. The point in question is whether the nurse coordinator collects and analyzes data for physicians and osteopaths to use in assessing nursing, or whether the nurses assess themselves as part of a generalized professional self-study.

Prospects for the Future

Concern over health care and public agitation for health insurance and comprehensive planning may have plateaued briefly in the early 1970s. It is certainly not at the frenetic level of the 1960s when medicare, medicaid, regional medical programs, and a host of other national and state legislation were burgeoning. In the first two years of this decade, the pace definitely slowed. We did see new legislation for controlling sickle cell anemia, Cooley's anemia, and drug abuse, and the National Health Services Corps was established. On the other hand, there were presidential vetoes of the Veterans Health Bill, the Social and Rehabilitation Services Bill, and the Older Americans Act (vetoed in 1972, but signed into law with lowered authorization levels in 1973). The watchwords in 1973 seem more often to be those of "budget ceiling," "costs," "inflation," and "taxes."

The programs of the sixties, viewed with objectivity, provide valid arguments for both the critics and the advocates of increased federal spending for health. Some of the categorical programs have been outstanding; some have missed widely their assigned mark. Some of the bureaucracies established by legislation have been remarkably efficient; some have been officious as well as effective.

As Congress suggests, perhaps this is the time for a serious, objective review of programs and accomplishments. Out of this, too, may come what Somers has persuasively proposed:

> There is a real urgency, a financial crisis that threatens the lives and well-being of many Americans as well as the viability of important segments of the health care economy. To say that a plan is not "perfect" is no excuse for inaction. We shall never achieve a "perfect" plan just by studying it or talking about it. We have to start moving.[11]

In the course of arriving at a comprehensive health plan, however, we must eschew either the monolithic approach or the continuation of stopgap, unarticulated, sometimes unrelated programs and plans that fragment and diffuse our efforts.

Nursing can take some consolation in looking beyond itself to the entire health care system. Out of the present politics of confrontation—with its vested interests, territorial rights, fears of change, and emotional reactions—there can, and must, evolve a more sane and responsive health care system, one that encompasses the characteristics that nursing has long advanced. In that comprehensive approach to maintaining health, preventing disease, and treating illness when it occurs, nursing's position will be as significant as the profession wills it to be and as responsible as the profession is willing to accept. Meanwhile, the kitchen might be mighty warm, and those who want to be involved in the cooking must resolve to pay the price—in controversy, debate, and arduous activity.

THE CHANGING VIEW OF—AND ON—AMERICAN WOMEN

Through the late sixties and early seventies, the American public became more and more aware that "women's lib" was a serious and intentioned effort to reexamine and recast the role of woman in American society. What had seemed to many—male and female—to be an aberrant minority claque assumed very different proportions as responsible leadership emerged, numbers grew, and programs became defined. The difficulties that this generation of liberators faced, however, were enormous. As Morgan put it:

> According to the Book of Genesis, God first created man. Woman was not only an afterthought, but an amenity. For close on two thousand years this holy scripture was believed to justify her subordination and explain her inferiority; for even as a copy she was not a very good copy. There were differences. She was not one of His best efforts.[12]

Despite the humorous touch, American women have found the road to economic and social equality a long, difficult, sometimes cruel, and frequently lonely one. Prior to 1920 when American women won the right to vote, our nation was ruled by a male electorate. Even at that, because of discriminatory laws and the systematic disenfranchisement of the Negro and other "unsuitables," the effective political control of the nation resided in the hands of an older, white male minority which conceded little in power to women. As political democracy spread, economic and legal autocracy remained. It is in these areas that the new feminist movement is now directing its energies.

Sexism and Health Care

Even before there was women's suffrage in the political scene, there were large numbers of women involved in the practice of health care in the United States. During the eighteenth, and much of the nineteenth centuries, women practiced the healing arts both in and outside the home. In fact, in our early history, the female practitioner likely enjoyed majority status in the medical scene.[13] Midwifery was an appropriate and accepted role for women, and as late as 1910 almost 50 percent of all babies born in the United States were delivered by midwives—many of them blacks and working-class immigrants.[14] As the nineteenth century lengthened, however, midwifery became less and less accepted among the wealthy though it continued to flourish for years among the poor classes. These female practitioners were of the "informal" variety, many without a formal education, and most without any form of license or certificate to practice. Through their work, however, real needs were filled and vital functions served.

With the emergence of American medical schools, and particularly after the Flexnerian reforms of those institutions, the "modern physician" came into more and more frequent competition and conflict with the "folk healers." Science and reform were pitted against art and tradition. By the same token, the "male" physician was arrayed against the "female" healer.

Nowhere was the battle more vehement than in the area of childbirth. Because this was the arena most reserved to the female health practitioner, it became the focal point of the physician's reform efforts. Despite the findings of a 1912 study at Johns Hopkins which indicated that most American physicians were *less* competent than midwives in the delivery of babies,[15] the attack mounted:

> Midwives were ridiculed as "hopelessly dirty, ignorant and incompetent." Specifically, they were held responsible for the prevalence of puerperal sepsis (uterine infections) and neonatal ophthalmia (blindness due to parental infection with gonorrhea). Both conditions were easily preventable by techniques well within the grasp of the least literate midwife (handwashing for puerperal sepsis, and eye drops for the ophthalmia).[16]

Instead of making these remedies better known, and working with the midwives for the purpose of extending improved care to the whole society, the medical profession set out systematically to eliminate the female practitioners. In the process, the sexist link of the health practitioners in America became even more pronounced as the male physician became the emergent figure.

By the end of the nineteenth century, medicine was, for all intents and purposes, closed to women as an occupational choice. Few medical schools accepted female applicants; the small number of women who completed their studies found local medical societies unwilling to accept them or to extend "professional courtesies" so that they might practice. Coupled with the virtual liquidation of the midwife and other female healers through the advent of state health practice acts which forbade them to function, this left nursing as the only really acceptable employment opportunity for women in American health care.

Women and Nursing in America

Unlike the midwife who was an independent practitioner, and the early female physicians who also practiced alone, the first nurses in America were "helpers" of the most basic variety.[17] A nurse was simply a woman who took care of neighbors or relatives, tending to their elemental needs and comforts. She was unschooled and untrained for her tasks except in the extension of the female, maternal aura in which she was viewed. Those nurses employed in hospitals prior to the Civil War came by force of circumstance to be the attendants of the old and dying—for those were the patients that came to the institution. Added to this, there was little of the social approbation later accorded nursing. Nurses of the time were frequently viewed as "a disreputable lot, prone to drunkenness, prostitution, and thievery."[18] Such an occupation was likely to have little attractiveness for most American women.

The advent of Florence Nightingale, and the introduction of her "different" type of nursing and her "trained" nurse, changed both the practice and the image of nursing in the United States. Out of the human wreckage of the Crimean War and the American Civil War, the nurse rose above the level of the unskilled, domestic servant to a functionary with important roles in treatment and alleviation. Accompanying this was a new regard in the eyes of her viewers. As Bullough considers it, the new nurse came "to bear the image of Florence Nightingale—strong yet compassionate, controlled in the face of suffering, yet seeking only to relieve the distress of her fellow man."[19]

Nursing, in the decades after the Civil War, found in a very real sense that the fellow man they served best was the predominately male medical profession. As a dependent and subordinate role player, "the nurse" became almost synonymous with "female." As one of the few honorable and appropriate occupations for women, it became an important vocational and social outlet, but largely for those individuals who would accept male dominance and control.

The social conditioning of nursing is evident in the transformation of its practitioners. In the first flush of "Nightingale training" many of the new schools drew their enrollments from the upper-middle and upper classes. Dorothea Dix, Isabel Hampton, Louisa Schuyler, and Euphemia Van Rensselaer were of the highest social strata—by birth, financial inheritance, or both. Nursing's acceptability to this elite undoubtedly restored its reputation, but they also imbued it with characteristics of their class and period. When nursing was more generally perceived to be a demanding, physically hard, and low-paid occupation, the elite classes dropped away and more and more of the new recruits came from the lower-middle and lower social classes. The values, however, that continued to be extolled were of the founders; femininity, gentility, decorum, obedience, and a serving graciousness were entrenched as nursing's characteristics.[20]

Women's Rights in America

The effective changes in nursing were spurred by women who were also involved in changing the roles of, or the opportunities for, women in America. In the words of one of the earliest declarations of women's rights, at the 1848 Seneca Falls Convention:

> *Resolved*, that the speedy success of our cause depends upon the zealous and untiring efforts of both men and women, for the overthrow of the monopoly of the pulpit, and for the securing to woman an equal participation with men in the various trades, professions, and commerce.[21]

Despite its critics and opponents, the Suffragette movement was strong and well-organized by 1890. Through a series of clashes and cases, women established their rights. With the expanded demands for feminine involvement in many occupations and services during the First World War, it became really a matter of time until voting rights were accorded in 1920. The depression and the Second World

War brought even more practical equality to women as they found more job opportunities and wider occupational choices available to them. The postwar era saw more and more women combining their domestic roles with full- or part-time employment at a growing variety of jobs.

Feminism as a movement, perhaps due in part to its earlier successes, became almost nonexistent during the fifties and early sixties. As Bird suggests:

> . . . instead of preparing themselves for professional careers . . . girls were marrying young and working at any job that would bring in money. In 1950 a record 11 percent of the students graduated from medical school were women, but by 1960 this figure dropped to 7 percent. The same thing happened in other professions, with the result that women lost ground or barely held their own in law, pharmacy, science, engineering and journalism.[22]

This trend, of course, could not be detected in nursing which had already been firmly entrenched as a female occupation. Over this same period of time, however, an increasing number of males began to enter the women's professions of elementary and secondary teaching, and a very few chose to become nurses.

The "calm" of the early sixties, however, gave way to the "sturm und drang" of the seventies. Women's lib, the first real women's movement after the Second World War, began to aim its sights not only on occupations and employment but on every facet of life. It has stressed that women should not only act as equals, but also think and feel as equals. And in this process, it has questioned every assumption about roles, relationships, and social expectations. What started as a political question, then spread to economics, has now become a critical examination of society—with nothing exempt and no one immune. What is to come, and how male-female relationships will be resolved, is far from clear.

Nursing and the Twentieth Century

As early as 1888, Ella V. Mark, a female physician, was challenging the societal expectations of the day concerning health practitioners. She argued:

> An experienced nurse is frequently more needed than a doctor; and to physicians a good one is a help which they only, can appreciate . . .[23]

There was considerable substance to her remarks. By 1900, the nurse training schools had begun to identify and utilize professional standards for education. Clinical experience took place under supervision in the hospital and related didactic instruction was carefully regulated. In comparison with many of the medical schools of the day, some totally lacking supervised clinical teaching, the schools of nursing were of fine quality.

Some medical historians note that around 1905, nurses and physicians each comprised about 35 percent of our health manpower, and that the average "trained" nurse compared favorably with the average "physician." Following the Flexner Report of 1910, however, the two professions grew apart. Medicine began to radically reform its educational patterns and institutions with emphasis on scientific growth, rigorous research, and high standards of scholarship. Nursing continued most of its education within the hospital and over the next several years initiated a limited, and sometimes tenuous, relationship with the collegiate community of America.

An inevitable result of the divergent educational courses was the imprinting of divergent social conditioning. Modern medicine became increasingly male with "hard" knowledge and skill; modern nursing became, if anything, increasingly female with "soft" art and skill. The scientific physician became the superordinate; the task-oriented nurse became more than ever the subordinate. Or so, at least, the common perception ran.

In reality, there have always been two competing elements in nursing. There have been the submissive females who are content, if not fulfilled, by acting as the handmaiden of the physician. On the other hand, from the advent of modern nursing, there have been those practitioners who see the profession of nursing as important and necessary to comprehensive health as that of medicine, and who see the two groups as equal and interdependent partners in the delivery of care. It is the ascendancy of the latter group in the face of the combined propulsion of increased concern over national health care provision and women's liberation that has characterized much of the interest in expanded and extended roles in nursing.

Schaefer points out this interrelationship in her analysis of nursing's professional commitment:

> Nursing is remiss in that, although it is the second largest women's occupational group, it has remained essentially uninvolved with the women's liberation movement.[24]

By the early seventies, however, nurses, if not nursing, were increasingly involved in the dialogue of "consciousness raising." The need for more health practitioners combined with the ever more frequent enunciation of nurses' desires for greater responsibility and authority. And it is in this context that the National Commission viewed the possibilities for new role relationships between medicine and nursing.

So long as nursing accepted the status and functions ascribed to it by a society which applied a "female" label to all its activities and capabilities, it is doubtful that much progress could be made in terms of significant role change. When societal need and professional self-worth combine, however, there is no prescriptive limitation that cannot be lifted. In the processes of implementing *An Abstract for Action* the Commission judged that time and tide were in concert.

PHYSICIAN AND NURSE: NEW ACQUAINTANCES

Out of the increased sensitivity to health care needs, and particularly in the face of stern pressure to create a national health insurance plan of comprehensive proportions, American medicine moved toward a reconsideration, not only of its own position and functions, but toward a recognition of the total contribution of significant "others" in the delivery of health care. As in most processes of social change, there had been hyperbolic statements and angry perceptions over the long historic interaction of physicians and nurses—the two largest health practicing professions.

To some women, there was no doubt as to the malevolence and oppressiveness of the physician:

> Our oppression as women health workers today is inextricably linked to our oppression as women. Nursing, our predominate role in the health system, is simply a workplace extension of our roles as wife and mother . .,. Doctors are the bosses in an industry where the workers are primarily women. Take away sexism and you take away one of the mainstays of the health hierarchy.[25]

On the other side of the coin, to some physicians there was no consideration of enlightenment, let alone equality. As one early president of the American Medical Association put it:

> Certain women seek to rival men . . . and the strongminded ape them in all things, even dress. In doing so they may command a sort of admiration such as all monstrous productions inspire, especially when they aim towards a higher type than their own.[26]

Fortunately in the decade running from 1963 to 1973, there was a considerable reassessment and rapprochement. In 1964, the American Medical Association and the American Nurses' Association sponsored the first national conference on nurse-physician relations in patient care.[27] This was followed by similar interprofessional meetings in 1965 and, again, in 1967.[28] From this came a variety of developments including the establishment of liaison committees between medicine and nursing at state and local levels, and a broadening of contacts and conferences between physicians and nurses working in the same or related fields of patient care.

By 1970, Bates was able to discern critical changes in the dynamic interactions of nurses and physicians in patient care while, at the same time, recognizing that underlying assumptions and perceptions militated against full role reconstruction. In her words:

> . . . When the physician thinks of the nurse, he views her as his technical assistant, and she is just that. . . . This relationship is characterized by medical authoritarianism on the one hand and nursing's acceptance of dependence or

> even deference on the other. The development of the full nursing role is thereby limited both by pressures from without and by timidity from within.[29]

The physician tended to view his primary role as bound up in diagnosis and treatment—the *cure* function. The nurse views her primary role as helping, comforting, and guiding—the *care* process. Both professions see an overlap in caring for the patients' physical and psychosocial needs, but both see their domains as generally separate and discrete.[30]

To some extent, this perceptual difference is occasioned as much by semantics as fact. Physicians make a "diagnosis"; nurses perform an "assessment." Physicians deal with "symptoms"; nurses respond to "discomforts." Physicians take a "history"; nurses gather "information." In these and many other ways, the two practitioners emphasize differences rather than express similarities.[31]

Whatever the real or imaginary distinctions in role performance, however, there is little doubt that new relationships and congruencies are emerging. In Figure 2-1, there is a schematic representation of the Bates formulation of traditional nurse-physician relationships in patient care.[32] Medical care is directed at meeting those patient needs for diagnosis and the onset of therapeutic care. The physician engages in some direct physical and assistive tasks, and in providing for the psychosocial needs of the patient. The nursing role is largely bound up in the physical and assistive tasks of caring for the patient, and there is activity in the psychosocial area of needs. There is some overlap, particularly in physical care tasks, but also some areas of unmet patient needs—especially those in the psychosocial area.

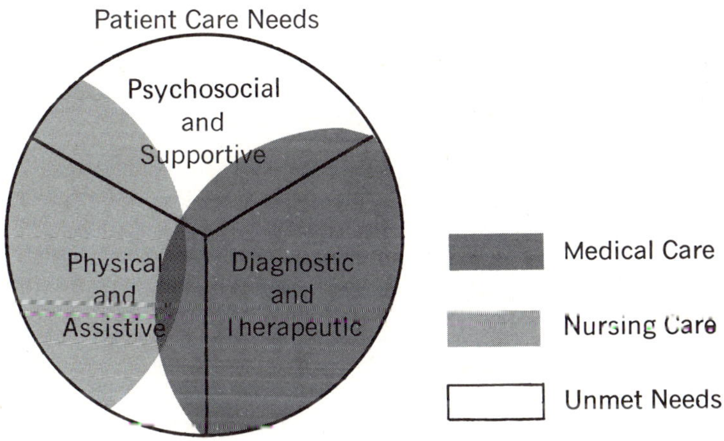

Figure 2-1. Schematic formulation of traditional nurse physician roles provided to meet patient care needs.

The patient is certainly having many of his critical needs met—and met professionally—yet he frequently harbors the feeling that everybody is too busy to listen to him, and he "doesn't know" what is going on. He becomes acutely aware of the lacks in the physical and assistive area because those are ones that impinge directly on his comfort and bodily needs.

The sixties were characterized by a great upsurge in demands for health care and by the simultaneous appearance of increased birth rates and longer life expectancy. The physician found that, in the midst of increased daily work pressures, he was often forced to limit and focus his attention to the physical disease, and reduce his concern for "the personal and social influences in relation to that disease."[33] Nursing, sometimes consciously, sometimes only by reflexive action, moved to heal the breach. In the mid-sixties, it was possible to detect a significant shift in role configurations. Figure 2-2 shows the result in schematic fashion.

As indicated in Figure 2-2, the retraction of medicine more sharply into the scope of diagnostic and therapeutic activities opened the way for an expansion of nursing into the unmet psychosocial needs area. That extension, however, was accompanied by a retreat from the traditional nursing activities in the physical and assistive area—practical nurses, aides and attendants began to appear in greater numbers acting in more diverse functions. Some of the "forsaken" tasks really were those directed to "comfort" more than "care" and were likely ones that nursing should have divested long before. On the other hand, the confusion of what constitutes nursing practice and the generalized aura that surrounds unplanned change, caused many physicians, a great number of nurses, and a considerable

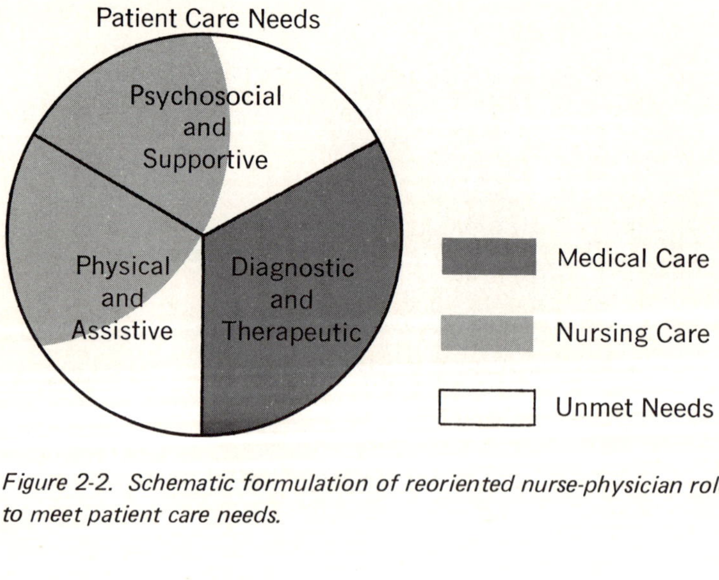

Figure 2-2. Schematic formulation of reoriented nurse-physician roles provided to meet patient care needs.

proportion of consumers to feel that nursing was abandoning the patient.[34] As a result, nurse practitioners in both episodic and distributive settings began to reconsider the roles they had taken up and those they had laid down.

As displayed in Figure 2-3, the emergent interdisciplinary, congruent roles of medicine and nursing represent a reformulation by both professions in an effort to provide comprehensive patient care through the best utilization of each. Medicine, as demonstrated in the resurgence of family and community medicine, is grappling with a broader perception of patient care which is more in keeping "with the doctor's liberal education and with medicine's ancient heritage."[35] In doing so, the physician has "moved back" into some of the areas he formerly delegated to others. Simultaneously, nursing has both extended its role into primary diagnosis and further into psychosocial care, and has reestablished its commitment to much of the physical and assistive treatment that it had once abandoned. Through the use of nursing teams, the professional care of the patient has been expanded to include many of the functions once identified almost exclusively in terms of ancillary workers.[36] The two professions have attempted to define that portion of assistive care which is essentially "comfort" rather than "treatment" and provide for that area by means of new organizational and personnel configurations.[37]

By no means was this joint approach to role reorganization universal. Quite the contrary. During the investigative phase of the Commission's activities, the staff was able to observe only a few instances of medical-nursing care that resembled the model shown in Figure 2-3. The probability, however, that these experimental approaches would come to represent the cutting edge of future change seemed very great. The diversity of the population served, the general satisfaction reported by

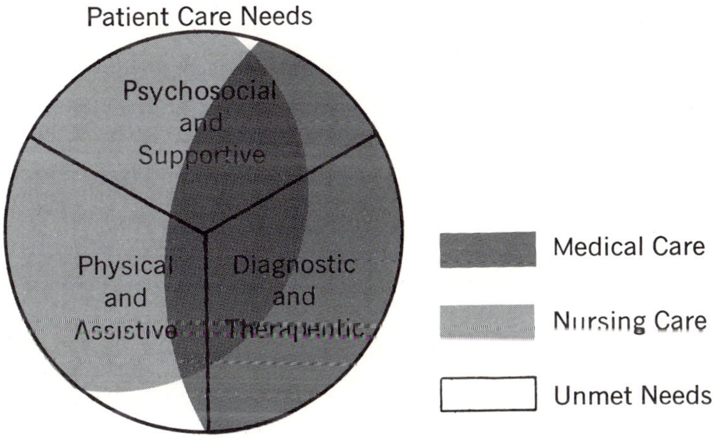

Figure 2-3. Schematic formulation of emergent nurse-physician roles provided to meet patient care needs.

those involved, and the observed effectiveness of closer interprofessional collaboration all argued for some general extension of the concept.

It was in the light of these beginnings that the Commission was encouraged, first to suggest many of its recommendations for joint professional approaches between medicine and nursing, and then to move toward the implementation of those proposals.

The dynamic interplay of new, or refocused, roles between medicine and nursing is not likely to result only in sweetness and light. As Bates sees the future trends:

> . . . both physicians and nurses may see these new nursing roles as competitive, and to be honest, I suspect we must say they are. Nurses will be competing with physicians for office space, for organizational support, for a fair share of the health care dollar, and for a fair voice in the decision-making process . . .[38]

If competition is inevitable, it is also something that is both normal and understandable. However, it is insufficient as a basis for formulating patient care. Bates goes on to propose:

> The nurse-physician team must not, of course, only be competitive; it must be collegial and collaborative. The team must consist of two professionals, each reasonably confident in his own field and each understanding and accepting the contributions and limitations of the other.[39]

This new relationship will not come easily or naturally because the professions of nursing and medicine have for too long tacitly accepted assumptions and behaviors that are incompatible with the new model. This means simply that change must be planned, consciously accepted, and jointly executed. The fact that some practitioners are already utilizing the model is proof that it can work; the challenge is to overcome the inevitable inertia accumulated over so many years by dint of our traditional roles and functions.

SUMMARY

Over the course of the implementation phase, the Commission and staff attempted to assess major trends in the environmental surround that would assist or impede the adoption of *An Abstract for Action*. Three general forces were identified as particularly pertinent: the developing support for national health insurance; the resurgence of women's rights movements in the nation; and the rediscovery by medicine and nursing of their mutual interdependence in the delivery of health care.

Despite the temporary economic downturn of the early seventies, continuing support for some form of comprehensive national health insurance has been generated among groups from all shades of political and social opinion. Several proposals are now before Congress, and additional bills are to be expected in 1973. The eventual provisions and benefits of such legislation are indeterminable, but there is common acceptance that health maintenance and disease prevention will be included as necessary health care along wtih treatment, cure, and restoration.

The heightened interest of women's rights coincides with the concerns over health care. The feminist leaders have voiced their dissatisfaction with both the care accorded women, and with the opportunities that women find in health careers. The combined thrust of these attitudes is to emphasize that we need more female practitioners of health care who are in responsible, authoritative positions.

The rapprochement of medicine and nursing, coming over roughly the same time period, provides a triune support for implementation of the National Commission's recommendations. Encouraged by the need for expanded health care, and sensitized by the growing restiveness of women to settle for dependent, limited roles, the two health professions have been exploring how they might best restructure their independent and interdependent functions so as to provide for quantitative and qualitative increments in health care delivery.

No hard and fast measures can be assessed for the individual or combined influence of these factors on the implementation of *An Abstract for Action*. It would seem, however, that singly and together these trends are supportive—and substantial. They represent a welding of societal demand for more care, together with a growing recognition of our underutilized resources in the form of the American female, at a time when medicine is willing to reconsider its traditional status and position within the health care system. Taken as a whole, then, we have many factors encouraging change—provided it is compatible with the goals expressed. In our considered judgment, the National Commission's objectives are closely related to these trends and the anticipated change processes should be mutually supportive.

FOOTNOTES

1. The National Commission for the Study of Nursing and Nursing Education. *An Abstract for Action*. Jerome P. Lysaught, Director. New York: McGraw-Hill Book Co., 1970, pp. 7-11.
2. Somers, Anne R. *Health Care in Transition: Directions for the Future*. Chicago: Hospital Research and Educational Trust, 1971.
3. ibid., p. 127.
4. Thompson, Julia. *ANA in Washington*. Kansas City, Mo.: The American Nurses' Association, 1972, p. 89.
5. "Essential Elements of a Health Care System: A Provisional Statement of the ANA Commission on Nursing Services." May 14, 1971. (mimeo).
6. "Recommendations for Inclusion in Position Paper on National Health Insurance." Legislative Committee, Council of Baccalaureate and Higher Degree Programs, NLN. May 8, 1973. (mimeo).
7. "Administration Gives ABC's on Funding Policies." *American Journal of Nursing*. 72:5:764 (May) 1973.
8. "Health Maintenance Organization and Resources Act of 1973, Report of the Committee on Labor and Public Welfare, together with Minority Views on S. 14." Washington, D.C.: U.S. Government Printing Office. April 27, 1973. p. 15.

9. "President Rebuffed on Health." *Washington Post*. 96:178:Al. June 1, 1973.
10. "Recommendations for Inclusion in Position Paper on National Health Insurance." op. cit.
11. Somers, Anne R., op. cit., p. 148.
12. Morgan, Elaine. *The Descent of Woman*. New York: Stein and Day, 1972, p. 1.
13. Ehrenreich, Barbara and Deirdre English. *Witches, Midwives, and Nurses: A History of Women Healers*. Oyster Bay, N.Y.: Glass Mountain Pamphlets, undated, p. 19.
14. ibid., p. 31.
15. ibid., p. 32.
16. ibid.
17. ibid., p. 21.
18. ibid., p. 33.
19. Bullough, Vern L. and Bonnie Bullough. *The Emergence of Modern Nursing*, Second ed. New York: The Macmillan Co., 1969, p. 106.
20. Ehrenreich, Barbara and Deirdre English. op. cit., pp. 34-35.
21. Hole, Judith and Ellen Levine. *Rebirth of Feminism*. New York: Quadrangle Books, 1971, pp. 434-435.
22. Bird, Caroline. *Born Female: The High Cost of Keeping Women Down*. New York: David McKay Co., 1968, p. 44.
23. Mark, Ella V. "Women as Guardians of the Public Health," in A.A.W. *Truth, Justice and Honor*. Papers read before the Association for the Advancement of Women, 16th Women's Congress, Detroit, Michigan, November, 1888. Fall River, Mass.: J. H. Franklin & Co., 1889, p. 52.
24. Schaefer, Marguerite J. "Toward a Full Profession of Nursing: the Challenge of the Educator's Role." *The Journal of Nursing Education*. 11:4:41-42 (November) 1972.
25. Ehrenreich, Barbara and Deirdre English. op. cit., p. 41.
26. ibid., p. 26.
27. "Medical and Nursing Practice in a Changing World: Proceedings of the First National Conference for Professional Nurses and Physicians." Sponsored by the American Nurses' Association and the American Medical Association. Williamsburg, Virginia, 1964.
28. "Nurse-Physician Collaboration Toward Improved Patient Care: Papers from the Second National Conference for Professional Nurses and Physicians." Sponsored by the American Medical Association and the American Nurses' Association. Denver, Colorado, 1965. *also* "The Sick Person Needs . . . Report of the Third National Conference for Professional Nurses and Physicians." Sponsored by the American Medical Association and the American Nurses' Association. Coronado, California, 1967.
29. Bates, Barbara. "Doctor and Nurse: Changing Roles and Relations." *The New England Journal of Medicine*. 283:3:130 (July 16) 1970.
30. ibid., p. 129.
31. Lynaugh, Joan E. and Barbara Bates. "The Two Languages of Nursing and Medicine." *American Journal of Nursing*. 73:1:66-69 (January) 1973.
32. The schematic representation in Figures 2-1 through 2-3 are based on the concepts presented by Barbara Bates in *The New England Journal of Medicine*, 283:3:129-133 (July 16, 1970). That journal did not publish the diagrams that Dr. Bates submitted with the article, and she graciously provided the National Commission staff with the original drawings she had developed. The figures used in this chapter are based on those earlier materials, and are somewhat modified by another conceptual rendering developed by Robert A. Hoekelman and Harriet Kitzman for the pediatric nurse practitioner program at the University of Rochester School of Medicine. The composite owes much to both these sources.
33. Bates, Barbara. op. cit., pp. 129-130.
34. Duff, R. S. and A.B. Hollingshead. *Sickness and Society*. New York: Harper and Row, 1968, pp. 374-375.
35. Bates, Barbara. op. cit., p. 130.
36. "Episodic Nursing Practice: Refinement and Expansion of the Roles." Rochester, N.Y.: The National Commission for the Study of Nursing and Nursing Education, 1971. (pamphlet). passim.
37. ibid., pp. 11-12.
38. Bates, Barbara. "Nurse-Physician Dyad: Collegial or Competitive?" *Three Challenges to the Nursing Profession: Selected Papers from the 1972 ANA Convention*. Kansas City, Mo.: The American Nurses' Association, 1972. p. 10.
39. ibid.

THREE

TOWARD CHANGE IN NURSING: ORGANIZATIONAL STRUCTURE AND INFORMATIONAL ACTIVITIES

While the National Commission had been enlarged in order to direct the implementation effort, and while its increased membership included leaders and practitioners of nursing and medicine, health management persons, educators and national policy spokesmen for health care, it was clearly recognized that even broader experience and more diverse points of view should be utilized in some systematic fashion.

Over the course of the investigation phase, the staff had received assistance from two standing committees, one composed of nurses and the other of multidisciplinary representatives, as well as a number of ad hoc groups formed to review findings, conclusions, and recommendations as these evolved from the study. So helpful were these critiques that the Commission and staff agreed some similar apparatus should be devised to ensure a continuing dialogue on the work of implementation. Because of the inherent differences in the activities of the two phases, it was anticipated that more standing advisory committees would be required and that their composition should be even more catholic than before. Over a period of several months, five standing committees were organized to provide counsel, commentary, and criticism to the staff and the Commission. Each of these groups had areas of particular emphasis, but all were afforded wide latitude in their discussions and suggestions. While instituted separately, some of the committees occasionally worked jointly on problems or concerns advanced by the staff.

ORGANIZATION OF ADVISORY COMMITTEES

As indicated in Figure 3-1, the five advisory committees were so organized as to work directly with the staff of the Commission in a free-floating fashion. Members of the groups received periodic reports and materials as well as news releases, publications, and commentaries. Preliminary agendas were distributed in advance of each meeting so that members would be informed of discussion areas and other topics might be suggested. Follow-up correspondence was invited and, on occasion, formal instruments were distributed to obtain reactions and suggestions. The membership and specific charge of each advisory group is treated in the following section.

Nursing Liaison Committee

In the planning and conduct of the original study, the American Nurses' Association and the National League for Nursing themselves had requested that the Commission and staff maintain rigorous independence and accord the nursing organizations those privileges proffered any other health associations. As a matter of procedure, the staff and Commission included the American Medical Association, the American Hospital Association, and other bodies on its advisory committees and in ad hoc discussion groups, along with spokesmen from nursing organizations. This added immeasurably to the objectivity and the breadth of analysis with which each recommendation was considered.

In the work of implementation, however, it was evident that many of the recommendations would require overt action on the part of the nursing organizations—indeed, some of the proposals required specific change within the "nursing establishment"—and that a much closer communication network needed to be established. The Nursing Liaison Committee was developed specifically to foster two-way dialogue between the Commission and those large organizations which were intimately involved in implementation activities. The sixteen members of the committee were:

Helen C. Belcher, Director, Nursing Education Project, Southern Regional Education Board.

†Margery Drake, Acting Executive Secretary, Conference of Catholic Schools of Nursing.

Carol Eady, Director of Nursing Education, Michael Reese Hospital and Medical Center, and President-Elect, National League for Nursing.

Jo Eleanor Elliott, Director of Nursing Programs, Western Interstate Commission for Higher Education.

Katherine Greenough, President, American Nurses' Foundation.

Eileen Jacobi, Executive Director, American Nurses' Association.

Martha Johnson, Director, Division of Nursing, American Hospital Association.

†Sister Francesca Lumpp, Director of Nursing, The Catholic Hospital Association, replaced Ms. Drake.

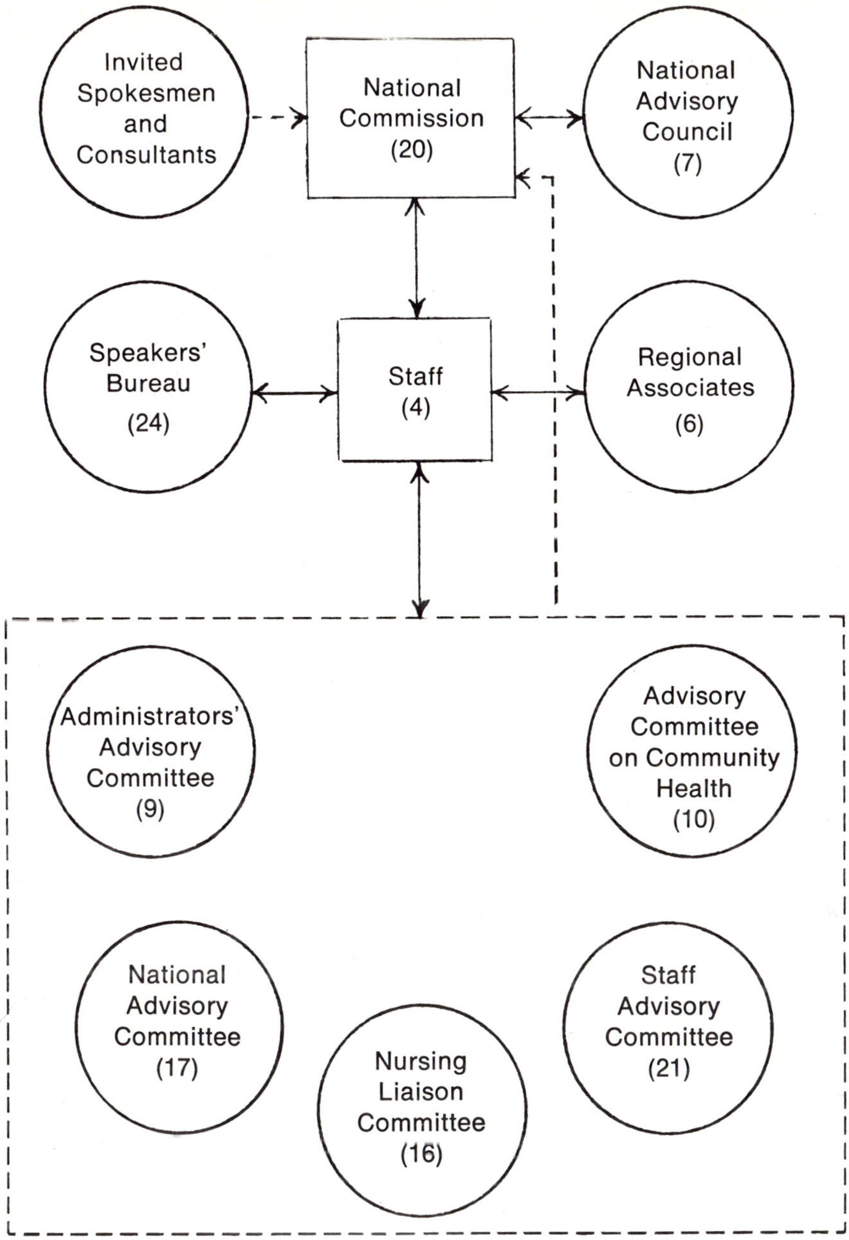

Figure 3-1. Schematic organization chart for implementation phase. Figures in diagram indicate numbers of members.

Susan McNeill, President, National Student Nurses' Association.

Naomi Patchin, Secretary, Committee on Nursing, American Medical Association.

*Hildegard E. Peplau, President, American Nurses' Association.

Eileen Ryan, Director of Nursing, New England Board of Higher Education.

Jessie M. Scott, Director, Division of Nursing, Public Health Service, U.S. Department of Health, Education, and Welfare.

‡Susan Taylor, Associate Director, American Nurses' Foundation.

Mary Ann Tuft, Executive Director, National Student Nurses' Association.

Margaret Walsh, General Director, National League for Nursing.

§Pearl Zemlicka, Chairman, Midwest Continuing Professional Education for Nurses (MCPEN).

Because these individuals were selected for their organizational offices, there was some turnover as indicated in the footnotes. Likewise, there were occasions when attendance at advisory committee meetings was delegated to officers or staff other than those formally appointed. For the most part, however, the listed individuals worked with the Commission staff. In addition to their participation in meetings of the committee, each member was in frequent contact with the staff about specific activities and organizational participation in the general process of implementation.

National Advisory Committee

Initiation of change in nursing patterns necessarily requires congruent adjustments in related fields and disciplines. To subject various projects and proposals to "reality testing" and to interdisciplinary consideration, a National Advisory Committee was established with representatives from nursing, medicine, allied health, higher education, and health administration. The individuals were selected because of their involvement in innovative approaches to practice and education and their commitment to developing better systems for the future. This committee has primarily assisted in formulating approaches to educational transition and role model developments in nursing practice. The seventeen members of this committee include:

Rachel Ayers, Director of Nursing, City of Hope National Medical Center, Los Angeles.

Ione G. Carey, Director of Education, Visiting Nurse Service of New York.

*Rosamond Gabrielson replaced Dr. Peplau on her election to the presidency of ANA.
‡Martha Pitel, Director, American Nurses' Foundation, replaced Ms. Taylor.
§Patricia Forni, Project Director, MCPEN, replaced Ms. Zemlicka.

Mary Jane Carter, School Nurse Practitioner, Albuquerque Public School System.

Lloyd C. Elam, President, Meharry Medical College, Nashville.

Mildred Fenske, Clinical Specialist, Vanderbilt University School of Nursing.

Loretta C. Ford, Chairman, Community Health Nursing, University of Colorado Medical Center.

John Rhodes Haverty, Dean, School of Allied Health Sciences, Georgia State University.

Howard Jacobson, Director, Macy Program, Harvard Medical School and Boston College Graduate School of Nursing.

Emylou Keith, Chairman, Executive Committee, The Study of Nurse Resources, Services and Education in Missouri.

Annette S. Lefkowitz, Director, School of Nursing, Northern Illinois University.

Israel Light, Dean, School of Related Health Sciences, Chicago Medical School/University of Health Sciences.

Janet Miner, President, Wyoming League for Nursing.

Ewald B. Nyquist, Commissioner of Education, The State Education Department, The University of the State of New York.

Mildred Quinn, Dean, College of Nursing, University of Utah.

Janice E. Ruffin, Clinical Specialist, Community Consultation Unit, Connecticut Mental Health Center.

Frances I. Waddle, Executive Director, Oklahoma Board of Nurse Registration and Nursing Education.

Gail L. Warden, Executive Vice President, Operations, Rush-Presbyterian-St. Luke's Medical Center, Chicago.

Again, individual members assisted the staff and Commission in projects and activities in addition to the scheduled meetings of the Advisory Committee. For example, Janet Miner was intimately involved in the development of the Wyoming Commission for Nursing and Nursing Education while Emylou Keith played a significant part in the establishment of the Missouri Committee for Nursing and Nursing Education. This active involvement in grassroots implementation assured the staff that the National Advisory Committee was able to maintain a continuing critical commentary on succeeding stages of the project.

Staff Advisory Panel

While the Nursing Liaison Committee provided an excellent entree to official organizations and their professional staffs, the Commission was desirous of having a supplemental source of information that would be comprised of nurse practitioners, nurse faculty and students, and clinical directors of nursing service—individuals who are actively engaged in the day-to-day concerns of nursing. The Commission felt that including in this group specialty practitioners from a wide variety of fields would ensure a high degree of relevance and a natural "sounding board" of nurse concern and opinion. There were twenty-one individuals appointed to the Staff Advisory Panel; at the time of acceptance, their positions were:

Carol Ann Alvord, Graduate Student, Indiana University School of Nursing.

Mary Baker, Undergraduate Student, Northeastern University School of Nursing, Boston.

Martha Barnard, Assistant Professor of Obstetrical and Gynecological Nursing, Department of Nursing Education, University of Kansas.

Teresa Chopoorian, Co-Director, Macy Program, Harvard Medical School and Boston College Graduate School of Nursing.

Joy Lynn Douglas, Director of Nursing Education, Methodist Hospital, Memphis, and Chairman of the Governing Council, Type VIII Membership of the American Hospital Association.

Christina Eberl, Community Nurse Practitioner, Buffalo, formerly with the Martin Luther King, Jr. Health Center, New York.

Marion Fleck, Coordinator of Health and Nursing Services, Albuquerque Public School System.

Nancy Gaspard, Associate Professor of Public Health Nursing, Boston College.

Sherry B. Grigg, Undergraduate Student, University of Virginia School of Nursing and, later, Nurse Practitioner, United States Air Force.

Joan Larkin, Undergraduate Student, University of Kansas School of Nursing and Nurse Practitioner, Omaha, Nebraska.

Harold MacKinnon, Director of Nursing Service, Jackson Memorial Hospital, Miami.

Marilyn Maxfield, Former President, National Student Nurses' Association and Nurse Practitioner, Salt Lake City.

Martha Mitchell, Assistant Professor of Psychiatric Nursing, University of Wisconsin at Madison.

Constance Monlezun, Graduate Student, Tulane University School of Nursing, Former Recording Secretary, National Student Nurses' Association.

Marcia Nobis, Nurse Practitioner, Oakland, California, Former Vice President, National Student Nurses' Association.

Muriel S. Pappert, Industrial Nurse Practitioner, New York Telephone Company.

Martha J. Parlapiano, Nurse Practitioner, Rockford, President, Association of Operating Room Nurses.

Beth Pearl, Nurse Practitioner, Phoenix, Former President, National Student Nurses' Association.

Carlita Peterson, Undergraduate Student, Grant Hospital School of Nursing, Columbus and Member of Committee on Breakthrough to Nursing.

Mary Jane Sands, Private Duty Nurse Practitioner, Pasadena.

Jacquelyn Smith, Assistant Administrator of Nursing Service, Goshen General Hospital, Indiana.

The Staff Advisory Panel was affectionately referred to as the "Young Turks" because, while lifetime and experience varied considerably, everyone in this group tended to approach each problem from a fresh point of view with relatively few "organizational givens." The dynamic interaction between students and faculty, practitioners and directors of service, generalists and specialists tended to bring light and occasionally some heat—to bear on a variety of situations. Nothing went unchallenged because it was customary or traditional. Yet proposals were constructive and the individual members assumed personal responsibility for testing their ideas.

Administrators' Advisory Committee

Because two out of every three active nurse practitioners is employed by a hospital, and because these institutions play such a key role in the utilization and career reward patterns of American nursing, the Commission indicated its desire to have one advisory committee composed of articulate spokesmen for the special concerns of health management. In addition, some hospital administrators play a key role in planning the evolution of nursing education, for the decision to maintain or relinquish hospital schools of nursing is pivotal in the development of an articulated system of educational institutions and levels.

Individual members of the Administrators' Advisory Committee were selected for their active involvement within their own professional organizations and their evinced interest in the problems of nursing education and practice. It was hoped that the committee could aid the staff in exploring changed patterns of utilization and reinforcement that would positively influence the attractiveness and satisfactions of a nursing career. At the same time, it was felt that the advisors could serve as a link between the Commission and various employer groups that would be affected by the recommendations of *An Abstract for Action*. At the very least, the committee could identify those points of concern among health administrators and articulate the feelings of many individuals who felt threatened by changing patterns in nursing practice and education. The nine members of the Administrators' Advisory Committee were:

Robert E. Adams, Executive Director, Research Hospital and Medical Center, Kansas City, Missouri.

H. Robert Cathcart, President, Pennsylvania Hospital Association and President, The Pennsylvania Hospital, Philadelphia.

Everett V. Fox, Administrator, Hospital Affiliation Contracts, New York University Medical Center.

Richard Highsmith, Administrator, Samuel Merritt Hospital, Oakland.

Gordon N. Johnsen, Administrator, Madison General Hospital, Wisconsin.

James E. Ludlam, President, American Society of Hospital Attorneys, and Practicing Attorney, Los Angeles.

Sister Mary Maurita, R.S.M., Executive Director, The Catholic Hospital Association.

Roy S. Rambeck, Executive Director, University of Washington Hospitals, Seattle.

Martin S. Ulan, Executive Director, Hackensack Hospital, New Jersey.

As anticipated, this committee verbalized a great number of concerns over the directions proposed by the Commission's recommendations. At the same time, however, data were examined unemotionally and a useful dialogue established between these individuals and the Commission staff. Areas of disagreement were narrowed as a result of discussion and points of common consensus were emphasized. In particular, positive progress was made through the participation of commissioners Stuart Marylander and Charles Paxson, themselves both hospital administrators, who met regularly with this committee.

Advisory Committee on Community Health

While the Administrators' Advisory Committee was, of course, heavily weighted in terms of large, complex health care facilities and their staffing problems, the Commission was equally concerned about the impact of the emerging institutions and systems for health care delivery. Health maintenance organizations, community care plans, and other "labels" are coming into common currency. There is, however, little yet in the way of systematization among these approaches; there is still considerable debate about the objectives to be served let alone patterns for reaching them. Nevertheless, it seemed essential that we obtain the aid of some individuals involved in the cutting edge of these changes.

To help the Commission and staff analyze current projects and demonstrations, and to predict the configuration of future systems, ten individuals were invited to serve on the Advisory Committee on Community Health. They were:

James B. Cobb, Director, Department of Community Health, American Medical Association.

Eli S. Egert, Director of Health Planning, University of Pittsburgh.

Frederick B. Hodges, Director, California State Department of Public Health.

Margaret C. Kauffman, Executive Director, Community Nursing Services of Philadelphia.

William F. Lee, Director, Veterans Administration Hospital, Fresno.

Margaret D. Lewis, Director, Visiting Nurse Service, Denver.

Katherine C. Neill, Director, Monroe County Public Health Nursing Division, Rochester, New York.

Eva M. Reese, Executive Director, Visiting Nurse Service of New York.

Scott K. Simonds, Professor of Health Education, School of Public Health, University of Michigan.

Vernon E. Weckwerth, Professor, Program in Hospital and Health Care Administration, School of Public Health, University of Minnesota.

This committee was the "youngest" of the advisory groups in terms of its appointment and activity span. Nevertheless, the implications of its area of study are profound and will have continuing impact on the future of American nursing and the implementation of Commission recommendations concerning practice and careers. In some ways, this advisory group was required to raise more problems than answers, but the parameters for consideration are of prime significance to the provision of all professional health care in our society over the coming years.

Comments on the Committees

It is, of course, impossible to single out the contributions of these seventy-three individuals (plus those other persons who helped over some portion of the three-year implementation phase). Many of them became much more involved and active than their commitment to serve on a committee would require; most of the advisors took deep professional interest in the obligations they accepted. In terms of interaction with the staff, these consultants consistently exposed problems, communication gaps, and tactical errors—but always with the positive purpose of facilitating the implementation effort. There were even occasions when individual advisors took great pains to propose ways to obtain the ends of certain recommendations about which they personally had some misgivings—recognizing that their own feelings should not be determinative of overall activities.

In total, these advisors provided hundreds of man-days to the Commission and its staff without salary or honorarium. Their effort contributed much to the implementation phase and to the strategies developed for carrying it out. Moreover, individual advisors took part in activities related to the Commission's recommendations and their realization at state and national levels.

DEVELOPMENT OF INFORMATIONAL PROCESSES

Because personal health is the very cornerstone of each individual's lifespace and, in the broad view, a primary national concern, there is no single "public" involved with the problems of nursing. Rather, each and all of the "publics"—citizens, health professionals, third party payers, and many more—have a great stake in what is done in nursing practice and education. In order to reach these groups and the opinion makers who influence them, the Commission, its staff, and advisory committees have engaged in the continuing round of efforts to report and interact on *An Abstract for Action* and its implementation.

The initial steps in this direction took place even before the formal start of the implementation phase. In February of 1970, a summary report of the Commission's findings and recommendations appeared in the *American Journal of Nursing.*[1] The same month, an abbreviated summary was published in *Nursing Outlook*, the official magazine of the National League for Nursing.[2] Still later, other journals of the nursing press provided their readers with reviews and commentary on the recommendations contained in the summary report.[3] Thus, a large segment of active nursing was at least alerted to the Commission's work well in advance of the final report's appearance in June of 1970. Thousands of the *AJN* reprints, together with a separate abbreviated version prepared by the Commission staff, were distributed over the following months.

Report and Information Meetings

In the period of time between the appearance of the summary report and the publication of the complete findings and recommendations of the Commission, a series of regional meetings was planned to announce and interpret the study and its findings. (A brief, but complete report on this activity is contained in *An Abstract for Action: Appendices.*[4]) The conduct of these meetings provided the Commission and staff with a baptism into the processes of implementation. Thirteen regional meetings were held. In addition to nursing organizations and institutions, invitations were extended to state governors, legislative leaders, medical and hospital representatives, lay persons active in health affairs, state boards of practice and licensure, health planning agencies, and a variety of other relevant groups.

The response was, in some respects, both encouraging and depressing. On the positive side, more than 1,475 individuals attended the thirteen meetings, and their participation was characterized by great interest, generally broad agreement with the Commission's work, and, on the whole, thoughtful presentation of uncertainty or disagreement. On the other hand, those who attended the meetings represented less than 15 percent of the total persons invited—although another 8 percent took the time to indicate their interest and explain that circumstances or conflicts prevented their attendance.

The first sobering realization to come from the regional meetings was that this process of public involvement and reporting must be carried on state-by-state and district-by-district. Over the first two-and-one-half years of the implementation period, then, the staff and advisory groups participated in a series of statewide informational meetings that extended the concept of the original report sessions. Through this means, we were able, over time, to reach many of the intended audiences.

As indicated in Table 3-1, the majority of states did participate actively in the report and information stage of the implementation phase; some of those states which did not conduct statewide informational meetings using commissioners or staff personnel developed their own alternative approaches to distributing information on state and national needs in nursing.

TABLE 3-1 STATEWIDE INFORMATIONAL MEETINGS CONDUCTED THROUGHOUT IMPLEMENTATION PHASE

States conducting meetings on implementation	44*
States not conducting informational meetings	7
	51**

*Some states planned and conducted a series of district meetings as well as statewide conferences.
**Total of 51 includes the District of Columbia.

Contact with Major Organizations

While the state and district meetings provided the staff, particularly, with grassroots reaction to the report and recommendations, it became clear very early that many nurses, physicians, and others were waiting to hear the reaction of national organizations to *An Abstract for Action* before committing themselves to implementation activities.

Beginning in the late spring of 1970, the Commission and the staff made overtures to a number of major organizations in the health and education fields. The associations were supplied with summary reports of *An Abstract for Action*, an invitation to address questions or comments to the Commission for reply, and a request to discuss possible cooperation in efforts to implement the report. Over the ensuing months, a number of responsive actions took place.

National League for Nursing. The NLN is an organization which works for the improvement of nursing services and education and its membership includes both nurses and others who share the desire for augmenting the quantity and quality of nursing manpower. There are currently some 15,400 individual members, over 90 percent of whom are professional nurses. In addition, however, there are more than 1,800 agency members distributed among six councils: Home Health Agencies and Community Health Services; Hospital and Related Institutional Nursing Services; Baccalaureate and Higher Degree Programs; Diploma Programs; Associate Degree Programs; and Practical Nursing Programs. Moreover, the League has forty-nine constituent leagues for nursing organized on state, area, and metropolitan bases.[5]

As one of the founding agencies of the National Commission for the Study of Nursing and Nursing Education, the National League for Nursing had, of course, followed the progress of the investigation phase quite closely. Commissioners and staff had met several times with various councils and staff groups from the NLN, and an abbreviated version of the report appeared in the February, 1970 issue of *Nursing Outlook*, official organ of the League.[6] It was anticipated, then, that some formal action would be taken by the League soon after publication of *An Abstract for Action.*

On March 13, 1970 the Council of Baccalaureate and Higher Degree Programs convened in Kansas City, Missouri, reviewed the summary report, and unanimously adopted a resolution which read in part:

> WHEREAS, The National League for Nursing and the American Nurses' Association supported both financially and professionally the National Commission for the Study of Nursing and Nursing Education; and . . .
>
> WHEREAS, This Council stands ready to work diligently to accomplish the recommendations of the Commission; . . . therefore, be it
>
> RESOLVED, That this Council endorse in principle the recommendations of the Commission as published in recent issues of the *American Journal of Nursing* and *Nursing Outlook* . . .[7]

Within the context of the resolution, however, the Council expressed one reservation having to do with the proposed level of federal funding for nursing. The National Commission had endorsed a level below that authorized by Congress and above that proposed by the Administration. The Council of Baccalaureate and Higher Degree Programs inserted a resolve in their endorsement statement to the effect that:

> RESOLVED, That this Council support federal funding at or above the level presently authorized in the nursing sections of the Health Manpower Act.[8]

With this single indication of concern, the resolution was forwarded to the staff of the National Commission.

Slightly more than one month later, on April 28, 1970, the Executive Committee of the NLN Board of Directors met in New York and unanimously issued the following statement:

> 1. The League supports the plan of the Commission to provide for implementation of the goals and principles of the Commission and its objective—to improve the delivery of health care to the American people, particularly through the analysis and improvement of nursing and nursing education.
> 2. The League further pledges its support by such appropriate services as may be available through already established service in the League offices.
> 3. The League will participate with other nursing and health groups in establishing a task force with the hope of finding ways and means of raising money to support the Commission's work.
> 4. The League also will provide $25,000 in 1972-73 for the Commission's work in implementing the recommendations of the study when more definitive program and budget plans of the Commission are forthcoming.[9]

While this decision of the Executive Committee certainly indicated positive support of the directions taken by *An Abstract for Action*, the action was underscored when the entire Board of Directors voted in February of 1971 to "endorse the *Abstract for Action* as it appeared in the *American Journal of Nursing*."[10] This step was taken to clarify the overall position of the national organization with regard to the report and its recommendations.

Because the League was organized with agency member councils, it was inevitable that certain recommendations of the National Commission would be viewed as threatening by some of the NLN agencies. This was particularly evident in the Council of Diploma Programs. At the biennial convention of the League in 1971, this Council formally proposed that the national organization and its Board of Directors "cease and desist" from further activities related to the implementation of the National Commission's report.

The NLN Board did not, of course, retract its commitments. Instead, it appointed a task force composed of members representing all the member agency councils, both supporters and dissidents, together with selected consumers of health care. This group was given the charge to study all recommendations in *An Abstract for Action* and prepare a report for the Board of Directors sometime in 1972.[11] Since the earlier actions of the National League had specifically addressed the contents of the summary report, it was felt that this more lengthy look was entirely appropriate and would serve to meet some of the entered objections. The task force met in January and again in April of 1972 and submitted its report to the Board on October 4, 1972. The Board, in turn, voted to receive the report and approve its distribution to the general membership for their consideration.*

While the task force was in the midst of its examination and report writing, the Council of Diploma Programs of the NLN convened in their annual meeting. At the sessions of April 6 and 7 of 1972, the Council voted "non-support" of eleven specific recommendations made by the National Commission and, at the same time, indicated that "collaboration at this time was not possible" in work toward the implementation of the Commission's report.[12]

Almost as a countermand to the independent action of the Council of Diploma Programs, the General Director of the National League for Nursing wrote on April 11, 1972,

> I am happy to inform you that NLN is prepared to implement its decision in 1970 to provide $25,000 in 1972-73 to the National Commission for the Study of Nursing and Nursing Education for the implementation of the Commission's report. . . .
>
> We look forward to hearing from you as soon as possible regarding the details of the Commission's plan for the final implementation stages.[13]

Perhaps the ambivalence that is seen in the ranks of the National League for Nursing reflects the approach-avoidance conflicts that have been recorded over the recommendations of each study of the profession dating back to 1923. Certainly, the contrast between acceptance and rejection among member agency councils mirrors the tension between change forces and adherents of the status quo. As one close observer analyzed it:

> What is said on this editorial page does not necessarily constitute any official position of the League; rather it represents the personal opinion of the editor or whoever's name is affixed to it. It would seem, though, that the Commission's activities would be of particular interest to NLN members. The Commission was charged, it will be remembered, to study "the present system of nursing education in relation to the responsibilities and skill levels required for high-quality patient care." The Commission's membership, like the League's, represents expertise in many fields, including both professional and community members. Finally, as was pointed out in *An Abstract for Action,* nursing 'holds within itself the key to whether or not the vast majority of our people will receive quality health care.'

*Note: A discussion of the NLN Task Force Report is provided on page 74.

> These recommendations didn't just come off the top of someone's head—they're the result of three years' intensive gathering and analysis of data. As such, they would seem to merit continuing open-minded consideration; controlled application, follow-up, and assessment of results; and a withholding of judgment until after trial.[14]

Although this editorial was not the "official position" of the League, it seems to pronounce the sentiment of the Board of Directors who pressed forward in their support of controlled application, follow-up, and withholding of judgment. Rather than wait for unanimity, the Board opted for change processes while providing the mechanism, through the task force, for ongoing review of the implications of the Commission's priorities.

As the editorial writers of *Nursing Outlook* saw the decision,

> It's unfortunate that this . . . decision to authorize such a task force was not made until early 1971.
>
> To our mind, however, none of this detracts from the value of such an analysis . . . Better late than never, we say . . .[15]

An earlier review would have been desirable; the fact remains, however, that the real alternatives presented to the National League for Nursing in 1970 were: (a) to do nothing until extensive study was undertaken, possibly followed by the development of a compromise, consensual position; or (b) to support the National Commission's implementation proposals in the confidence that good outcomes would be lasting and poor results could be discarded. The Board of Directors of the National League for Nursing demonstrated that, if they were to sin, it would be by commission rather than omission, and they supported the implementation process.

It is a commentary on the basic correctness of the Board's position that, in the detailed review, "many of the NCSNNE recommendations . . . were endorsed without question by the task force."[16] (Recommendations about which the task force had questions will be pointed out and discussed in Chapters 4, 5, and 6.) To their credit must go the recognition that months and years might have been wasted only to determine that most of the Commission's recommendations should have been implemented as quickly as possible. Because of the cross-currents within the organization, the overall support provided the Commission and staff throughout the implementation phase is quite remarkable.

American Nurses' Association. The ANA is the largest professional association of registered nurses in the United States with an individual membership of around 160,000. Established in 1896, the Association is commonly viewed as the world's oldest professional organization of women—although, of course, membership is unrestricted by considerations of sex, nationality, race, creed, or color. The ANA is comprised of fifty-three state and constituent associations, including the

District of Columbia, Guam, and the Virgin Islands. These groups are further composed of more than 800 district groups which meet local needs and concerns.[17]

The purposes of the ANA are threefold: to foster high standards of nursing practice; to advance nursing education in the delivery of nursing services; and to promote the welfare of nurses to the end that all people will have better health care. In organizing to achieve these ends, the Association has a number of commissions and congresses including those on: Nursing Education, Nursing Services, Nursing Practice, Research, Continuing Education, and Economic and General Welfare.

Together with the National League for Nursing, the ANA had assisted in the establishment and funding of the National Commission, and, like the NLN, had followed the progress of the investigation with interest. The Research and Statistics Department, for example, cooperated with the Commission staff in the assemblage of baseline data during the investigation phase of their work; moreover, there were a number of joint meetings of staff personnel and discussions with members of commissions and congresses on matters pertaining to their expertise. Thus, there was little in the way of a surprise to most ANA officials when the summary report and recommendations of the National Commission appeared in the February, 1970 issue of the *American Journal of Nursing.*[18]

In May of 1970, the House of Delegates, highest authority in the ANA, took up the matter of the Commission report at its biennial convention. Having studied the summary report, but not yet having had an opportunity to examine the complete set of findings and recommendations, the House eschewed a lengthy discussion of details and quickly moved that its members endorse "the second phase of the work of the Commission and . . . make a financial contribution toward the progress of implementation."[19] With only scattered questioning and no dissension, the delegates voted overwhelmingly in favor of the motion.

At this point in time, it was common knowledge that the ANA was in the midst of a severe financial crisis which had caused it to reduce staff and curtail services to its own members and commissions. Thus, the inclusion of the reference to "financial contribution toward the progress of implementation" was considerably more salient than might appear on the surface. It was obvious that the organization could not, at the time of the convention, specify any particular amount, but it was highly significant that the delegates saw the Commission's report as a matter of highest priority.

Following up on the start made by the House, the Board of Directors and the ANA staff discussed both the recommendations and the implementation planning over the next several months. On March 17, 1971, for example, the Executive Director of the ANA wrote the National Commission:

> The ANA Board of Directors finds the Commission's study useful in that it presents in broad strokes some of the problems facing nursing and

points directions in which the profession should move. They believe that the thrust of the Commission should go forward, and they look forward to reviewing the complete report . . .

The Board considers it extremely important that the report be studied throughout the organization at all levels . . . and urges that any efforts toward implementation of these recommendations be approached through the state organizations so as to build on ongoing activities and relationships. . . .[20]

By the fall of 1971, the ANA Board of Directors was prepared to carry out the decision of the preceding convention, and empowered the Executive Director to inform the Commission:

The ANA Board of Directors, meeting in September approved the Finance Committee recommendation that the amount of $25,000 be provided in the 1972 ANA budget for the National Commission for the Study of Nursing and Nursing Education.[21]

While the path toward understanding and support may seem relatively uneventful as compared with some of the happenings within the National League for Nursing, there were specific recommendations that caused concern and animated discussion. In May of 1971, following extensive study and review, the Board of Directors endorsed the four central recommendations contained in the summary section of *An Abstract for Action* and expressed ANA's substantial agreement with the Commission's findings and recommendations. There was one caveat underlined, however, and that concerned the Commission's statements about federal funding. The ANA Board, like the NLN Council of Baccalaureate and Higher Degree Programs, felt that the National Commission should have called for much higher levels of federal support than it did. As the ANA put it:

ANA, which has a policy of seeking public funds for the expansion and improvement of nursing education, expressed the belief that the fourth [central] recommendation would be more helpful had the references to Congressional authorizations for fiscal 1970 been omitted since these authorizations were not adequate in either types of support or amount of money to meet anticipated nursing manpower needs.[22]

If the report of the National Commission thus caused concern because of what it said, there were other organizational components of the American Nurses' Association that were equally upset at the things the report did not say. The Commission on Economic and General Welfare of the ANA studied *An Abstract for Action* and felt constrained to pronounce:

The Commission (E&GW) believes these . . . recommendations fail totally to reflect acceptance of the essential, fundamental principle to which

> ANA is committed—that is, collective participation by nurses in establishing their conditions of practice and employment. What is endorsed tacitly is perpetuation of the unilateral paternalistic establishment of "conditions to promote opportunity for excellence in nursing practice" by hospital administrators.[23]

In this case, and in some other instances of upset, the National Commission and its staff sought to resolve differences of interpretation and clarify points of uncertainty. Over time, this was sufficiently successful that general consensus and cohesion were achieved. As Hildegarde Peplau, then President of the American Nurses' Association, viewed the state of the situation:

> The report makes many illuminating and important points about nursing today and where it should go in the years ahead. It is especially gratifying to have an independent commission reiterate or verify so much of what organized nursing has been saying in the past few decades. Much of ANA's philosophy and programs that it has pioneered are reflected in this report.[24]

In elaborating on the action of the ANA Board of Directors endorsing the central recommendations of *An Abstract for Action*, Dr. Peplau went on to comment:

> The work of the NCSNNE, the report and the implementation phase can make a significant contribution to the advance of nursing. There should be no confusion about ANA's recognition of the value of pronouncements by an independent, autonomous Commission that corroborate so much of what organized nursing has long recognized as essential to progress. Nor should there be confusion about the value that can be derived from a report that provides specific recommendations for action from a Commission that intends to stay in business to get actions on its recommendations. ANA has much to gain from such support of its own programs and goals.[25]

This definitive action of the American Nurses' Association demonstrated its basic concern and commitment toward implementation and its willingness to let points of dispute be tested over time. Like the National League for Nursing, the ANA opted for the overall thrust of the National Commission's proposals and refused to be diverted by the presence of specific disagreements.

Other Nursing Organizations. While the ANA and NLN occupy a central position in any analysis of American nursing, it is also true that many other organizations are comprised of, and speak for, nurse members. Specialty practice groups, student associations, educational bodies, and many other organizations play an increasingly vital part in the development of nursing policy, and the nurses involved in these structures are one of the publics that the Commission was deeply concerned to reach. Beginning with the publication of *An Abstract for Action*, and continuing throughout the implementation phase, every opportunity was taken to initiate dialogue with the more specialized interest groups in nursing, and the results of these contacts were uniformly positive.

The Council of the Conference of Catholic Schools of Nursing, for example, represented in 1971 the great majority of nursing schools under the administrative control of Catholic institutions. These schools included both collegiate and diploma programs. Having engaged in discussions with NCSNNE staff representatives over the period of the investigation, and having studied the final report and recommendations for several months, the Council adopted a policy statement which said, in part:

> The National Commission has taken an independent look at the totality of nursing and its concerns and related the issues so identified to the social system that provides the whole spectrum of health care for the American public. The Commissioners have made every effort to insure an objective report free from bias and the influence of pressure groups, including the nursing profession itself. . . .
>
> The Council of CCSN has drawn certain inferences from a study and analysis of this report that are particularly relevant to the attainment of the revised purpose and objectives of the Catholic Hospital Association . . . Therefore, the Council commends the recommendations contained in the report, *An Abstract for Action*, to the CHA Board of Trustees and the membership of the Conference of Catholic Schools of Nursing to serve as guidelines for developing and/or supporting programs related to nursing.[26]

While the Council statement carried no reservations or equivocations, the newly formed American Association of Deans of College and University Schools of Nursing was more guarded. Meeting in October of 1971, the deans endorsed in principle the report and recommendations of the National Commission. The group, however, expressed some concern over the implications of certain recommendations for "current and futuristic movement of nursing education into institutions of higher education." The Association established a committee to meet with the staff of the National Commission and explore these specific areas, and, in a series of two sessions, these matters seemed to have been satisfactorily resolved.[27]

Beginning in the 1950s, and with increasing acceleration, nurses banded together into professional societies related to their areas of clinical specialization. These "specialty practice groups" were first regarded as splinter organizations which diverted energy and manpower from the two established nurse associations—the ANA and the NLN. As time passed, there was greater recognition that these societies served special and different ends and that one could, indeed, be an active member of both a specialty practice group and a more broadly aimed professional organization.

By the 1970s, there were some fifteen specialty practice groups, and the National Commission sought to enlist their aid in the implementation of its recommendations. A number of these groups responded positively, but pointed out that their own formative problems and small membership prevented any extensive involvement. The more established organizations, however, moved quickly in support. Three of the specialty practice groups passed formal resolutions of endorsement and others worked informally through their organizational networks. None of the specialty groups opposed the proposals set forth in *An Abstract for Action.*

The Americal Association of Industrial Nurses became the first specialty practice group to comment publicly on the Commission report, and in October of 1971 their Board of Directors voted their "endorsement and support" of the recommendations. This statement was not intended to be a simple token of help. As indicated by their executive director,

> This action came as the result of careful study of the Commission's recommendations by the members of the Board and . . . We are interested to learn how AAIN can contribute to the implementation of the recommendations and, again, offer our complete cooperation.[28]

Sometime later, the Association of Operating Room Nurses became the second specialty practice group to announce a formal stand on the National Commission's work. The Board of Directors in October, 1972 adopted a statement which read, in part:

> Within the pattern set by other professional organizations, and appropriate to the aims and purposes of AORN is our commendation of the work and recommendations of the National Commission for the Study of Nursing and Nursing Education.[29]

At almost the same time, the Executive Committee of the Department of School Nurses of the National Education Association adopted a formal statement of support. The resolution included the statement that:

> The National Education Association Department of School Nurses has developed educational programs, drafted statements of philosophy and functions, and implemented model programs for the expanded role of the School Nurse consistent with the directions proposed by the National Commission in its implementation efforts . . . [therefore] the Department of School Nurses will take all appropriate action toward the implementation of the recommendations.[30]

These announcements of encouragement and assistance from nurse practitioners in a variety of fields were instrumental in emphasizing the broad base of support that could be found at nursing's grassroots. Moreover, the leadership of these groups, supplementing the contributions provided by the ANA and NLN, instilled the hope that some greater consensus might be developed among all nursing organizations—not only toward the implementation of the Commission's report, but toward the continuing solution of other problems as they might arise. Indeed, in this sense, *An Abstract for Action* could serve as an example that agreement and cooperation might be reached and that nursing organizations could be supportive rather than divisive in attaining professional aims.

Two other nursing organizations require mention for their activity in behalf of the National Commission's work. The American Nurses' Foundation is a tax-exempt organization whose function is to develop financial support for nursing research and, then, to disseminate funds alone or conjointly with other foundations or associations, to finance and promote specific research projects. The ANF had played a crucial role in the establishment of the National Commission prior to the investigation phase; its Board of Directors voted in 1966 to provide up to $50,000 to aid in establishing an independent study of nursing. This support financed the development of research proposals and background papers which, in turn, facilitated the granting of monies by the Avalon Foundation and the W. K. Kellogg Foundation. Having been a key to initial erection, the ANF continued its interest and encouragement. In the spring of 1971, it commented:

> It is of interest to the American Nurses' Foundation, whose central concerns are the promotion and support of nursing research, that throughout the Commission's recommendations the need for research and the consequent need for funds and personnel are stressed. . . .
>
> The American Nurses' Foundation Board of Trustees has supported the work of the Commission by agreeing to take an active part in a task force for the purpose of raising additional funds to finance the Commission's implementation phase.[31]

The need for a fund-raising task force was obviated by the support proffered by the ANA, the NLN, and the W. K. Kellogg Foundation, but this overt action on the part of the ANF Board of Directors certainly had a salutary effect on the assuredness with which the National Commission could plan a full program of implementation activities.

The second nursing organization to play a key supportive role throughout the implementation phase was the National Student Nurses' Association. This organization of over 40,000 members felt that it could best play its part in implementation through an educational program aimed at student nurses across the country. Using the pages of its magazine, *Imprint*, the NSNA published a four-part series on the students' view of the National Commission report. The articles addressed the general background and findings, and then individual analyses of the recommendations on nursing practice, nursing education, and nursing careers. In addition, the NSNA involved the National Commission in forums at successive national conventions in order to foster dialogue on the implications of the report for current and future students of nursing.

Following the conclusion of the series, the editor of *Imprint* underscored the importance the NSNA attached to student involvement and understanding in these words:

> It seems inconceivable, with the acclaim given the so-called "Lysaught Report" and the number of nursing schools across the country in the process of revamping their educational curricula, that nursing students are not acquainted with the recommendations that are influencing the changes. Yet are you? . . .
>
> No other profession begins and ends in a vacuum. Social trends and political forces play a vital part in their existence. Yet, we as nursing students, in a profession which is so closely tied to humanity, people and social change, are educated in a technological vacuum. Nursing students, you and I have not read *An Abstract for Action*, or *Nursing Reconsidered*, by Esther Lucile Brown. So, how can we discuss the issues intelligently?[32]

While certainly not all nursing students read the National Commission's report, and likely fewer than those did so voluntarily without some professional assignment, one of the highlights of the implementation phase was the interaction with student nurse groups across the country. Unlike their experienced elders who often asked, "Why change?" these individuals were more apt to query, "Why not?" If their directness can sometimes prove disconcerting, their sincerity is singular, and their involvement is intense.

American Medical Association. Among the "publics" which the National Commission was required to address is that of the medical practitioner. These are the individuals who work more closely than anyone else with the nurse in the care setting. Historically, the nurse and the physician long labored almost exclusively together in the treatment of illness and disease. As the number and variety of health aides increased, functional patterns necessarily changed, but the primacy of the relationship between the medical and the nurse practitioner continued.

It seemed essential to the National Commission that medicine be involved in any effort directed at changing the role of nursing because, by definition and by fact, any change in one role requires a related change in congruent roles. Thus, if a nurse expands her functions in patient care, she inevitably affects what the physician does—either by doing some things that the medical practitioner has traditionally performed in the past, or by originating new demands for consultative assistance.

Lack of communication and joint planning is reflected, first of all, in the fragmentation of patient care, then in the frictions and frustrations of professional jockeying. To prevent this kind of waste, the National Commission sought to involve medicine and, in particular, the largest single organization of medical practitioners, the American Medical Association, in the developmental phases of both the investigation and the implementation. Contacts were maintained with the Council of Medical Education and the Committee on Nursing of the AMA, and with other bodies on an ad hoc basis. With the publication of *An Abstract for Action*, however, the Committee on Nursing became the primary discussant concerning the report and any appropriate AMA response. At the invitation of the committee, the NCSNNE staff attended their fall meeting in 1970 to discuss the recommendations and their implementation. Following that meeting, the committee chairman, Dr. Charles L. Leedham, wrote:

> I want to take this opportunity to thank you on behalf of the members of the Committee on Nursing for your presentation at the November 28 meeting in Boston. We appreciate your courtesy in responding to our questions and in sharing information . . . The Committee is in agreement about endorsement of the four major recommendations of the Commission and will ask the Board of Trustees of the AMA to endorse them. After the Board has had an opportunity to assess the recommendations and take appropriate action, the Committee on Nursing will then consider plans for future activities.[33]

Shortly after the first of the year, the matter was placed before the AMA Board of Trustees, and their resultant action was swift and positive. In February, the trustees voted that "the recommendation of its Committee on Nursing be approved, the four [major] recommendations of the National Commission be endorsed,"[34] and further, that the AMA Committee on Nursing have the responsibility for implementing these recommendations within the structure of AMA.

This decision not only underscored the philosophical acceptance of *An Abstract for Action*, but paved the way for continuing interaction and planning with the Committee on Nursing to secure the realization of such proposals as the National Joint Practice Commission between organized medicine and nursing.

American Hospital Association. Whereas the physician is the closest care colleague of the nurse, the hospital administrator is the primary employer—approximately two-thirds of all practicing registered nurses are employed in the hospitals throughout our nation. Just as the AMA is the largest single organization of physicians, so the American Hospital Association is the preeminent spokesman for the more than 7,000 hospitals distributed across the United States.

Like the National League for Nursing, the AHA is composed of institutional and personal members whose interests span a broad range of health activities. In addition to hospitals and in-patient facilities, the institutional members include the Blue Cross plans, comprehensive health planning units, home care facilities, and hospital schools of nursing. Personal members include hospital attorneys, engineers, volunteer service people, trainers, personnel administrators, nursing service directors, and seven other categories of specialization.

In the face of such diversity, the Association, in September of 1970, established a ten person advisory panel under the chairmanship of David B. Wilson, M.D., then director of the University of Mississippi Medical Center to study *An Abstract for Action* and suggest any appropriate action to be taken by the American

Hospital Association regarding the National Commission's recommendations.[35] Membership on this advisory committee included physicians, administrators, educators, nurse educators, and nursing service directors. The study group met twice—in late September and early November—and at the conclusion of the second session adopted a formal statement on the report and the recommendations of the National Commission. The introductory paragraph stated:

> The National Commission for the Study of Nursing and Nursing Education has issued a report . . . that deserves the attention of those engaged in the delivery of health care to the public and of those engaged in the preparation of practitioners to provide that care. Although the focus of the report is on nursing, the point is made clear that the problems of nursing and nursing education must be viewed from the standpoint of the delivery system of health care and not as isolated entities within the health field.[36]

The report then addressed the important relationship between the nurse and the hospital in enhancing the provision of care and stressed the need for broad participation on the part of other professional groups in influencing what nursing and nursing education should be now and in the future. The preamble concluded with this statement:

> The report has identified troublesome problems and issues in nursing and nursing education, some of which have been pointed up in previous studies. The American Hospital Association believes that now is a propitious time to reemphasize the old issues and to identify urgent new ones for action and constructive solution.[37]

The advisory committee then went on to address the central recommendations of the National Commission report, and said:

> In regard to recommendations proposed by the Commission, the American Hospital Association believes the following:
>
> 1. Nursing should be viewed as a profession, and the scope and practice of nursing in the health field should be expanded to achieve professionalism.
>   *a.* Research in nursing practice and education should be given greater support in terms of commitment, finances, and interprofessional cooperation.
>   *b.* The scope of independent nursing practice in the clinical aspects of patient care should be extended.
>   *c.* The competencies associated with the emerging terminology of 'clinical nurse' and 'master clinician' used to describe the highly competent nurse practitioner should be recognized and clearly defined.
>   *d.* Relationships between physicians and nurses as copartners in patient care should be fostered.
>
> 2. Local hospital practice committees have the greatest potential for influencing nursing practice. Joint practice commissions on state and national levels would serve a useful purpose by supporting actions at the local level,

recommending such actions for general adoption, stimulating research, and influencing legislation.

3. Master-planning commissions on nursing education are needed and should be coordinated insofar as possible with health and manpower planning agencies and with commissions on higher education.

4. The concept of episodic and distributive nursing care, as defined and emphasized in the report, is a useful one because the hospital is concerned with the totality of health services and is now the major health resource in most communities. However, career patterns related to episodic and distributive nursing care should emerge from a completed basic nursing program.

5. The improvement academically and organizationally of all programs in nursing education should be vigorously and emphatically pursued, and the establishment of new programs associated with systems of higher education should be encouraged.[38]

This positive analysis, so accepting of the basic thrust of *An Abstract for Action*, was forwarded to Dr. Edwin L. Crosby, then executive president of the AHA, who, in turn, laid it before the Board. Subsequently, it was approved as a statement of and for the American Hospital Association on the recommendation of its General Council and the Council of Professional Services.

The action of the General Council paved the way for direct contact with state hospital associations, AHA staff personnel, and specialty groups within the Association on activities related to the implementation of the National Commission's report, and materially aided in the understanding and acceptance of the recommendations by hospital people.

There was dissonance, of course, among some elements of the AHA membership groups. Particularly, the Type VIII institutional members, the Hospital Schools of Nursing, found the Commission's educational recommendations threatening and the advisory committee's statement that " . . . new programs associated with systems of higher education should be encouraged . . ." to be less than satisfying. On the whole, however, the American Hospital Association had spoken in unmistakably supportive terms and lent its weight to the implementation program.

Licensed Practical Nursing. There are in the United States today more than 345,000 licensed practical nurses with a high percentage—perhaps 75 percent—actively employed in nursing activities. By simple interpolation this would indicate that roughly 40 percent of the staff nurse positions are occupied by licensed practical or vocational nurses.

At the early organizational meetings of the National Commission, it was agreed that the staff should examine generic problems and issues related to nursing and health care. In view of the limitations on time and resources, however, the commissioners directed that primary focus be placed on the registered nurse with the expectation that findings and recommendations would broadly encompass all nurses and all nursing practice. The concerns of the registered and practical nurse, from all indications, might vary in degree but not in kind and a thorough investigation of nursing roles, education, and careers should produce generalizable findings and recommendations over the entire spectrum included within the term *nursing.*

As a practical matter, the site visits, interviews, and discussion meetings had to include licensed practical or vocational nurses, and practical attention was given to the educational opportunities available to practical nurses wishing to become registered nurses.[39] The staff, however, did emphasize its observation and analysis of the latter group in accordance with the directive of the Commission. Such an approach was certain to disappoint licensed practical nurses and their principal organizations—all of whom believed that more stress and attention should be given the work of the practical nurses.

The public reaction of the LPN organizations was considerably less enthusiastic than that of RN groups. In April of 1970, the National Association for Practical Nurse Education and Service discussed the summary report and recommendations of the National Commission, and its Assembly adopted a resolution which stated in part:

> WHEREAS, No study of nursing is comprehensive and realistic without the inclusion of practical/vocational nursing . . .
>
> RESOLVED, That this Assembly go on record as opposing any study which does not include practical/vocational nursing education, and further
>
> RESOLVED, That a copy of this resolution be forwarded immediately to the National Commission for the Study of Nursing and Nursing Education.[40]

On receipt of this communication, the staff of the National Commission offered to meet with the Executive Committee of NAPNES to discuss the full report and recommendations with the aim of identifying specific points of misunderstanding or disagreement. On September 12, 1970 that meeting was held, and an exchange of views occurred. No particular portions of the report were singled out for disapproval by the Executive Committee, but there was strong feeling that more involvement should have taken place.

In February of 1971, the National Commission received a statement on its report from the Executive Board of the National Federation of Licensed Practical Nurses. While expressing concerns similar to those advanced by NAPNES, the conclusion of the NFLPN Board was less sweeping and more positive. The statement included the observation that . . .

> . . . it is not feasible to design a system of nursing service and nursing education that will meet future needs without a plan to incorporate the utilization of the practical nurse.[41]

Having admonished those involved in the implementation of *An Abstract for Action* not to overlook the practical/vocational nurse, however, the statement continued . . .

> The report has identified problem areas and real issues in nursing and nursing education, and the National Federation of Licensed Practical Nurses, Inc., believes it is time to move ahead to develop some constructive solutions to the mounting problems in nursing.[42]

The NFLPN Executive Board then made five specific proposals related to the National Commission recommendations:

> 1. The concept of episodic and distributive nursing care as presented in the report is realistic in terms of total health services. Therefore, we believe that practical nursing, as a supportive service, should be developed and expanded simultaneously with the development of nursing as a profession.
> 2. Practical nursing education programs should be evaluated in terms of basic nursing, and a study be made of the functions of the licensed practical nurse in today's health care system.
> 3. A realistic basic nursing program should be defined in relation to patient needs, and developed as a career pattern to provide horizontal and lateral [sic] mobility in the health services.
> 4. Relationships between nurses and physicians should be fostered as co-partners in patient care.
> 5. State Planning Commissions on nursing and nursing education should be a coordinated plan developed by all health groups and agencies related to health care, including manpower planning agencies.[43]

These comments, along with expressions of interest and concern from the Council of Diploma Programs of the National League for Nursing were forwarded by staff to the National Commission which reviewed them and directed that further information be developed on the impact of *An Abstract for Action* on licensed practical nursing along with recommendations for alternative action to be taken by the Commission based on staff findings.*

Health and Education Associations. One of the emphases in *An Abstract for Action* is the consideration of statewide and regional planning for nursing education in order to make best use of limited resources as well as optimizing the pattern of institutional offerings. It was particularly gratifying, then, that three interstate compacts for education took specific action to support the work of the National Commission.

On April 1, 1971, the New England Board of Higher Education unanimously approved the following resolution:

> The New England Board of Higher Education endorses the recommendations and findings of the National Commission for the Study of Nursing and Nursing Education and supports the role of the New England Council on Higher Education for Nursing as a vehicle for regional implementation of said findings.[44]

*See Appendix E, The National Commission and the Licensed Practical Nurse.

Approximately two weeks later, the Council on Collegiate Education for Nursing of the Southern Regional Education Board commended the National Commission for its efforts to promote the improvement of health care; the Council,

> . . . expressed its support and commitment to work with the Commission toward implementation of its recommendations, especially those related to the development of varied models of statewide planning, multidisciplinary collaboration, and curriculum innovation.[45]

On October 5, 1971, the third interstate association announced its endorsement in these words:

> The organization of the Midwest Continuing Professional Education for Nurses (MCPEN) supports the recommendations relative to continuing education as stated in the report of the National Commission. . .[46]

Still another significant voice was raised in support of *An Abstract for Action* in July of 1971 when the American Public Health Association announced:

> The report of the National Commission to Study Nursing and Nursing Education has been reviewed by the members of our Council on Health Manpower and, based on their recommendation, has been endorsed by our Executive Board in behalf of the American Public Health Association.[47]

Because the APHA membership is multidisciplinary and includes consumer and public representation as well as that from the health occupations, the action by their Executive Board underscored the willingness of those outside nursing to become involved in the concerns of that profession to enhance the delivery of health care.

REVIEWS, COMMENTARIES, AND PUBLICATIONS

At the same time that contacts were being made with organizations and associations concerned with nursing and its evolving patterns, information was being provided to the public and to nurses through a series of independent reviews of *An Abstract for Action.** While many of these raised questions and concerns over particular aspects of the report, on balance most were positive and advocated that controversial aspects be settled by trial and evaluation. For example, Sorenson, writing in *Nursing Research,* raised the question of specialized educational patterns in this way:

> Is the implication that all baccalaureate programs should have two tracks from which students may elect, depending upon whether they wish to

*See Appendix A.

> prepare for distributive or for episodic care? . . . The answer calls for research into different kinds of nursing programs and how they prepare the practitioner for what she is going to be facing in the delivery of health care.[48]

There was general consensus that nurses should examine the report closely. Smith suggested, "No published work in the last decade should command more considered attention from the nursing community than *An Abstract for Action*. . . . The importance of this study cannot be overstated. It addresses itself to the difficult and perplexing issues in nursing that confront us today."[49] In a similar vein, Kelisch states, "This study . . . will be required reading for nurses, health workers, and other individuals in the forefront of the struggle to achieve nursing excellence."[50]

Some saw the role of the report as that of a catalyst. As Murry indicates, ". . . this book is strongly recommended and it should be required reading for every professional nurse. Those who do not agree with the conclusions and projections may be stimulated to offer alternative approaches."[51]

The most dramatic, and acerbic, contrast to these reviews appeared in "An Appraisal of *An Abstract for Action,*" prepared by Christy, Poulin, and Hover.[52] In a lengthy analysis of the report, these writers found little that was positive, much that was biased, and some that was highly dangerous in their opinion. In particular, the appraisal criticized the historical accuracy of the National Commission report, the methodology employed in aspects of the investigation, and the interpretation placed on some of the specific recommendations.

Perhaps the flavor of the critique is best expressed in two of the summary sections. In one, the writers stated:

> We believe that the Commission produced a report that promoted their own preconceived ideas. Relatively recent issues in nursing, such as the differentiation among preparatory programs, were not investigated. We agree that the report contains a restatement of some long-standing needs recognized by nursing and some recommendations long aspired to by nursing. However, additional recommendations not previously supported by nursing were based upon inadequate and improperly interpreted data, opinions of the commissioners, and opinions of health professionals other than nurses.[53]

In the other, the comment was made:

> We question the wisdom of implementing any recommendation not carefully scrutinized and endorsed by the ANA.[54]

Whatever the intent of the appraisal, it assuredly produced a considerable reaction. The *American Journal of Nursing* carried a number of letters to the editor devoted to the article in subsequent issues. Some of the letters were supportive of the critical analysis; others were in sharp disagreement; a few were simply appreciative of the fact that debate had been entered into by those who were concerned about the directions and impact of the recommendations contained in *An Abstract for Action.*

As an example of the first type of reaction, King wrote, "The authors are to be commended for their objective, scholarly, and constructive critique of the most recent study of nursing and nursing education in America."[55] Relatedly, Betson suggested that the appraisal was ". . . an absolutely marvelous critique of the original report. Every nurse should be aware of the biased and inexcusable errors brought to light in this article."[56]

The second category of reactions was far less complimentary. In a semi official reply to the appraisal, the director of the National Commission undertook a point by point response to a number of specific criticisms. He then wrote:

> The question that is really being raised is whether the integrity, good faith, and fair intentions of the Commission are to be believed . . . Such a deep-held suspicion of anything, and everything, emanating from outside nursing is a conspiratorial theory, and a perceptual and semantic block, that admits of no discussion, and allows for no correction . . .
>
> Let the recommendations of the National Commission be judged on their merits, not on the basis of whether nursing originated them or not.[57]

Another critic of the appraisal, Young, phrased her feelings in this way:

> I find myself wondering at the authors' basic intent. The same lack of objectivity and accuracy of which they accuse the author of the report pervades most of their criticism . . . Have we resolved our problems in nursing practice and nursing education so well that we can dismiss a major study on the basis of minutiae? We should remain open-minded and spend our energies on more positive efforts.[58]

Lambertsen expressed her concern over the appraisal in these words:

> Certainly one does not quarrel with the right and privilege of any individual to question recommendations of any report or study but one would expect that in taking issue supporting data would be presented . . . The appraisal has the tone of a frenzied personal vendetta rather than a socially responsible critique.[59]

Other commentators questioned the interpretation given specific recommendations by the authors of the appraisal, their generation of assumptions, and the essentially teleological arrangement of their arguments.

Perhaps, however, when all was said and done, it was the content of the third category of reactions that proved most useful. In a carefully reasoned argument, Cleland wrote:

> I believe it would be more appropriate to view the Lysaught report as tenable hypotheses some of which may eventually be disproved. Perhaps by

> analogy it would be helpful to consider the risks involved in tentatively accepting these recommendations. Christy et al are concerned about Type I error—acceptance of one of these recommendations which may be proved false. This is the bias of the historian whose retrospective view can be very precise. Where action for the profession of nursing is concerned, I tend to worry more about Type II error—rejection of a recommendation when it is true. In a practical sense, what are the risks of accepting a recommendation and trying to implement it? If the recommendation proves valid, we can take some giant strides toward improved patient care and greater role satisfaction within the profession. If the recommendation is not valid, it can be disproved with a few trials in a few settings with no great harm. The alternative is not to act.[60]

From a different viewpoint, Resnik addressed the overtones of the argument when she remarked:

> How refreshing to see in print a strong stand on a nursing issue—whether it is right or wrong, scholarly or emotional . . . I also have felt the discomfort expressed by the authors in the lack of negative reactions to the report, but for different reasons. Usually, when we nurses did not agree, our strategy was a silent, behind-the-scenes, blocking tactic—a most elusive but effective way to perpetuate the status quo . . .[61]

With the preponderance of reaction taking the form of a willingness to "try" the recommendations, the large-scale debate over the appraisal tended to fade. Its appearance had generated discussion, and this, in turn, emphasized the need for continuing attention by the Commission and its staff to the explication and explanation of specific recommendations contained in *An Abstract for Action.*

One participant in the discussion generated by the appraisal, Schlotfeldt, proposed a specific approach to the resolution of the controversy. She suggested that:

> Forthright statements of agreement/disagreement explicating the ANA's official position with regard to each recommendation (along with reasons) would likely unite the profession in its support of most of the commission's recommendations . . . The commission members and staff should have ANA's appraisal of the report.[62]

No specific action was taken by the American Nurses' Association in pursuance of this recommendation, but the idea was brought to life by a different organization in 1971. The National League for Nursing, faced with disagreement among its councils over *An Abstract for Action*, appointed an eleven-member task force to study the implications of the NCSNNE Report.* The group met for one day in January, and two days in April, of 1972. Its completed work was received by the NLN Board of

*See page 57.

Directors in October of 1972 and subsequently released through the medium of *Nursing Outlook.*[63]

The task force went through each of the National Commission's recommendations in the areas of: roles and functions, education, and careers. Each recommendation was restated, then, the committee either accepted or rephrased it according to their interpretations, viewpoints, and/or predilections.

The entire document runs to twenty-one pages of text; its approach, however, can be illustrated by means of the following selected section:[64]

> *Chapter 7: Summary and Conclusions*
>
> The four summary recommendations on pages 156-161 [*An Abstract for Action*] were modified according to the revisions previously discussed for specific chapters.
>
> 1. *The federal Division of Nursing . . . grant funds or research contracts to investigate the impact of nursing practice. . . .*
>
> The Recommendation was endorsed as stated.
>
> 2. *Each state have, or create, a master planning committee that will take nursing education under its purview. . . .*
>
> The word "deadlines" was removed.
>
> 3. *A National Joint Practice Commission, with state counterpart committees be established. . . .*
>
> This Recommendation was modified to suggest that representatives of licensed practical nurses and health management executives be included in the early efforts of the joint practice commission.
>
> 4. *Federal, regional, state, and local government adopt measures for the increased support of nursing research and education. . . .*
>
> This Recommendation was endorsed as stated.

As indicated in this sample, much of the report consists of an exercise of amanuensis punctuated by substitution, query, and occasional asides. For example, in reacting to the National Commission's recommendation that a joint committee be established between the ANA and the NLN to consider changing accreditation procedures, the task force remarked rather testily:

> As with several previous Recommendations, the Task Force questioned the source of data contributing to the development of this one.[65]

The remarkable aspect of this statement is that the task force *at no time* during its three days of deliberation, or at any point before or between those meetings, contacted the National Commission or its staff to question, or request information about, data, sources, or any related materials. This lack of communication was apparent, for example, when the task force addressed such concepts as episodic and distributive care. In their words:

> The Task Force spent a considerable amount of time discussing this Recommendation . . . The specific meaning of the terms . . . was ambiguous to the committee and created confusion when implications and implementation were considered . . . The notion of two career patterns, as suggested by the Commission was NOT rejected, but it does need to be clarified and made more explicit.[66]

If the task force was having difficulty in comprehending these concepts, there were readily available elaborative materials in the form of two NCSNNE monographs which expand on and illustrate episodic and distributive practice. Again, the task force did not request these materials, nor, apparently, did they acquire them through other channels.

In yet another passage, the task force, "... acknowledged that since it did not possess all the data available to the Commission, it may not have interpreted [a Recommendation] ... as intended by the Commission."[67] In this particular instance, however, the expressed shortcoming did not interfere with the task force determining that the recommendation under discussion be deleted on the basis of its own "thoughtful deliberation."

The report of the task force, whatever its methodological or procedural limitations, represented the first, " . . . formal, organizationally-sponsored critique of what has come to be known as the Lysaught report."[68] As such, it performed a useful function, and contributed to both the development of greater consensus about many recommendations and to the specificity of concern or disagreement over the remainder. As the editor of *Nursing Outlook*, Edith P. Lewis, viewed it:

> Many of the NCSNNE recommendations, it will be noted, were endorsed without question by the task force. The most significant areas of disagreement seem to have been with the meaning and implications of those now familiar words, "episodic" and "distributive," and with the position that "strong and vital" hospital schools of nursing should, by due process, convert themselves into degree granting institutions . . .
>
> The task force recommendations, it should be noted, do not represent official NLN position, since the League Board of Directors neither approved nor disapproved the [Task Force] report but, rather, voted to distribute it to the membership for consideration. There is also the question of how much impact this report—coming three years after the fact, as it were—can have, since the Commission's work is already well into the implementation stage. It's unfortunate that this critique was not developed sooner after the Commission's published report. . . .[69]

From the standpoint of the National Commission, the report of the task force was a valuable reminder that many of the recommendations in *An Abstract for*

Action require continuing explanation and that no concept, definition, or interpretation could be taken for granted. To those who had hoped for a broad-scale rejection of the National Commission's recommendations, however, the report of the task force proved to be a great disappointment. The NLN Council of Diploma Programs had voted nonsupport for eleven recommendations of *An Abstract for Action.*[70] The NLN task force showed a proclivity to indulge in some editing and rephrasing of several of those same recommendations to make them more suitable to its tastes. In only one case, however, did the task force actually suggest the deletion of a recommendation—assumedly an action equivalent to nonsupport.

The National Commission had recommended that: Those hospital schools that are strong and vital, endowed with a qualified faculty, suitable educational facilities, and motivated for excellence be encouraged to seek and obtain regional accreditation and degree granting power. Although aware that two schools had already undergone such transformation, the task force "recommended the deletion of this recommendation," in large part because the members disapproved of "a college just for nurses," and felt that a student's education should be provided through, "multiple and diverse situations and associations."[71] What the task force apparently did not know—and did not undertake to find out—is that both the cited institutions became multipurpose colleges with students in fields other than nursing.[72] This point is made only to illustrate the hazards of substituting subjective feeling for objective information.

From the beginning of the implementation phase, the staff of the Commission was concerned about the generation of informational materials to the nursing profession, related health groups, and to particular publics as these became involved.

A computerized mailing list of more than 9,500 individuals was developed so that we could contact national and state health organizations, heads of educational programs, directors of nursing service, planning and manpower agencies, and individual leaders of implementation activities. Information and press releases could be sent on either a general or selected basis to these recipients.

Specialized mailings were also prepared from time to time. For example, the physician members of the National Commission prepared a joint letter, together with selected enclosures, for their professional colleagues in an effort to acquaint them with *An Abstract for Action*. The letter and materials were sent to: state medical societies, deans of medical schools, medical directors of teaching hospitals, directors of regional medical programs and comprehensive health planning bodies, and selected national leaders. Comparable mailings, prepared in conjunction with the health management and nurse members of the Commission, were sent to thousands of other leaders in health education and care delivery.

Special articles were prepared for the "health press." During the implementation period, the Commission staff authored papers for publication in: *Nursing Outlook, The Journal of Continuing Education in Nursing, The Journal of Nursing Administration, Federation Bulletin, American Journal of Public Health, The Sur-*

gical Team, The Journal of Nursing Education, Today's Education, and a number of other journals. These, together with articles authored by persons not directly related to the National Commission, produced a wide familiarity with the general content of the report and the nature of the recommendations.

A series of sixteen pamphlets was developed and printed by the National Commission to elaborate on particular concerns that grew out of the implementation phase.* Some of these related to specific recommendations such as the expansion of episodic and distributive nursing practice; some were in the nature of "background" papers intended to explain misconceptions about the costs of nursing education or the need for research into nursing practice. Over the thirty-six months of implementation, more than 130,000 of these pamphlets and reprints were distributed to nurses, other health professionals, and interested lay persons.

DESIGNATION OF THE TARGET STATES

Verbal communication and publications might satisfy the need to inform persons about the changes proposed by the National Commission, but it became clear early in the implementation phase that there was a companion need to begin involvement in, and demonstration of, the practical tasks of carrying out the recommendations.

Early in 1971, the Commission staff conducted a survey of the 48 continental states to assess their interest in and readiness for participating in an effort to secure progress in implementing *An Abstract for Action.* Employing the resources of our various advisory committees and the consultant aid of the federal Division of Nursing, states were viewed in terms of the following criteria:

1. Selected states should represent a broad range of geographic, economic, and social patterns;
2. Selected states, as a group, should include the most significant health and care delivery problems, such as urban concentration, rural separation, adequacy of facilities etc.;
3. Selected states should have recently completed, or be currently involved in, studies and assessments of nursing needs and resources so as to provide a sound data base for decision making;
4. Selected states should have initiated some overt activities related to the proposals for change recommended by the Commission.

Using these guidelines, the staff attempted to develop a rank order of choices. Because of the constraints imposed by the criteria, this became a more arbitrary task than had been anticipated. Geographic closeness, for example, militated against the selection of some states which otherwise might seem to suit all the requirements. At the same time, rumors that some form of selection process was underway prompted a number of states to "volunteer" for inclusion and this caused considerable anxiety among other states that they might not be fairly evaluated. To

*See Appendix A.

provide some safeguard against errors of both omission and commission, the preliminary rankings were reviewed with the consultants from the Division of Nursing and with nurse leaders from the Interstate Compacts for Higher Education. From this discussion, there was derived a final listing of states for consideration by the National Commission; in April, 1971 nine states were officially designated as "model" or "target" states for purposes of implementation. These were: California, Georgia, Illinois, Kansas, Maine, North Carolina, Pennsylvania, Texas, and Wyoming.

In addition to the geographic dispersion of the nine states, as shown in Figure 3-2, there is also a distinct regional relationship. The nine target states come from eight different Department of Commerce areas; the South Atlantic region contains two target states, the East-South-Central none, and all other regions are represented by one designated state. Taken together, they represent a microcosm of all the health care delivery problems that have beset our society over recent decades. Within the model states exist the urban ghettos of large cities and sparsely populated rural areas far removed from health centers. Within these states there are wide variations in population-practitioner ratios, in the availability of institutional resources, and in economic and social patterns. Within the states, too, there are varying postures of awareness and reaction concerning health problems.

Some of the differences in personnel and facilities among the target states at the time of their designation can be seen in Tables 3-2 and 3-3. The ratio of nurses and physicians to the population is, of course, only one gauge of health care potential, but the marked differences between states like Georgia and California in

TABLE 3-2 SELECTED HEALTH CARE PERSONNEL AND FACILITIES DATA WITHIN THE TARGET STATES

Target State	RN/100M	MD/100M	BRN/100ADP	%RN Empl.
California	312	170	13.6	61.4
Georgia	156	95	13.5	67.7
Illinois	330	122	8.2	60.9
Kansas	303	98	11.2	62.3
Maine	414	92	3.0	61.8
North Carolina	244	94	11.8	77.1
Pennsylvania	395	131	9.3	57.6
Texas	188	106	12.8	64.0
Wyoming	379	92	9.9	74.3

Sources: *Facts About Nursing, 1970-71 Edition.* New York: American Nurses' Association, 1972; and *Health Resources Statistics, 1970.* Washington, D.C.: PHS Publication No. 1509, 1970.

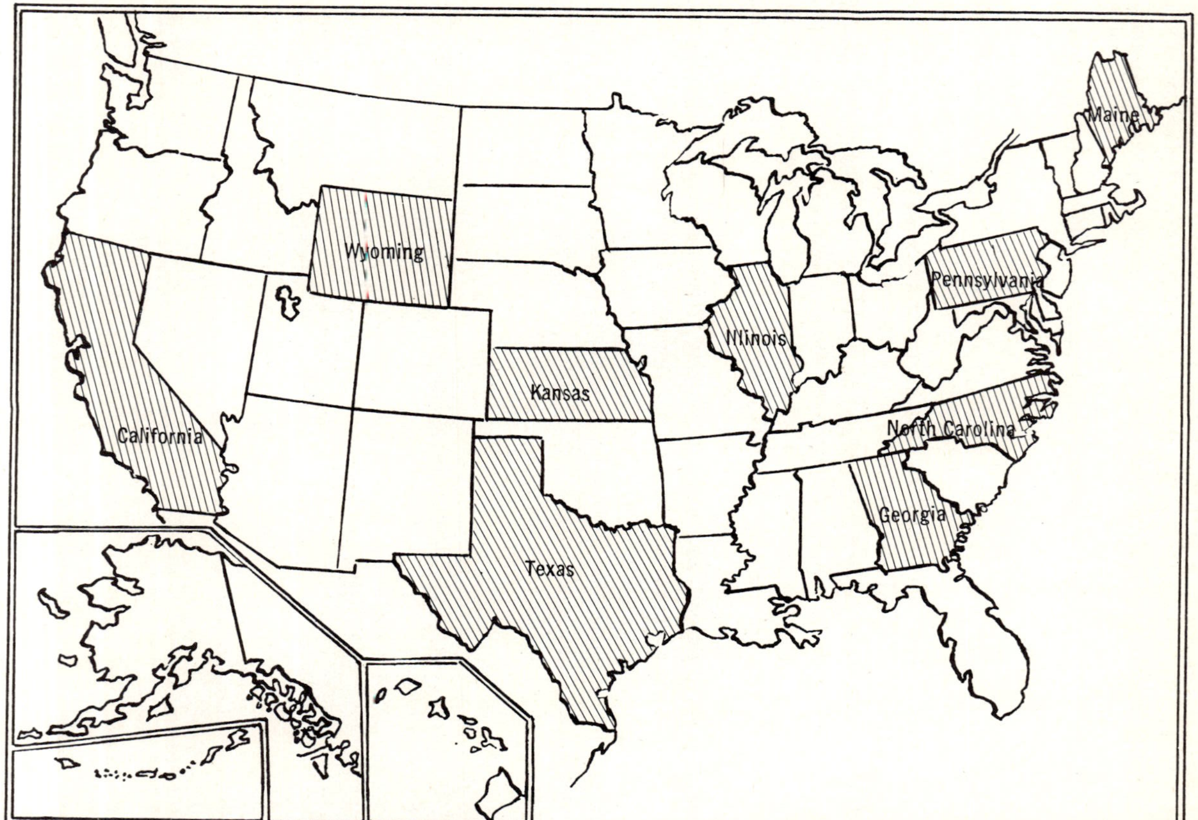

Figure 3-2. The target states designated for implementation activities by NCSNNE.

this regard necessarily affect any planning for change. Similarly, the ratio of bedside nursing personnel per 100 average daily patients (BRN/100ADP) in hospitals is only one comparison that speaks to the allocation of personnel, but the marked differences among states illustrate the variation in approaches that need to be considered and questioned. Finally, the percentage of employed registered nurses is an indicator of not only how well we are retaining one group of skilled personnel, but also a reminder of the manpower pool that remains to be tapped if a concerted effort to redevelop the health care delivery system is mounted.

While Table 3-2 displays considerable difference from one state to another, it cannot indicate the internal variation within each of the target states. Despite the favorable ratio of nurses and physicians to population in California, for example, there are some counties within the state that are almost destitute of health practitioners. Similarly, there are considerable differences in the distribution of all health workers between urban centers and the rural areas in each of the states.

Table 3-3 is a selected comparison of educational facilities for the preparation and advanced training of health practitioners within the target states. Obviously, some of these states are donors, and others donees, in the sense of preparing qualified practitioners for the nation as a whole. California and Pennsylvania together, for example, contain more than 15 percent of our entire complement of medical schools. Maine and Wyoming, in contrast, are entirely dependent upon physicians educated and trained outside their own borders; the two states without medical schools also have the lowest physician to population ratio. (The limitation

TABLE 3-3 SELECTED DATA ON EDUCATIONAL FACILITIES FOR HEALTH PROFESSIONALS WITHIN THE TARGET STATES

	RN Preparatory		RN Graduate		
Target State	Total Inst.	Non-Coll.	Masters	Doctoral	MD/DO
California	82	13	6	1	8
Georgia	26	8	2	0	2
Illinois	78	44	5	0	6
Kansas	22	14	1	0	1
Maine	6	4	0	0	0
North Carolina	42	19	3	0	3
Pennsylvania	117	91	2	1	8
Texas	44	14	2	0	4
Wyoming	2	0	0	0	0

Sources: *Facts About Nursing, 1970-71 Edition.* New York: American Nurses' Association, 1972; and *Health Resources Statistics, 1970.* Washington, D.C.: PHS Publication No. 1509, 1970.

to this extrapolation is clearly indicated in the case of North Carolina, however, which has three medical schools yet still possesses a comparatively low ratio of physicians to population. There are, of course, a host of factors underlying each of the cited figures.)

Table 3-3 indicates the disparity in numbers between preparatory programs and those designed for advanced clinical skills in all the states, and also shows the variation in progress toward a collegiate system of nursing education. While Wyoming has only collegiate programs today, 78 percent of the preparatory institutions in Pennsylvania are outside the collegiate system. In terms of statewide planning, there are also concerns about the sheer number of preparatory nursing programs when one considers the limitations on resources, finances, prepared faculty, and appropriate clinical facilities. That there can be different approaches to these problems was implicit in the very concept of nine individual state laboratories. The National Commission's purpose was to determine empirically through the cooperation of the target states what commonalities and what uniqueness might be discovered in a concerted approach to enhanced health care.

With the designation of the target states in April, 1971, a series of follow-up communications was generated. In each model state, the governor's office was officially notified and their replies, without exception, were interested and positive. Notifications were also sent to the major health organizations in each state, and there was general endorsement of the concept that nursing, medicine, health management, and others should become involved in the task of implementation. In each state, and in every case, this resolution toward involvement was seen as a commitment to an overall, developmental approach with assurance that the state committees themselves would select the specific activities and priorities to be undertaken, as well as the pace to be established in each area of concern.

As a result, individualized approaches were taken in the nine states. Most planned a series of multidisciplinary information meetings to inform nurses and others within the state of the report and recommendations of the National Commission and their own designation as a model laboratory for implementation. Several of the states had, from their studies of nursing needs and resources, already constituted interdisciplinary committees involved in nursing affairs; others took this opportunity to approach state medical and hospital associations asking them to help nurses in forming joint approaches to planning and practice.

In the face of many obstacles, and with little in the way of resources to call upon, the nurses in the nine states made remarkable progress in organizing, aided by the timely support of medicine and hospital administration. Table 3-4 indicates the status of target state implementation at the end of the first eight months of effort.

By December of 1971, all nine states had been able to establish some definite form of leadership through an ad hoc or steering committee, and each state had made some progress toward forming and legitimating a master planning committee for nursing education and a joint practice committee to consider practitioner roles in health care delivery.

TABLE 3-4 SUMMARY OF TARGET STATE IMPLEMENTATION ACTIVITIES
APRIL 1–DECEMBER 1, 1971

Target State	Ad Hoc or Steering Committee	Master Planning Committee	Joint Practice Committee
California	Operational	Operational	Operational
Georgia	Operational	Operational	In process
Illinois	Operational	Designated	Unorganized
Kansas	Operational	In process	In process
Maine	Operational	Designated	Designated
North Carolina	Operational	Designated	Designated
Pennsylvania	Operational	Designated	Designated
Texas	Operational	Operational	In process
Wyoming	Operational	Designated	In process

Source: Lysaught, Jerome P. "From Abstract into Action: Progress Report from the National Commission for the Study of Nursing and Nursing Education." *Nursing Outlook.* 20:3:173-179 (March) 1972.

In the following months, through the help of a financial grant from the W. K. Kellogg Foundation, small amounts of "seed money" were provided to the target states to facilitate the organization of committees and to assist in the distribution of educational materials related to the states' activities. In addition, consultant help and material support was provided by the National Commission staff, and, in the fall of 1972, a national meeting of target state representatives was held to exchange information and experiences and to plan further activities related to implementation.

Through continued effort, slow but steady progress took place within each of the states. Sometimes the work of implementation was affected by wholly unexpected circumstances. In Georgia, for example, Governor Carter had designated the Georgia Educational Improvement Council to be the statewide master planning agency for nursing education. This group was moving rapidly when the Council itself became caught up in a massive reorganization of state agencies. The planning group had to mark time until the governor could reassign that primary responsibility to the Office of Comprehensive Health Planning. Again, in California, the Coordinating Council for Higher Education had been formally requested by the state legislature to prepare a master plan for nursing education. This Council established an advisory group which satisfied all aspects of a master planning committee and thus was endorsed by the steering committee in the state. Just as progress was being made on the content of the master plan, the legislature retracted its charge to the Council, and activity, for the time being, ceased. Significantly, in each state where obstacles or problems have been encountered, focus has simply shifted to another aspect of implementation where progress can continue while difficulties are being resolved.

As a result of these target state activities, two outcomes have emerged. First, there is the distinct development of mechanisms within the nine states for the accomplishment of change in nursing well beyond the termination of the National Commission. The continuing progress over the period since December 1, 1971 is displayed in Table 3-5. Moreover, a ripple, or contagion, effect has been seen in the fact that states other than the designated laboratories have been able to profit from the examples and initiate their own planning and joint practice committees to effect change. Appendix C provides a summary of progress within all the fifty states and the District of Columbia.

Despite the accomplishments to date, each of the nine target states is still in the early stages of identifying and solving their critical problems in nursing education and practice. That they have already come so far, however, is proof that others can as well. That they still have far to go is only a recognition that we have done little in the past in terms of genuine interdisciplinary planning and development. Through the remainder of the implementation period, the target states will continue to amass information on change processes that will stand them and others in good stead over the coming years.

FURTHER ORGANIZATIONAL EFFORTS

The distribution of the target states plus the increasing efforts at organization in other states across the country dictated the development of additional assistance

TABLE 3-5 SUMMARY OF TARGET STATE IMPLEMENTATION ACTIVITIES APRIL 1, 1971–April 1, 1973

Target State	Ad Hoc or Steering Committee	Master Planning Committee	Joint Practice Committee
California	Operational	Inactive	Operational
Georgia	Operational	Operational	Operational
Illinois	Operational	Operational	Operational
Kansas	Operational	Operational	Operational
Maine	Operational	In process	In process
North Carolina	Operational	Operational	Operational
Pennsylvania	Operational	Operational	Operational
Texas	Operational	Operational	Operational
Wyoming	Operational	Operational	Operational

that could be readily available. Rather than increase the size of the Commission's staff, it was decided that individuals residing in the several regions be officially designated as Regional Associates to aid in implementation efforts. The central staff would work closely with these persons, keeping them fully informed of decisions and developments, and, from time to time, would participate with them in larger meetings or more complicated problem solving. The country was broken down into seven geographic areas, as indicated in Figure 3-3, and six Regional Associates were named to work with them (the central staff maintained basic responsibility for one area to ensure that it was seeing problems similar to those encountered by the Associates). While there was a general effort to use Regional Associates within designed areas, it frequently happened that whichever advisor was available and in first contact with a state would continue in a consultant relationship despite regional boundaries. And, in some cases, several of the advisors would, over time, work with particular states. The Regional Associates and their general areas of concern were:

Myrtle K. Aydelotte, Director of Nursing, The University of Iowa Hospitals, *Great Lakes Region.*

Virginia Z. Barham, Nursing Consultant, Kaiser-Permanente Medical Centers, *Southwest Region.*

Luther Christman, Dean, Rush College of Nursing and Allied Health Sciences, *Southeast Region.*

Grace L. Deloughery, Dean, Center for Nursing Education, Spokane, *Northwest Region.*

Maryann E. Pierleoni, Nurse Practitioner, Kansas City, *Midwest Region.*

Charles H. Russell, Dean of Instruction, Mattatuck Community College, *Northeast Region.*

The central office staff assumed primary responsibility for the *Middle Atlantic Region.* Included within each of these assigned areas was at least one target state, while an effort was made to have some degree of geographic proximity and relatedness of health care concerns. In the last analysis, however, availability of these volunteers and the travel commitments of the commissioners and the staff were often determinative of assignments and follow-up.

Just as the Regional Associates were instituted to extend the reach of the staff in meeting requests for aid, so, as the tempo of implementation activities increased, there was a need to provide even more assistance to the states and their internal districts. Requests for information and presentations came so frequently that, in 1972, a speakers' bureau was established. Composed of twenty-four volunteers from the advisory committees to the Commission, the group held a two-day training session in the fall of 1972 to discuss common questions and concerns, and to preview an audio-visual presentation that was devised to provide an overview of the National Commission's report and recommendations. Over the remainder of the implementation period, these individuals continued to meet with

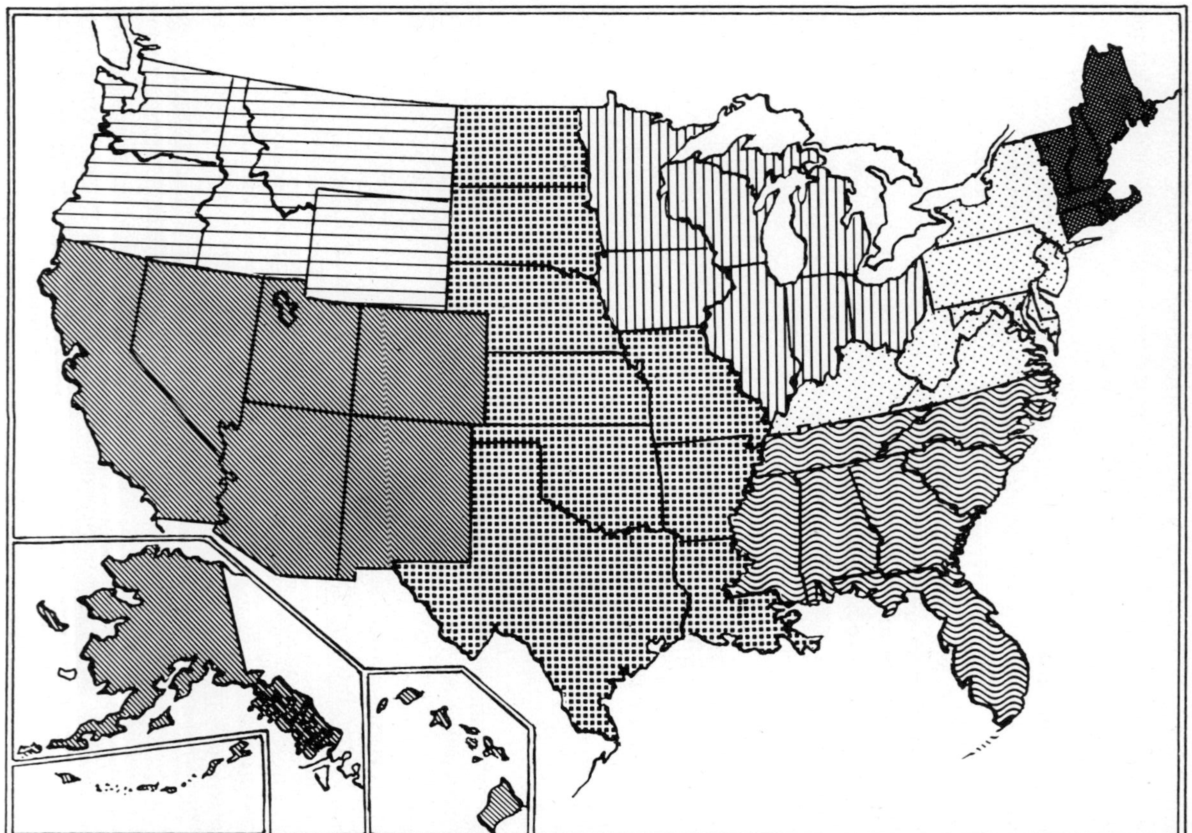

Figure 3-3. Regional areas designated for implementation purposes of the NCSNNE.

student groups, nurses' organizations, and other concerned bodies to explain and encourage acceptance of the Commission's proposals.

In terms of the general organization of efforts for implementation (see Figure 3-1), a final group of persons should be mentioned. From time to time, the National Commission invited individual spokesmen and consultants to meet with them to discuss particular aspects of health care, joint practice, or education. These persons were not involved in the advisory committees or other assisting groups, but did volunteer their help in providing insight and experience to the Commission. Included among these advisors were:

Robert A. Hoekelman, Chairman, The National Joint Practice Commission.

Shirley A. Smoyak, Vice Chairman, The National Joint Practice Commission.

Margaret G. Tyson, Project Director, Department of Nursing, Columbia University.

Harriet H. Werley, Director, Center for Health Research, Wayne State University.

Ruth S. Young, Executive Secretary, The Nurses' Association of the American College of Obstetricians and Gynecologists.

This utilization of outside resources and commentary gave the Commission and staff one more opportunity of comparing analyses and trends as these were viewed by advisory panelists and by independent observers.

SUMMARY

In order to bring a wide range of opinion and expertise to bear on the problems of implementation, five advisory committees were appointed to work with the Commission and the staff on a variety of concerns. These advisory groups included:

The Nursing Liaison Committee—composed of leaders from national nursing organizations, interstate educational compacts, and the student nurse association.

The National Advisory Committee—a multidisciplinary group of recognized leaders in health and education.

The Staff Advisory Panel—the "Young Turks" of nursing—students, faculty members, and practitioners who were intimately involved in many of the grassroots problems of implementation.

The Administrators' Advisory Committee—health administrators recognized for their leadership in hospital associations and for their interest in nursing education and practice.

The Advisory Committee on Community Health—an interdisciplinary group involved in the cutting edge of changed health care and health maintenance systems.

These several committees, comprising more than seventy individuals, met occasionally with the staff and with individual commissioners to discuss problems, activities and priorities related to the implementation program. Their voluntary donation of time and consultant help was a major contributing factor to the progress achieved by the Commission in its mission of change.

During the first months of the Commission's second phase, a major effort was mounted to contact and inform the professions and organizations that would be most intimately affected by the proposed developments in nursing. Beginning with the American Nurses' Association and the National League for Nursing, co-sponsors of the original plan for the investigation, *An Abstract for Action* received nursing's organizational support. What was perhaps more surprising to those who have long worked in the health field, was the ready willingness of the American Medical Association and the American Hospital Association to become involved. Their support of the central thrust of the Commission's report emphasized the broad recognition of a need for change—and a consensus on the general direction in which that change should lead.

Other nursing organizations, interstate educational compacts, health associations, and statewide bodies joined the supportive elements. Only two groups evidenced disaffection. Licensed practical nurse organizations indicated they wanted to be included in any of the implementation planning, and expressed reservations about the Commission's report until they saw its implications for their own members. The organizations of hospital schools of nursing were, of course, dismayed by the Commission's recommendations to establish, for once and all, a collegiate system of nursing education. Even these elements, both licensed practical nurses and hospital schools, found much in the report, however, that they could support and approve.

Critical reviews, critiques, and commentaries were generally positive about the Commission's report. Most analysts, even while indicating concern about specific recommendations, reserved judgment pending experimental trial and resultant acceptance or rejection. One major exception to this proved to be an appraisal that found almost nothing of value—and a great deal that was dangerous. On balance, this review was at such extreme variance from every other published expression that discussion simply moved on. The one organizational review, that by the NLN task force, tended to accept most of the recommendations while rephrasing others to make them more palatable or innocuous.

As concerns and misconceptions did appear, the Commission and its staff arranged for a steady stream of communications to elaborate on, or clarify, the report and its recommendations. More than fifteen journal articles, sixteen monographs, and thirty press releases were prepared in the period of implementation—as well as the volume of *Appendices* to the original report. In addition, more than twenty-five other articles, reviews, and monographs, authored by non-Commission spokesmen, appeared in the health and education press addressing the implications of the report and its recommendations. Through these means and others, including special mailings and computerized information lists, frequent efforts were made to encourage action.

With the organization of the communication plan and network, it became more and more apparent that some form of demonstration laboratory would be necessary to determine the optimum ways of going about change. Much of the Commission's implementation involved action at the state level to secure educational planning and new functional relationships between nursing and medicine. In order to experiment with how best to secure change, the Commission in April of 1971 designated nine states as "models" for purposes of implementation. Selected for their broad range of economic, geographic, social, and health care patterns, the nine states contain elements of almost every problem that besets our nation in terms of the health system. These model states include: California, Georgia, Illinois, Kansas, Maine, North Carolina, Pennsylvania, Texas and Wyoming.

Over the succeeding months, the Commission, its staff, and the advisory committees worked with state groups to establish first some catalytic agencies and then some more permanent arrangements to plan and guide change. In two years, all of the nine states have made substantial progress, yet each of them still faces great challenges. Their successes and their failures, however, represent a learning experience not only for themselves but for all their fellows. Out of these nine laboratories can come the distilled knowledge that will permit even faster progress in years to come by other states.

As a result, first of the target state activity, and then the resultant upsurge of interest in other states, the Commission found that it had to add two additional organizational entities. The first was a small group of regional associates who worked intimately with the Commission staff in aiding and supporting the target states and others as they became more and more involved in implementation. When the pace continued to quicken, a speakers' bureau whose talents were much deeper than that contained in the name, was established. This group of volunteers also was completely knowledgeable about the Commission's work and plans, and represented that body in state and district meetings across the country.

Finally, to ensure that the implementation period continued to be aided by outside analysis and exchange of ideas, a number of consultants and spokesmen were requested to meet with Commissioners and advisory groups on a frequent basis to criticize and to comment upon the implementation plans and priorities. Their contribution ensured a healthy give and take as well as a simple form of check-and-balance.

FOOTNOTES

1. "National Commission for the Study of Nursing and Nursing Education: Summary Report and Recommendations." *American Journal of Nursing*. 70:2:279-294 (February) 1970.
2. "Summary Report and Recommendations, National Commission for the Study of Nursing and Nursing Education." *Nursing Outlook*. 18:2:46-47 (February) 1970.

3. See Appendix A, "Publications Related to *An Abstract for Action*," for a listing of articles, reviews, and critiques.
4. The National Commission for the Study of Nursing and Nursing Education. *An Abstract for Action: Appendices.* Jerome P. Lysaught, Director. New York: McGraw-Hill Book Company, 1971. pp. 401-409.
5. *Facts About Nursing, 1970-71 Edition.* New York: American Nurses' Association, 1972, pp. 258-260.
6. "Summary Report," op. cit.
7. Personal communication with enclosure from Laura C. Dustan, Chairman, Council of Baccalaureate and Higher Degree Programs to Jerome P. Lysaught, Director, NCSNNE, dated March 23, 1970.
8. ibid., see enclosure.
9. Personal communication from Margaret E. Walsh, Secretary and General Director, NLN, to Jerome P. Lysaught, Director, NCSNNE, dated April 29, 1970.
10. Personal communication from Margaret E. Walsh, Secretary and General Director, NLN, to Jerome P. Lysaught, Director, NCSNNE, dated February 23, 1971.
11. "Report of the Task Force to Study the Implications of the Recommendations Presented in *An Abstract for Action*." *Nursing Outlook.* 21:2:111-118 (February) 1973. See particularly the introductory statement on the history and composition of the task force.
12. Personal communication from Frances K. Peterson, Director, Department of Diploma Programs, NLN, to Jerome P. Lysaught, Director, NCSNNE, dated May 15, 1972.
13. Personal communication from Margaret E. Walsh, General Director, NLN, to Jerome P. Lysaught, Director, NCSNNE, dated April 11, 1972.
14. Lewis, Edith P. "Editorial: In Perspective." *Nursing Outlook.* 20:3:163 (March) 1972.
15. Lewis, Edith P. "Editorial: Lysaught Report Revisited." *Nursing Outlook.* 21:2:93 (February) 1973.
16. *ibid.*
17. *Facts About Nursing, 1970-71 Edition.* New York: American Nurses' Association, 1972. pp. 254-257.
18. "National Commission," op. cit..
19. Stenographic transcript of proceedings, 1970 American Nurses' Association, prepared by Horne & Shell, Inc., New York, New York and provided to the NCSNNE by the ANA, in part, as a record of business related to the report of the National Commission. pp. 211-214.
20. Personal communication from Eileen M. Jacobi, Executive Director, ANA, to Jerome P. Lysaught, Director, NCSNNE, dated March 17, 1971.
21. Personal communication from Eileen M. Jacobi, Executive Director, ANA, to Jerome P. Lysaught, Director, NCSNNE, dated October 27, 1971.
22. "ANA Approves NCSNNE Report's Four Central Recommendations." *ANA in Action*, 3:3:14 (Fall) 1971.
23. "Statement of the Commission on Economic and General Welfare on the Findings and Recommendations of the National Commission for the Study of Nursing and Nursing Education." Enclosure to a memorandum from Alice L. Ahmuty, Director, to Executive Directors, State Nurses' Associations, dated October 7, 1971.
24. "ANA Board Endorses *An Abstract for Action*." News release prepared by the NCSNNE for general distribution, dated June, 1971. p. 1.
25. ibid. p. 2.
26. "Statement of the Council of the Conference of the Catholic Schools of Nursing on the 1970 Report of the National Commission on [sic] the Study of Nursing and Nursing Education," dated January 9, 1971. (mimeo).
27. Personal communication from Madeleine Leininger, President, AADCUSN, to Jerome P. Lysaught, Director, NCSNNE, dated November 23, 1971.
28. Personal communication from Dorothy M. Saller, Executive Director, AAIN, to Jerome P. Lysaught, Director, NCSNNE, dated September 23, 1971.
29. "Endorsement of the NCSNNE Report by the AORN." Action of the Board of Directors dated October, 1972 and transmitted by letter from Martha J. Parlapiano, President, AORN, to Jerome P. Lysaught, Director, NCSNNE, dated November 7, 1972.
30. "Resolution of the Department of School Nurses, National Education Association, Regarding the National Commission for the Study of Nursing and Nursing Education." Accepted by DSN Executive Committee, dated September 1972, and transmitted by letter from Oreta O. Norris, Administrative Director, DSN-NEA, to Jerome P. Lysaught, Director, NCSNNE, dated September 15, 1972.

31. "Abstract for Action: Nursing Commission Reports." *Nursing Research Report.* 6:1:5 (March) 1971.
32. Schumann, Mary Jean. "Imprint Editorial." *Imprint.* 19:5:8 (December) 1972.
33. Personal communication from Charles L. Leedham, Chairman, AMA Committee on Nursing, to Jerome P. Lysaught, Director NCSNNE, dated December 11, 1970.
34. Personal communication from Ernest B. Howard, Executive Vice President, AMA, to Jerome P. Lysaught, Director, NCSNNE, dated March 2, 1971.
35. "Minutes of the Advisory Panel to Review the Report of the National Commission for the Study of Nursing and Nursing Education." AHA, Headquarters Building, Chicago, September 29-30, 1970. (mimeo).
36. "Statement on Report of National Commission for the Study of Nursing and Nursing Education." *Hospitals.* 45:10:131 (May) 1971.
37. ibid.
38. ibid.
39. See, for example. "Appendix P. Career Enhancement Programs for the Licensed Practical/Vocational Nurse." The National Commission for the Study of Nursing and Nursing Education. *An Abstract for Action: Appendices.* Jerome P. Lysaught, Director. New York: McGraw-Hill Book Company. 1971. pp. 395-399.
40. Personal communication from Rose G. Martin, Executive Director, NAPNES, to Jerome P. Lysaught, Director, NCSNNE, dated April 15, 1970.
41. "Statement on Report of the National Commission for the Study of Nursing and Nursing Education." Approved in February 1971 by the Executive Board of The National Federation of Licensed Practical Nurses, Inc., dated March, 1971. (mimeo).
42. ibid., p. 1.
43. ibid., p. 2.
44. Personal communication from Alan D. Ferguson, Director, NEBHE, to Jerome P. Lysaught, Director, NCSNNE, dated April 13, 1971.
45. Press release of the Southern Regional Education Board, Atlanta, Georgia, dated April 16, 1971. (mimeo). p. 1.
46. Personal communication from Pearl Zemlicka, Chairman, MCPEN, to Jerome P. Lysaught, Director, NCSNNE, dated October 5, 1971.
47. Personal communication from Thomas R. Hood, Deputy Executive Director, APHA, to Jerome P. Lysaught, Director, NCSNNE, dated July 2, 1971.
48. Sorenson, Gladys. "An Abstract for Action." *Nursing Research.* 20:2:173-174. March-April, 1971.
49. Smith, Kathryn M. "An Abstract for Action." *American Journal of Nursing.* 71:4:814-818. April, 1971.
50. Kelisch, Beatrice J. "An Abstract for Action." *Library Journal.* October 15, 1970.
51. Murry, Ruth N. "An Abstract for Action." *Nursing Outlook.* 19:6:380 (June) 1971.
52. Christy, Teresa E., Poulin, Muriel A., and Julie Hover. "An Appraisal of *An Abstract for Action.*" *American Journal of Nursing.* 71:8:1574-1581 (August) 1971.
53. ibid., p. 1581.
54. ibid.
55. King, Imogene M., "Letters." *American Journal of Nursing.* 71:10:1914 (October) 1971.
56. Betson, Carol, ibid. p. 1914.
57. Lysaught, Jerome P., ibid. pp. 1914-1918.
58. Young, Lucie S., "Letters." *American Journal of Nursing.* 71:11:2124 (November) 1971.
59. Lambertsen, Eleanor C., ibid. p. 2118.
60. Cleland, Virginia S., "Letters." *American Journal of Nursing.* 71:10:1918-1919 (October) 1971.
61. Resnik, Barbara A., ibid. p. 1914.
62. Schlotfeldt, Rozella M., "Letters." *American Journal of Nursing.* 71:11:2124 (November) 1971.
63. "Report of the Task Force to Study the Implications of the Recommendations Presented in *An Abstract for Action.*" *Nursing Outlook.* 21:2:111-118 (February) 1973.
64. Report to NLN Board of Directors, Task Force to Study the Implications of the NCSNNE Report." September 12, 1972. (mimeo). pp. 20-21.
65. ibid. p. 11.
66. ibid. p. 4.
67. ibid. p. 10.
68. Lewis, Edith P. "Editorial: Lysaught Report Revisited." *Nursing Outlook.* 21:2:93 (February) 1973.
69. ibid.

70. Personal communication from Frances K. Peterson, Director, Department of Diploma Programs, NLN, to Jerome P. Lysaught, Director, NCSNNE, dated May 15, 1972.
71. "Report of the Task Force to Study the Implications of the Recommendations Presented in *An Abstract for Action.*" op. cit. p. 114.
72. "From Diploma School to College: Two Case Studies on Changing Patterns Within Institutions for Nursing Education." Rochester, N.Y.: NCSNNE, 1970 (pamphlet).

FOUR
TOWARD CHANGE IN NURSING: ROLES AND FUNCTIONS

Over the past several years, a common thread of concern for health care has emerged from several distinct, but related, variables. The first of these is the growth in numbers of people to be served. Since the Second World War, our steadily expanding population has contributed to an increased need for health service. So, too, has our societal determination to bring *all* our population within the system—thus ensuring that the poor, the disadvantaged, and the isolated receive care. Moreover, the very success of our system to date has significantly, if variably, lengthened life expectancy and thus increased the "people pressure" on practitioners and facilities involved in the delivery of care. The combined impact of the very young, the very old, and the heretofore neglected, presents us with whole classes of clients who need more than average amounts of health care at the very time we are experiencing difficulty in maintaining our traditional provision of services.

Economics, also, has served to stimulate the demand for expanded care over this same period of time. The increased insurance coverage of our population through both private and public plans is, for all practical purposes, a blank check or promissory note to meet health care needs in our society—whenever and wherever they arise. Logic and logistics aside, most analysts agree that, by 1975, almost 100 percent of our people will be covered by prepaid health insurance and will have expectations about care availability far beyond our present capacity to deliver. Add to this the disconcerting point that more Americans, encouraged by their program for basic protection, are spending increasing amounts of discretionary income on cosmetic or marginal treatment, and we find ourselves facing capillary collapse because the system is simply insufficient for the flow required.

A third confounding variable relates to the growing complexity and interdependence of care transmission. Labor statisticians now recognize more than 125 different health occupations, encompassed within twice that number of job titles. The growth of knowledge, technology, and specialization has been reflected in the proliferation of functions and personnel so that care is compartmentalized, decision making diffused, and, on occasion, responsibility remitted. Garfield has documented much of this in diagrammatic fashion.[1] In the early nineteenth century, a care system might have been illustrated as in Figure 4-1. The simple dyadic relationship meant that the practitioner, who might have been a physician, a midwife, a barber-surgeon, or any of a variety of healers, was in direct and personal contact with the patient. While shortcomings were pronounced in terms of both knowledge and treatment, there was a functional elegance in the ability to communicate and handle problems.

Before the end of the century, however, the beginnings of scientific medicine and formalized nursing had brought a recognizable division of labor into health practice. At one point, perhaps in 1900, almost 75 percent of our American practitioners were physicians and nurses, nearly evenly divided in numbers, with the remainder sprinkled among aides, attendants, and other helping groups. The relationship in the provision of care at this time most frequently resembled Figure 4-2. Our dyad had become a triad. Of particular significance, however, is the fact that, while our number of principals increased arithmetically, their social interactions and communication pathways had grown geometrically. While it may have been possible for the nurse and the physician to know what the other was doing, each additional component added to the system over the ensuing years has made it more and more difficult to ensure that the patient's needs are being effectively and efficiently met. No one ever set out to develop a pattern of 125 occupations, together with a factorial set of relationships, in order to deliver health care. No one,

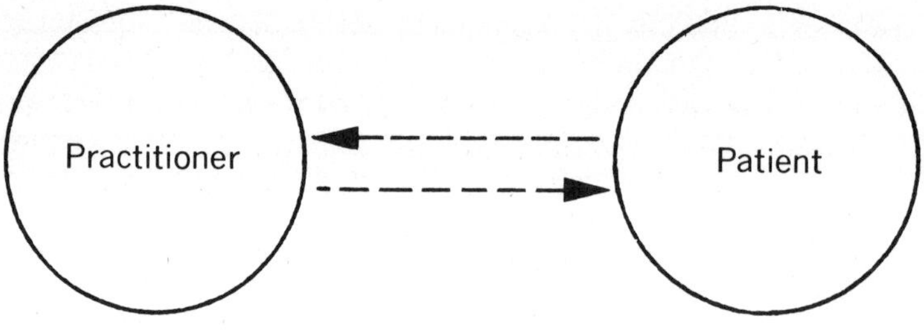

Figure 4-1. Early practitioner-patient relationship.

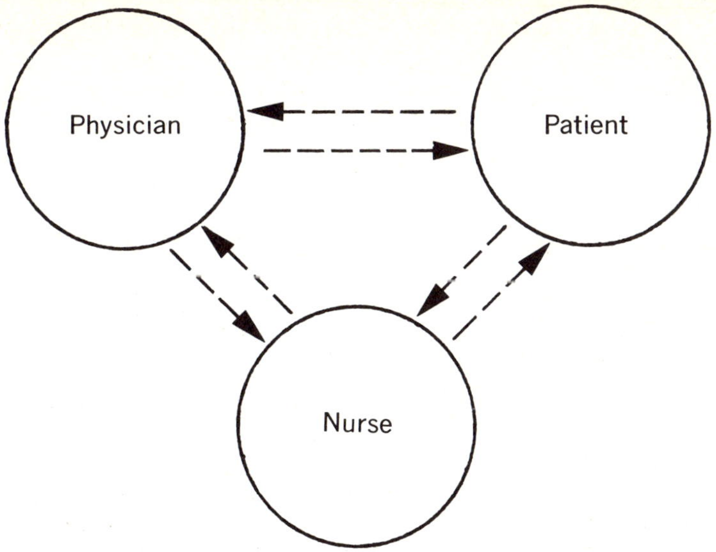

Figure 4-2. The physician-nurse-patient relationship.

either, wishes to return to the "good old days" of 1900 with its limitations in science and application. Most everyone would agree that we need to make sure we know where we are, where we are going, and how best to get there. And this, in turn, requires that we examine the impact of our system, or non-system, and the functional relationship of our care practitioners.

To meet the health problems posed by increased population, changed economics, and organizational complexity is difficult. To do so under the twin pressures of time and rhetoric presents a dilemma. To do it without clear understanding and communication between our two largest bodies of health practitioners—our nurses and physicians—is patently impossible.

One of the very obvious things that we must do is to see that all of our health professionals are used to the very highest level of capacity—both to ensure that the public derives the greatest immediate impact from their service and to ensure that the practitioners are unencumbered in their efforts to utilize their skills, hard won through education and experience.

In this regard, more and more people are beginning to see that our reserve of 1,400,000 nurses—active and inactive, currently and formerly licensed—comprises our largest single potential for effecting real advances in health care. They represent the largest pool of health personnel, educated and equipped to perform at a critical level of clinical skill. Just as importantly, we know that large numbers of them have been underutilized or misutilized in our traditional approaches to health care provision.

In order to get at the underlying problems that affect the practice of nursing, literally to unleash the latent power that resides in this great body of personnel and to redirect the nurse-physician relationship into more congruent pathways, the National Commission proposed a series of seventeen recommendations. The highest priority was given to the development of new communications and planning arrangements between the two primary practitioner groups, American nurses and physicians.

THE NATIONAL JOINT PRACTICE COMMISSION

Emphatic corroboration of the need to expand the functions and role of the nurse, while emphasizing joint approaches to the actual change processes, is seen in the report of the Secretary's Committee to Study Extended Roles for Nurses. This group has stated:

> We believe that the future of nursing must encompass a substantially larger place within the community of the health professions. Moreover, we believe that extending the scope of nursing practice is essential if this Nation is to achieve the goal of equal access to health services for all its citizens . . . Moreover we are aware that there are complex and often delicate questions of professional attitudes involved in any consideration of nurses functioning in extended roles. It would be naive to gloss over the fact that working relationships between physicians and nurses are often less than ideal with results that are disadvantageous to both professions, but more importantly to their patients.[2]

The secretary's committee put its finger squarely on the problem when it emphasized, not only the need to change roles, but to do so through the involvement of *both* medicine and nursing. Fortunately, this recognition coincided with a reawakening to the problems and promise of cooperation between the two professions that has been taking place for some time. At the national level, the American Medical Association and the American Nurses' Association have been laboring to develop better communications and understanding. Within the individual specialty areas, nurses and physicians have attempted to clarify new roles and educational standards for changing patterns of practice.[3] In a number of the states, the two professions have issued combined statements on practice and engaged in joint efforts to modify health practice acts in the light of evolving functions and relationships.[4]

Each of these developments is encouraging and commendable, but the urgency of our health concerns is such that accelerated movement toward change is a simple necessity. In addition, we need a designated mechanism that will provide continuity, concerted planning, follow-up, and dissemination of results if we are to achieve any fundamental realignment of practitioner roles and functions. For all these reasons, the National Commission urged:

> A National Joint Practice Commission, with state counterpart committees, be established between Medicine and Nursing to discuss and make recommendations concerning the congruent roles of the physician and the nurse in providing quality health care . . .[5]

Formation of the NJPC

With the inauguration of the implementation phase of the Commission's work, information meetings were arranged with a large number of medical and nursing groups. By the spring of 1971, the governing boards of the American Nurses' Association and the American Medical Association had taken overt action to endorse and support the summary recommendations of *An Abstract for Action* including one urging the establishment of a National Joint Practice Commission. In early summer, at the suggestion of our advisory committees, it was agreed that we should initiate overtures to these two organizations asking them to serve as joint sponsors of the project. In retrospect, the reasons for choosing these organizations were quite simple:

> 1. The ANA and the AMA are the two largest organizations of nurse and physician practitioners;
> 2. Both these organizations had for some time initiated and participated in a variety of interprofessional liaison activities; and
> 3. Both organizations had now formally endorsed the concept of a joint practice commission thus indicating at least a beginning commitment to implementation.

The NCSNNE staff contacted the leadership of the ANA Congress for Nursing Practice and the AMA Committee on Nursing for their assistance in planning concrete actions toward the establishment of a National Joint Practice Commission. On August 4, 1971 the members of these two groups met jointly to discuss the desirability and practicality of such an organization.

At this session, the participants reviewed the experience of prior, related activities such as joint care conferences, interagency and state liaison committee work, and their own organizational efforts. The participants then reviewed the structure of their parent bodies and the relationship of their committees to that overall organization pattern. Consideration was given to the form and placement of a joint practice group, its composition, and its purposes. Out of all these considerations, and following both joint and separate sessions, the nurses and physicians agreed that a National Joint Practice Commission was desirable and that it should be established according to a common set of shared understandings.

In a "Memorandum of Agreement" drafted by the participants, the following specific provisions were enumerated:

> 1. The National Joint Practice Commission . . . would be established to

discuss, study, and make recommendations concerning the congruent roles of the physician and the nurse in providing quality health care to our nation's people.

2. In doing so, it is agreed that the NJPC would examine the roles and functions of *both* professions and make recommendations for new or altered practice by *both* professions.

3. In arriving at its objectives, the NJPC would work in cooperation with state counterpart committees, specialty group task forces (or such other means as the Commission itself might choose) to develop statements on joint practice, proposals for model health practice acts, position papers on licensure, etc.

4. As early as practical, too, the NJPC would invite participation, in the studies on congruent roles, from health management people, representatives of other health care groups, and representatives of consumers of health service.[6]

The participants then turned their attention to the composition and organization of the proposed body. There was no hesitancy in reaching agreement that the Commission should be composed of equal numbers of nurses and physicians. It was also agreed that the majority of members from each profession should be identified as practitioners—for this purpose being defined as one who engages in direct patient care activities approximately fifty percent of the time—and that some members of the Commission should also be members of the ANA Congress for Nursing Practice and the AMA Committee on Nursing so as to ensure close communication between and among all the involved parties.

As a final point, the participants agreed to take before their respective governing boards the details of the memorandum and request that formal action be taken to approve the "understandings" and appoint individuals to serve as the first members of the NJPC. By separate action of the two boards in September, 1971, the NJPC came into existence and steps were initiated to nominate and designate the individuals who would serve on the Commission.

Over the fall of 1971, the AMA and ANA set about their individual processes for designating the commissioners. With the acceptance of the charge by the persons concerned, that body was initially comprised of the following persons:

Nurse Practitioners	*Medical Practitioners*
Genrose J. Alfano, New York	*Thomas F. Dillon, New York
Patricia Devine, Kansas	A. Alan Fischer, Indiana
Marilyn J. Howe, California	Robert A. Hoekelman, New York
Nancy Melvin, Arizona	Joseph W. Marshall, Idaho
*Anna B. Sherlock, Arizona	William H. Muller, Jr., Virginia
Shirley Smoyak, New Jersey	*Robert A. Murray, Texas

*Over the first eighteen months, the following changes took place in the membership of the NJPC: Daniel W. Beacham, Louisiana, replaced Thomas F. Dillon, New York; William M. Deyerle, Virginia, replaced Robert A. Murray, Texas; Dorothy Butler, Ohio, replaced Anna Sherlock, Arizona.

Virginia Stone, North Carolina | Otto C. Page, Oregon
Barbara Taylor, Massachusetts | James W. Walker, Florida

On January 20-21, 1972, the first meeting of the NJPC took place in St. Louis, Missouri and was hosted by the NCSNNE. The members reviewed the antecedent actions and the charges forwarded by the governing boards of AMA and ANA, as well as the findings and recommendations that had led to the creation of this new organization.

The decisions of the parent boards provided the NJPC with basic guides to its objectives and activities. It was apparent, however, that the parent bodies had delegated to the group itself a wide latitude over decisions on internal organization, staffing, finance, and operations. Temporary officers were elected and ad hoc committees appointed to study and report back on four areas of immediate concern:

1. Structure and organization;
2. Experimentation in joint nurse-physician roles;
3. Developments in state level joint practice relations; and
4. State and national communications and planning.

With the help of staff from AMA, ANA, and the NCSNNE, these subcommittees prepared questionnaires, gathered material, and conducted preliminary planning sessions prior to the second meeting of the entire body in April of 1972. By means of their interim activities, immediate progress on organization proceeded.

Objectives of the NJPC

Through the use of a structured conference technique, the individual members of the NJPC generated a set of specific organizational goals. These were then discussed and rank-ordered in a set of priorities based on common agreement and understanding. Arranged in summary fashion, these are the objectives of the Commission.[7]

1. To identify, define and examine health care needs.
   a. Identify unmet health care needs, nationally and regionally, which are amenable to medical and/or nursing care.
   b. Identify social, educational, and economic barriers which now prevent or impede quality health care.
   c. Define affordable quality health care for the United States.
   d. Examine types of health care delivery systems together with related priorities in use in varied geographic and regional areas.
2. To examine the roles and functions in medical and nursing practice in order to define new and altered patterns.
   a. Examine the authority, responsibility, and operation of each profession in terms of current and projected practice patterns.

b. Identify the independent and interdependent roles and functions of medicine and nursing with particular attention to transitional areas affected by changing practice patterns.
c. Identify the responsibility that medicine and nursing are willing to assume in fulfillment of the determined health care needs of the nation.
d. Identify the changes in medical and nursing practice needed to improve the quantity and quality of health care.
e. Examine how, and to what extent, medicine and nursing can change to meet health care needs.

3. To improve the communications between medicine and nursing to advance joint planning and action.
a. Identify ways of enhancing communications between the two professions at national, state, and local levels.
b. Identify means of improving joint planning in the provision of health care.
c. Foster and improve working communications and joint planning between medicine and nursing in order to enhance the delivery of health care.

4. To propose changes in educational patterns and relationships that would enhance the new role functioning of nurses and physicians.
a. Investigate interdisciplinary teaching programs and other educational approaches that could lead to improved understanding of role functioning and practice between nurses and physicians.
b. Study and recommend continual modification in the preparation and continuing education of nurses and physicians that would relate to changing health care needs and delivery patterns.
c. Study the present motivation modalities that affect medical and nursing student selection of specialties for practice.

5. To address the traditional problems which affect nurse-physician relationships in order to establish enhanced role functioning.
a. Examine the issues that affect collaborative nurse-physician relationships such as sex, social class, and professional status.
b. Study other colleague relationship problems for the purpose of proposing new means and approaches for enhancing collaboration of nurses and physicians.

6. To encourage and assist in the development of state counterpart joint practice committees.
a. Outline the methods and procedures for the establishment of statewide joint practice committees.

7. To identify and address ensuing problems related to basic role reorganization.
a. Identify problems that may arise because of role changes, in such areas as legal custom and education, and seek to solve them.
b. Identify problems in understanding and acceptance by professionals of changed medical and nursing roles and seek to gain acceptance.
c. Provide models and demonstrations aimed at resolving problems in practice roles and functions.

This multifaceted set of purposes obviously is an ambitious long-term commitment. Many of the specific objectives are developmental and evolutionary. For these reasons, then, the NJPC is involved in programming operational systems that can begin to contribute to their ultimate goals.

Program of the NJPC

Continuing activities of the NJPC have included the completion of organizational structure and development of initial task forces to work on problems of joint concern to medicine and nursing.

Structure of the NJPC. At its second meeting, the NJPC elected permanent officers for initial terms. Robert A. Hoekelman was chosen chairman and Shirley A. Smoyak was selected to be vice chairman. A subcommittee on organization developed drafts for articles of incorporation and by-laws; after their modification by the group, these were forwarded to the governing boards of AMA and ANA and subsequently approved with some modification. These documents will now serve as the basis for governance and the securing of financial support. Detailed reviews of projected budgets and plans for acquisition of staff personnel are now underway.

Development of Task Forces. In order to carry out its charges, the NJPC early decided that it would have to work through committees or task forces created, not to conduct research, but to review completed demonstrations, projects and literature related to particular areas of health care, and then formulate generalizations and recommendations for altered practice relationships between nurses and physicians.

These task forces were intended to be multidisciplinary, with exact composition varying in accordance with the problems under scrutiny. Each would include a member of the NJPC and be supported by the Commission staff. While no clear set of priorities existed for the selection of primary targets, the NJPC agreed that three central concerns for early action were: care of the aged, rural health, and interdisciplinary learning patterns for nurses and physicians. Each of these fields has received attention in the past and there is a considerable amount of data and material available, but no clear directions exist for the optimum allocation of nurse-physician manpower in the reduction of the problem areas.

It is the intention of the NJPC, through the establishment of these task forces, to implement those recommendations which emerge as most promising and to encourage continuing attention to the remaining impediments. As progress is made in these first three fields, additional task forces will be designated to examine changed role patterns in other areas.

STATEWIDE JOINT PRACTICE COMMITTEES

Second only to the priority given the NJPC in the planning of implementation activities was that part of the National Commission recommendation which called for the "development of state counterpart committees." Even while negotiations were beginning for the establishment of the NJPC, the NCSNNE staff prepared, "A

Guide for Establishing Statewide Joint Practice Commissions."[8] This document acknowledged that the National Commission's interest in joint practice stemmed largely from the development of the liaison or ad hoc committees which had been active in some twenty states over the period of our investigation. These state groups had prepared joint statements on specific aspects of practice, provided for needed dialogue between physicians and nurses, and in some cases, had been involved in considerations of proposed amendments to health practice acts.

These committees had evidenced their contribution to improved practice, but they had also shown some shortcomings. To begin with, they existed in less than half of the states and the majority of nurse-physician associations at this level were uninvolved. Secondly, these committees for the most part had addressed narrow areas of common concern. For example, a number of the "liaison" committees had issued statements on such specific interventions as the initiation of intravenous injections. Finally, there was commonly voiced concern that more practitioners should be involved in the dialogue between physicians and nurses—rather than association staff persons, educators, administrators, etc.

With these considerations in mind, the National Commission essayed to assist in forming state joint practice committees based on the pattern assumed by the National Joint Practice Commission. Helped by the staff from AMA and ANA, communications were instituted with all the state associations urging them to become involved and to begin to structure interdisciplinary practice groups in a form compatible with the NJPC.

Where liaison committees or ad hoc groups already existed, the National Commission suggested only those modifications that would bring practitioners into more basic dialogue. Where no precedent or organization existed, efforts were made *ab initio* to establish a viable body. Particularly within the nine target states, there was a drive to establish a statewide joint practice committee in order to learn the problems and the processes so they might be shared as other states moved toward the same end.

As the NJPC became more and more functional in its own right, it took up the communications effort and urged that state medical societies and nursing associations work together toward the establishment of joint practice committees. In order to generate a tangible target date for many of the states, and in order to encourage a concerted attack upon common problems, the NJPC announced in August, 1972 plans for a National Conference of State Joint Practice Committees to be held the following November. The call for the meeting indicated that it was intended to:

> . . . provide an opportunity for state representatives to explore common issues and share both progress and problems they have experienced in developing joint discussion of professional roles and functions. In addition, the meeting will afford a means of communication between the states and the NJPC on activities, issues, and plans for the coming year.[9]

The response to the invitational meeting so far exceeded expectations that its actual conduct was imperilled. An original budget was developed in anticipation of fifteen to twenty states participating. When twice that number had indicated their intent to take part, reconsideration was required. At the outset, the NJPC had planned to cover all expenses. With special aid from the AMA, ANA, and NCSNNE, it was possible to assure the states that all the direct conference costs could be covered, but that each state would have to assume responsibility for the transportation costs of its representatives.

This unanticipated event required an early commitment from all the states, including many in which only the most preliminary joint discussions had taken place. Its effect was to encourage even greater participation by the nurses and physicians. When the conference convened on November 9, 1972, there were representatives present from 47 states; 37 of these had both nurses and physicians in attendance. Over the next two days, the NJPC Commissioners and the state delegates exchanged information and views on a variety of subjects, with a series of presentations given on: the development of statewide committees; descriptions of expanded joint practice in various care settings; legal implications of extended joint practice; and joint educational programs for altered practice functions.

As a result of the NJPC activities and the conference follow-up, there has been an increased activity in the organization of statewide joint practice groups. By April 1, 1973, the state of development had reached the levels indicated in Table 4-1.

As shown in the table, more than half the states had operational or beginning joint practice committees between medicine and nursing less than fifteen months after the inaugural meeting of the National Joint Practice Commission. Some of these represent shifts in the composition of previously established liaison committees; most of them, however, are newly designated planning bodies. In a small number of states, physician and nurse planning is still tied to "Allied Health" or similar types of standing arrangements; in only three states is there no organizational approach, as yet, to the concerns of joint roles in health care practice.

TABLE 4-1 STATUS OF IMPLEMENTATION: STATEWIDE JOINT PRACTICE COMMITTEES

Category of Status	Number of States*
Operational state joint practice committee	27
State joint practice committee in process	3
State liaison committee	14
Other committee or organization	4
No organized body	3

*Total of 51 includes the District of Columbia.

Because of their newness, most of these state joint practice committees are still in their own organizational stages, attempting to establish ground rules and mechanisms by which to proceed. Of those committees which have gotten past the preliminary stage of organization and into the work of planning, there is the common experience of grappling now with the reality of working together as partners and fellow members rather than as "nurses" and "physicians." Years of separation and organizational rivalry are not overcome by one session, or two, of cooperative discussion. Only through continued experience and long-term commitment can we begin to achieve the mutual confidence required for change processes.

There are an increasing number of state joint practice committees which have given evidence that change can be accomplished. The California Joint Practice Committee, using the "Report of the Secretary's Committee to Study Extended Roles for Nurses," has formulated related statements on practitioner roles in primary, acute, and long-term care. The committee's recommended statements have been forwarded to the California Medical Association and California Nurses' Association boards for consideration and approval. Relatedly, a resolution has been introduced in the state assembly to utilize ensuing joint practice statements as the basis for determining and defining health care practice in that state.

The North Carolina Joint Practice Committee has developed guidelines for six task forces to explore joint role relationships of nurses and physicians in nurse-manned clinics, school health services, occupational health care, emergency health care, maternal and infant care (including midwifery), and long-term care (including that in nursing homes). The state committee has examined a number of role modification approaches including: physician assistants, family nurse practitioners, and nurse midwives. The implications of these altered practice roles have been considered for their effect upon nursing education and liability insurance coverage for those engaged in expanded role practice. The committee has met with representatives of the State Board of Pharmacy and the State Pharmaceutical Association to discuss recommendations of the Legislative Research Commission's Committee in relation to proposed changes in the Pharmacy Act.

In other states, too, the pace has quickened. The Illinois Joint Practice Committee has formulated proposals for change in the state's licensing laws, and these have been referred to the sponsoring organizations for appropriate action. The Michigan Joint Practice Committee has taken up the task of enhancing interdisciplinary educational opportunities at the basic, preparatory level between medicine and nursing. The Wyoming Joint Practice Committee has appointed task forces to prepare statements on emergency room care and home health care.

Within the individual states, beginning activities generally reflect local priorities. In combination, however, the work of the several state committees mirrors the national concerns for more coordination and planning to solve our grave problems of health delivery. Through a continuing interplay of national and state joint practice workings, we are beginning to develop interdisciplinary action that could be decisive in the construction of a new and better system.

EPISODIC AND DISTRIBUTIVE NURSING PRACTICE

From the beginnings of modern nursing in the United States, the practice of the profession has been intimately bound up in the development of the hospital system. Conditioned by the daily concern for the acutely ill, and by the occasional devastation of war, disease, and natural disaster, hospitals and nursing grew up together. The first nurses practiced in hospitals; the first schools of nursing were located in hospitals; the largest single employers of nurses continued to be hospitals; and the most pervasive image of the American nurse is that of a white-garbed female in a hospital setting.

This long and close relationship, however, obscures two very fundamental points:

> 1. Nursing practice is, by both definition and fact, far broader than the traditional concerns of the hospital for the treatment of grave illness, injury, or disease. Nursing has long included elements of health maintenance, disease prevention, and nonacute patient care.
>
> 2. Acute, or episodic nursing practice, is not synonymous with either "general nursing" or "hospital care" even though this institution is the most common location for the provision of that care because of the concentration of personnel, resources, and equipment.

Many competent observers of our current health care system have expressed their concern for the development of a total plan for care covering the complete range of patient needs. As the Citizens Commission on Graduate Medical Education stated:

> Many physicians who are not content with the provision of a repair service when illness strikes share the dream of a more encompassing and far-reaching health service. Their goal is to prevent illness, to maintain each patient in as near optimum health as can be achieved. Sanitation, immunization, public health measures, dietary instruction and physical fitness programs are all steps in this direction. But there are other steps to be taken.[10]

Certainly one of the other steps to be taken is to utilize more fully the capacity of nursing, the largest of our health practicing professions, in the expansion of our health care system to include the maintenance of health and the prevention of disease as well as the treatment and cure of maladies.

It has been estimated that perhaps fewer than 12 percent of our actual health care problems are those related to cure, while more than 88 percent of the problems people encounter are really ones of care—education for health, periodic examination, dietary advice, long-term, nonacute regimens.[11] Yet, paradoxically, the greatest resources and, by far the institutional bulk of our health care system, are directed at the episodic or cure aspects of the problem. The education and emphasis of most physicians and nurses is aimed at the treatment and amelioration of maladies and affliction, and the structural nucleus of our health care system—the hospital—has been molded to the exigencies of cure type cases.

While the vast majority of our population at any one time can be classified under the general terms of "well" or "mildly unwell," a diagrammatic comparison of our allocation of nurse resources clearly shows how poorly our traditional strategy of health delivery matches the nation's needs. Figure 4-3 compares the proportionate distribution of nurse manpower to indicated consumer needs.[12]

It is eerie that data indicate almost 89 percent of our full-time nurse practitioners engage in episodic concerns while only 11 percent are involved in such areas as public health, occupational health, school nursing, and related care activities. Certainly, the use of any comparison such as this is hazardous. No one would argue that nurse hours spent in the care of the acutely ill patient should be the same as those for the mildly unwell. The sheer, inverse nature of the relationship, however, is persuasive of our need to examine our entire structure of nursing roles and functions.

Recognizing that we have such a tremendous stake in the maintenance of health and the prevention of catastrophe, our National Commission urged that two companion patterns of nursing practice be established:

> 1. One career pattern (episodic) would emphasize practice that is essentially curative and restorative, generally acute or chronic in nature, and most frequently provided in the setting of the hospital and the in-patient facility.
>
> 2. The second career pattern (distributive) would emphasize the nursing practice that is designed essentially for health maintenance and disease prevention, generally continuous in nature, seldom acute, and most frequently operative in the community or in newly developing institutional settings.[13]

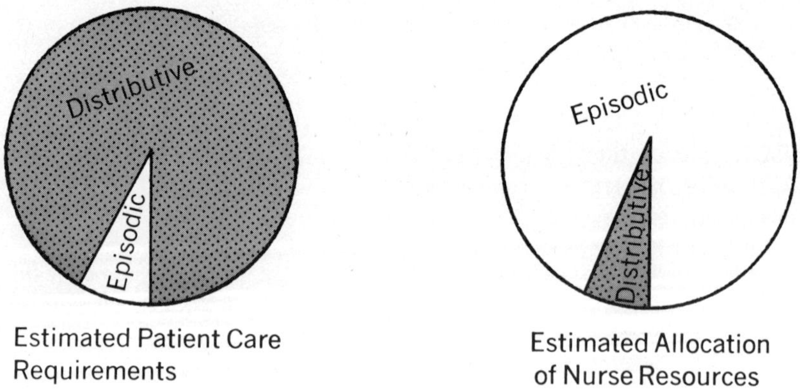

Figure 4-3. Diagrammatic comparison of consumer needs and nurse resource allocation for episodic and distributive care.

It is no accident that Secretary Richardson's committee to examine the future role of nursing concluded, one year after the publication of *An Abstract for Action*, that one of nursing's greatest contributions to health care could come from a realignment of traditional roles and functions. That committee wrote:

> One of the most important opportunities for change in the current system of health care involves altering the practice of nurses and physicians so that nurses assume considerably greater responsibility for delivering primary health care services. The term primary care as used in this paper has two dimensions: (a) a person's first contact in any given episode of illness with the health care system that leads to a decision of what must be done to help resolve his problem; and (b) the responsibility for the continuum of care, i.e., maintenance of health, evaluation and management of symptoms, and appropriate referrals.[14]

Whether one prefers the term *distributive* or *primary* in describing this form of nursing practice, there is no distinction between the expressed concerns or the intended thrust of these two recommendations. Both see the need for considerably increased emphasis on the nonacute, nonepisodic parameters of health care. Both see the immense possibilities for nursing to become the prime professional contributor to a changed strategy of national health care.

An Interactive Model for Nursing Practice

In its investigation into the characteristics of nursing practice, the National Commission early discovered that the tradition of hospital nursing had so colored most of the educational programs and service commitments that many individuals in and out of the profession simply assumed that preparation for acute, episodic care is, in truth, preparation for all nursing practice. So pervasive is that assumption, that to question it assumes all the dimensions of heresy, and many may miss the incongruity of a statement such as the one made in a letter to the editor of the *American Journal of Nursing*:

> The authors criticize the report's recommendations for the "episodic" and "distributive" tracks in nursing education. I heartily concur. I have just finished an exciting summer doing public health nursing as the final course for my B.S. degree. I could never have met the challenges without my generalist background preparation. If I hadn't first learned to care for the ill individual, I could never have given adequate care to the well individual.[15]

What have we done in nursing to conclude we must learn to care for the ill before we can care for the well? Is it not at least as plausible that one can learn to work with and care for the well in preparation for treating the ill? Or is it not possible that one can have preparatory experience of a nature that permits concentration in either distributive or episodic care to be built on a foundation of truly "general" nursing?

Our findings and data indicated that patient condition ought to be at least as important as patient location in the proper determination of treatment. Moreover, the nature of nursing care demanded in a specific instance varied in predictable ways, dependent upon the environmental setting and the general state of health of the consumer. From these empirical findings, the National Commission generated a conceptual model to account for the interactive variability noted in the process of site visits and observations.[16] The parameters of that model are shown in Figure 4-4.

On one dimension, we find *patients* grouped according to general health condition, from the well patient who may need some form of screening, routine immunization, or counseling, through the mildly unwell person who requires rehabilitation exercises, a continuing dietary regimen, or the like, to the acutely unwell individual who has suffered an injury, a critical illness, or some other form of malady. On a second dimension, we find the *environmental setting,* in which the hospital or other in-patient facility is simply one of a variety of settings for the provision of care. There is the outpatient facility, the neighborhood center, the health maintenance organization, and the community clinic. Also, there is the home, the office, the factory, the school, and a host of other settings. Finally, there is the full range of *nursing behaviors,* including assessment or diagnosis, actual intervention or treatment, and instruction of the consumer, his family, or other health workers in the continuation of a determined regimen for care.

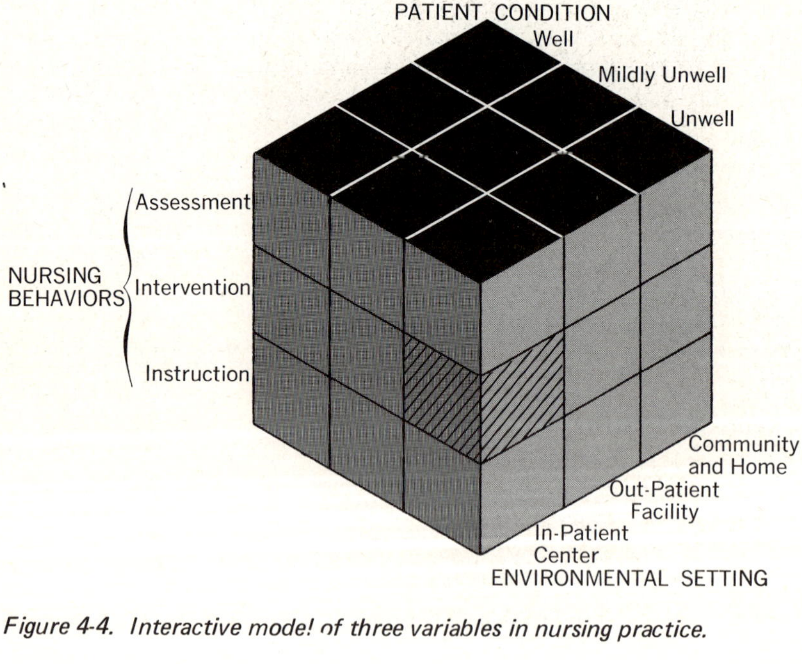

Figure 4-4. Interactive model of three variables in nursing practice.

It is long past due for us to confront seriously the distinction between *cure* and *care* in our arrangement of a health delivery system. Cure and episodic pratice relate essentially to the treatment and management of illness or injury once incurred. Its results are very visible, frequently very satisfying to both practitioner and patient, and occasionally involve the dramatic. Who can forget the publicity attached to transplant surgery and the attendant evidence of excitement and interest? Who can deny the exhilaration of the successful intensive care unit struggle to combat myocardial infarction?

Care is far more pervasive since it begins with wellness and bends its efforts toward the sustaining of that condition. Its results are seldom visible except over long periods of time. While its outcomes may be satisfying, they are seldom attributable to any single practitioner or health worker. And, though its results may be determinative of an individual's life span or the economic solvency of a health plan, they are seldom likely to be cast in heroic proportions. More often, the approach is in quiet subdued tones—the person who plans fluoridation for the city water supply may do more for prevention of tooth decay than all the dental surgeons of the metropolis, but does society even recognize this contribution?

If we reexamine our "cubistic" model for nursing practice, we can come to the somewhat depressing conclusion that most of our preparation, and much of our utilization, of practitioners is centered around the medical cure model, which is aimed at the episodic treatment of the hospital patient through a set of nursing interventions. This is important—and, of course, vital in many situations. But that particular correlation of variables represents in optimum fashion only one cube of twenty-seven compassed by the model. This does not mean everything we have done is wrong. It does mean that we must take serious stock of what we have labeled "general nursing" and recognize we have for too long emphasized one part of nursing practice and largely appended other roles to that area. Distributive care is too important to be treated as an afterthought. Both episodic and distributive roles must be emphasized; both are needed and both are vital.

In its reflections on the problems of our times, the secretary's committee commented:

> Our system is still largely operating on the Hippocratic principle that the doctor or nurse must wait until the patient seeks help before they set about to minister to his needs. Despite some limited efforts to the contrary, the health care system still operates on a "come and get it" basis. Yet some of the greatest advances in the health field, especially in the areas of disease prevention and health maintenance, depend upon the health care delivery system reaching out to those people who do not see the need or lack the opportunity to "come and get it."[17]

Again, the committee drew a sharp contrast between the success of our scientific advancement in the development of tools for enhancing health and the limited encroachment we have been able to make on our old problems.

> It has been said that biomedical science has advanced further in the last three decades than in all prior history. . . . And, equally important, progress in biomedical technology has not been matched by a necessary change in the underlying philosophy of the provision of health care.[18]

If there is need for further indication of consensus on these points, it may be found in Esther Lucile Brown's *Nursing Reconsidered: A Study of Change*. She notes in her inquiry into evolving professional roles in both institutional and community settings that:

> Nursing is currently undergoing large and dynamic alteration. . . there is now opportunity to fashion a new role in which nurses with greater professional competence will be more active participants in coordinated efforts to plan and provide better care for the seriously ill, and to extend preventive, rehabilitative, and counseling services to those large segments of the population for whom such attention has been minimal.[19]

Finally, there is the cross-cultural or, perhaps, pan-cultural confirmation of the need to change our approach to nursing functions in the World Health Organization Working Group report on *Trends in European Nursing Services.* They report:

> There is widespread concern in Europe over the shortage of suitably qualified nurses to cope with the increased and highly diversified demand for health services.[20]

And so, after years of viewing one portion of the practice spectrum as the "general core" of nursing, the profession must now develop a plan for meeting the full range of consumer needs subsumed by the term *health system.* The terminology used to marshal the arguments for such an expanded view of nursing's proper province is varied, but the conceptual component is consistent. Whatever system one utilizes, it is still apparent that nursing roles must broaden and more emphasis must be placed on *care* along with, but not in place of, cure.

TABLE 4-2 COMPARISON OF TERMS USED TO DELINEATE SPECIALIZED AREAS OF EXPANDED NURSING PRACTICE

Source	Practice Area 1	Practice Area 2
Traditional terminology	General practice	Public health
Esther Lucile Brown	Institutional care	Community care
The secretary's committee	Acute care	Primary and long-term care
World Health Working Group	High risk care	Community care
The National Commission	Episodic care	Distributive care

While some may view the National Commission's application of terms as a pedantic exercise in neology, it seems apparent to us and to many of our advisors that the traditional terminology masked much of the need for fundamental reassessment because of the semantic haze evoked by such terms as *general nursing* and *public health nursing*. Indeed, an extrapolation of the interactive model does show that episodic and distributive practice are far more than "nice" synonyms. They are a denotation of what practice must become rather than a definition of what practice is or has been.

Interestingly enough, the specialty practice groups in American nursing, developed some years ago—through pragmatism—a system of selective care concerns that is generally amenable to a schema utilizing episodic and distributive formulations. Figure 4-5 is one way of illustrating a partial separation of functional specialization.

This rational division of labor cuts through the tortuous theoretical formulations that have for so long conditioned the nursing profession's approach to full

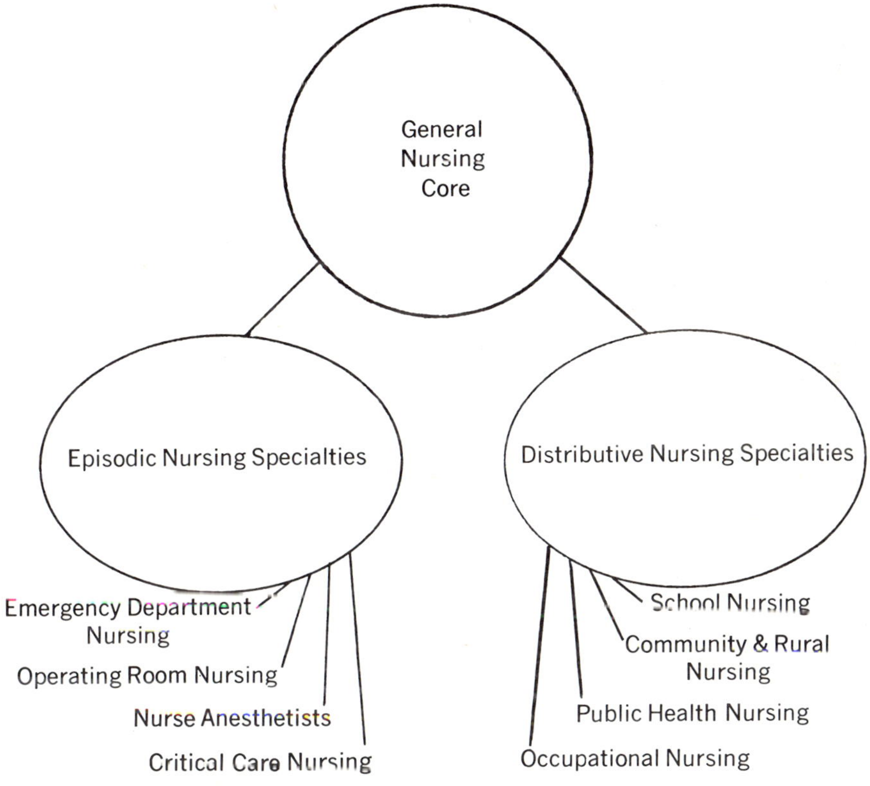

Figure 4-5. Sample separation of nurse specialty groups by areas of professional practice.

care coverage. By recognizing the entire panoply of nursing's role and functions, we may now begin to expand both episodic and distributive practice, most assuredly to the benefit of our consumers and clients, and therefore to the benefit of nursing as well.

Expanded Roles in Episodic Practice

The fact that nursing education and service have long emphasized the primacy of acute patient care is no guarantee that episodic practice exists in any sort of ideal state. While the secretary's committee observed:

> The role of the nurse in acute care is in many ways more clearly defined than it is in other areas of health care.[21]

They hastened to add:

> The nurse's role in acute care has, by tradition, been somewhat restrictive in many clinical settings, perhaps by virtue of the fact that the physician is recognized as the chief health practitioner in these settings. It should be anticipated that nurses, and head nurses in particular, will become increasingly free of managerial functions. This will provide opportunity for nurses to assume responsibility for the clinical management of patients.[22]

This proposal to better utilize the nurse comes at a most propitious time. In her examination of changing nurse roles in the institutional setting, Brown wrote:

> One of the most conspicuous changes in nursing is the increasing demand for nurses with the specialized technical skills and judgment to provide the continuous and intensive nursing observation and intervention required by post-surgical patients in recovery units, and acutely ill or severely ill surgical and medical patients in a growing variety of intensive-care units.[23]

Thus, the recognition that we must use nurses more productively in episodic practice comes at a time when nursing, itself, has begun intensively to develop those skills and knowledges that will permit the individual practitioner to meet greater challenges and perform at higher and expanded levels of practice.

Perhaps the clearest way to describe the directions in which we must go is to provide three brief case examples of current innovative use of nurse clinicians in the episodic setting.[24] These sketches can only begin to illustrate the role enlargement that must be fostered over the full range of patient care requirements.

> *Case Number 1.* Gwen Marshman is a nurse clinician in the orthopedic service at Strong Memorial Hospital in Rochester, New York.[25] She sees each patient who is admitted on that service at least once. At that first meeting, she may begin preparing the short-term patient for pre-operative exercises, and plan continuing follow up for the long-term patient. Subsequently, she will see patients from twice a day to three times a week.

She is directly involved in the application of large casts and complex tractions and at these times, provides for the emotional support of the patient rather than the technical assistance of the physician. She develops plans for continuing nursing care, and instructs both staff and patients in the management and treatment of the malady.

Her role is viewed as that of a care coordinator, working with house officers and staff nurses, to provide continuity in patient care regimens, and the highest level of treatment consistent with needs. While an outstanding practitioner in her own right, she is involved in planning, teaching, and evaluation of care.

Case Number 2. Cathy Baldy is a nurse clinician in hematology at the Henry Ford Hospital and Clinic in Detroit.[26] Her case load includes patients with leukemia, lymphoma, hemophilia, sickle cell anemia, and multiple myaloma plus general medicine referrals from hematologists and other nurses. At any given time, she will be working with thirty-five to forty acutely ill patients—in the hospital, in outpatient clinics, and in their homes.

She makes rounds with the hematology service, plans patient management, and writes nursing prescriptions that appear on the medical chart of the patient. Her work involves patient care, patient and family teaching (for example, recognition of symptoms of infection and pacing of rest activity), and discharge planning which includes the utilization of community resources available to the patient.

As a nurse clinician, she is expected to provide a role model for the staff nurse, and serve as an instructor for enlarging the skills of students and other nurses in the assessment, planning and management, as well as the provision, of high quality care.

Case Number 3. Joan Templeton is a nurse clinician on the Bothin Burn Unit of St. Francis Memorial Hospital, San Francisco, California.[27] This is a ten-bed intensive care unit.

The nurses perform burn hydrotherapy, apply and change burn dressings, participate in the initial application, and subsequent changes, of heterographs (porcine skin), and collaborate with the physician in assessment of the readiness of tissue for grafting.

As part of the national effort to develop data on burn cases, the nurses also keep extensive research records on patient progress, therapeutic intervention, and other relevant indices.

While serving as a role model, and as a clinical instructor for staff and students in the unit, the clinical nurse also coordinates various activities of ancillary services with the nursing staff in providing physical, occupational, and diversional therapy based on the progress and prognosis of the patient.

In these and many more instances, we find nurses functioning as full partners in an expanded care team, taking responsibility for decision making and care provision in ways that differ significantly from the traditional boundaries of nursing practice.

The Secretary's Committee to Study Extended Roles for Nurses suggests that many nurse practitioners in the acute setting will in the future, customarily:[28]

1. Secure and record a health and developmental history and make a critical evaluation of such records.
2. Perform basic physical and psychological assessments and translate the findings into appropriate nursing action.
3. Discriminate between normal and abnormal findings on physical and psychosocial assessments.
4. Make prospective decisions about treatment in collaboration with physicians.
5. Initiate action and treatments within protocols developed jointly by medical and nursing personnel—such as adjusting medication, ordering and interpreting laboratory tests, and prescribing certain rehabilitative and restorative measures.

If such developments are encouraged through participatory planning and joint decision making by medical and nursing practitioners, then we have the foundation for the development of a whole new era in episodic, or acute, patient care. The first to benefit will be the clients—the patients and their families. But, too, we will have made a significant start on the establishment of a truly satisfying career in nursing practice that alone can solve our perennial problems of manpower shortages, limited utilization of practitioners, and unmet health care needs of our society.

Expanded Roles in Distributive Practice

Just as the clinical nurse in the episodic setting must break away from tradition in order to extend her role, so, too, the clinical nurse in the distributive setting faces restrictions, conventions, and limitations that must be overcome if any true expansion of practice is to occur. As the National Commission has stated:

> Many observers have felt in the past that nurses were miscast when they went into school systems, industrial organizations or even physicians' offices. Seldom, it seemed, were their capacities utilized, nor could the individual practitioner exercise most of the clinical skills with which she had been prepared.[29]

With the growing recognition, however, that health care is a lifetime proposition and that health maintenance and disease prevention are significant portions of the total care system, we see significant departures in the kinds of activities in which nurses engage in the distributive area of care.

To illustrate some of the widespread changes occurring throughout the country, a series of vignettes may serve as indicators.[30] Because of the breadth of concerns and services included in the definition of distributive practice, however, it is impossible to highlight the wide assortment of emerging nurse roles.

> *Clinical Liaison Nurse*. In order to help provide comprehensive, integrated, and uninterrupted care to the long-term patients of Rancho Los Amigos, a new category of practitioner, the Liaison Nurse, was developed.[31]

This person is selected on the basis of advanced study in a clinical specialty combined with the experience of community health practice. Moreover, the individual must have the ability to be comfortable implementing the care ordered by a physician while recognizing and practicing the independent functions of nursing at a high level of expertise.

The Liaison Nurse has no shift assignment, and no restriction on area of activity within the hospital or the community. Her professional function is to follow the patient as needed from service to service, and into the home or residence, to assure a continuity of care and the management of the prescribed regimen.

To carry out this responsibility, the Liaison Nurse is involved in Admission Conference and Care Planning meetings with the staff nurses to develop a sound assessment of patient needs and a plan for nursing care. The Liaison Nurse engages in actual patient treatment, continuing assessment, and progress evaluation. Also, it is expected that this nurse will serve as a clinical role model and instructor for the nurses, occupational and physical therapists, and other members of the care team. Teaching also extends to patient self-care and instruction for family members, friends, or community health workers involved in patient assistance.

Discharge planning is another function of the Liaison Nurse role. This normally entails an inspection of the facilities in which the patient will be housed and the recommendation of needed equipment. Recovery and/or adjustment programs are determined. This is followed, as needed, by visits, telephone conferencing, and continuing clinic liaison to monitor progress and patient condition.

Clinical School Nurse. New problems are emerging within our schools. Misuse of drugs, venereal disease, pregnancy, child abuse, and learning disorders are all conditions that society now perceives to be mounting. In an effort to control them, administrators and classroom teachers have begun to "rediscover" the school nurse. In a pilot program devised by the Denver Public Schools and the University of Colorado Schools of Medicine and Nursing, school nurses are provided four months of intensive advanced work in child care and school health.[32] Emphasis is placed on: physical examination; physical, psychosocial, and personality processes; interviewing techniques; and parent counseling.

Upon completion of the formal theory and clinical practice, the school nurses return and have continuing consultation on routine health evaluations, utilization of referral resources, and the development of a comprehensive well-child care program. In addition to handling minor ailments, the school nurses assess learning problems (such as perceptual difficulty or acquired deformities) and attempt to anticipate children's needs for emotional support, medical treatment, or other therapy.

The instructional component of the school nurses' role has widened immeasurably. The nurses provide inservice education programs for the school faculty, and have increased both student and parental contact for tutorial teaching. Reflecting the quietly dramatic change in emphasis is the decision to add school health aides to the Denver system so that the scheduling, office work, and other administrative tasks, formerly performed by the school nurse, can be accomplished. The nurse, nowadays, is too busy practicing her profession to keep up with the non-nursing components.

Clinical Community Nurse. The Dr. Martin Luther King, Jr. Health Center seeks to provide health care to an entire community of 12,000 families, a total population of perhaps 45,000 people. It emphasizes preventive care and health maintenance, using ambulatory care in clinic and home whenever possible. Acute care, in-patient facilities are available, of course, on need.

The heart of the center operation lies in the development of eight Primary Health Care Teams designed to serve a broad range of client health needs.[33] Each team serves approximately 1500 families, and consists of two public health nurses, six family health workers, one internist, and one pediatrician. Moreover, each team has ready access to: a full-time dentist; a part-time psychiatrist; a midwife; a health advocate (an individual trained by lawyers, educators, and community organizers to serve as an ombudsman); and the many specialty services and clinics at Montefiore Hospital.

Within the team, the physicians emphasize curative treatment, the nurses concentrate on health maintenance and disease prevention, and the family health worker is involved with the social health issues such as welfare payments, school dropouts, housing adequacy, etc. The team meets weekly for an extended lunch to discuss problems, initiate planning, and expand the cooperative aspects of the work.

Each of the nurse practitioners is viewed as the team coordinator for care and treatment of 750 families. In this capacity she formulates family care plans, performs routine care, and makes necessary referrals. She supervises the work of three family health workers, interacts closely with the physician team members, and has contact with the back-up health practitioners.

It is in her own clinical role that the nurse coordinator has found tremendous pressure for enlargement. In the beginning, the nurse was expected to concentrate on well baby and maternal care. The needs of the families soon established that this was far too narrow an approach. Reflecting the impoverishment of the community in terms of health care, there were demands for chronic disease maintenance, treatment of emotional problems, routine child and adult preventive care and assessment, crisis management, pre- and post-maternal care, a myriad of therapeutic services. It was clear that the nurse coordinator had to become a broadly competent primary care practitioner serving as a generalist and the decision coordinator for the entire system.

A resounding theme in these developments is that the clinical nurse practitioner, supported by professional colleagues and varied care facilities, can vastly expand and deepen our health care system's impact. In rural areas and urban ghettos, in school and industry, in extended care or preventive screening facilities, the new model of the nurse clinician is our best hope for providing the quantity and quality of care that our people require. And most importantly, the nurse is equipped to ensure that care is dispensed with dignity, humanity, and concern.

Toward New Care Dimensions

While there is certainly some general core of knowledge and experience that all nurses should command, it is increasingly evident that scientific advances, clinical knowledge, and the variety of patient needs and environmental settings will combine to demand differentiation and increased specialization in nursing practice. Throughout the implementation phase, the National Commission has endeavored to emphasize that one of its priorities is to see the reestablishment of nursing practice as the first and proper end of that profession. In doing so, we have necessarily sought to "stimulate nursing, the other health professions, and the consumer public to the possibilities of enlarged emphasis on distributive care." This, however, must be seen in the context that nursing, and society, have frequently seen all non-episodic care as an appendage or sideshow to the true practice of the profession.

It is not only essential that we obtain nurse practitioners for "wellness" and "illness", but also critical that we encourage the thrust of nurse clinicians toward extended roles in both episodic and distributive care. *An Abstract for Action,* the report of the secretary's committee, and Esther Lucile Brown's study of changed practice in both institutional and community settings, all concur in both the reality of extended roles and their necessity. We shall know that we have reached our common goal when, in the words of the National Commission:

> . . . nursing patterns . . . are so organized that recognition, reward, and increased responsibility . . . are based on increasing depth of knowledge and demonstrated competence to perform in complex clinical situations.[34]

In short, we need more nurse clinicians in both episodic and distributive settings who can perform in extended role functions as partners and colleagues of physicians and other health workers. From these practitioners, ultimately, will come the solution to our health delivery problems hastened by the advice and recommendations of our joint practice committees at national, state, and local levels.

PERSONAL AND PROFESSIONAL GROWTH THROUGH PRACTICE

The fourth priority of the National Commission in terms of the implementation of its recommendations in the area of nursing roles and functions revolves around the reexamination of traditional utilization patterns in nursing service so as to increase the involvement of nurses in direct patient care throughout all kinds of settings and facilities.

It is not satisfactory to plan for enlarged practice roles, or to extend the scope of nursing practice into new dimensions, if at the same time, we do not take additional steps to:

1. Reduce the non-nursing functions of the individual practitioner commensurate with enlarged practice demands.
2. Develop a rational career pattern that emphasizes growth and continuation of practitioner commitment.
3. Reorganize our institutional systems in such ways as to foster and encourage expanded practice roles.

One of the first surprises that a person encounters in examining the utilization patterns in nursing is that the more experience and qualifications a nurse might possess, the less likely it is that she or he is going to be directly involved in patient care. The grouped results of numerous studies on nursing practice are displayed in Figure 4-6.

Our present general patterns of nurse utilization—at least within the institutional setting—mean that staff nurses frequently spend less time in direct patient care than licensed practical nurses, aides, orderlies, or even student nurses. Because the outstanding staff nurses are subject to promotion to head nurse, then to supervisor, we can see that our conventional wisdom tends to direct our best practitioners away from the patient while encouraging care to be provided by those less qualified and prepared.

While the beginning nurse practitioner may have tremendous interest and dedication to patient care, the system soon begins to exert its conditioning influences. Recently, Treat and Kramer reported the results of a study involving nursing service in both hospital and public health settings.[35] They analyzed questions asked by and of practitioners and sought to determine whether there were differences in the patterns of staff nurses and supervisors. The results are shown in Figure 4-7.

While the nurses' questions range over the three areas of patient care, personnel, and systems maintenance, with a variation from 30 to 38 percent, the supervisors' questions are predominantly weighted, three to one, in terms of systems maintenance over patient care. This, of course, is a documented example of common phenomena that beginning nurse practitioners experience in the work situation.

If this circumstance only impinged upon the nurse, it would be difficult enough to ignore. But the constant pressure to "nurse the system" before the patient, has predictable results on the quality of care. The fact, as Anderson observes, "that nursing was shaped . . . as an arm of administration rather than a clinical department . . ."[36] inevitably has taken its toll. It reaches its conclusion in comments such as those by Duff and Hollingshead: "The registered nurse . . . knew

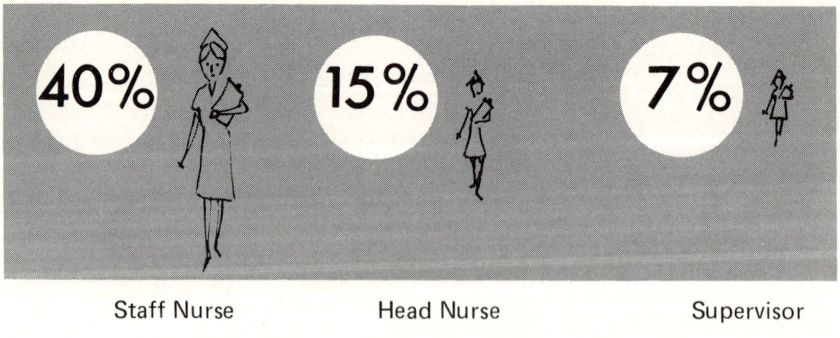

Figure 4-6. Percentage of time devoted to patient care by various nursing levels.

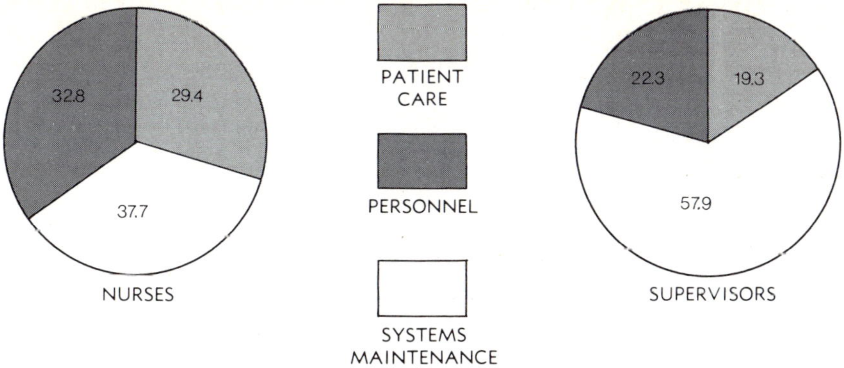

Figure 4-7. Comparison of question categories employed by nurses and their supervisors.

comparatively little about the medical problems of patients and almost nothing about their personal problems. . . . Under these conditions, the patient and nurse could not develop a problem-solving relationship."[37]

To combat the present system of promotion, which inexorably draws the qualified practitioner away from the patient or client, the National Commission has examined, encouraged, and promulgated the development of new models for nursing care that embody the potential for personal and professional growth through practice and nurse-patient involvement. One conceptual model, equally adaptable to both episodic and distributive practice, is shown in Figure 4-8.[38]

The staff nurse, through educational preparation and guided clinical experiences, would begin to function as a care provider, with limited skills in patient data collection, in assessment, and in preparing, executing, and evaluating patient care plans. With the assistance of a clinical nurse who would function as care team leader, and with the consultant aid of a master nurse clinician who is an outstanding practitioner, the staff nurse would grow in knowledge and experience in all aspects of the nursing role.

The clinical nurse would evolve from the ranks of the staff nurse. Through in-service and continuing education, deepened clinical experience, and the preceptorial guidance of the master nurse clinician, those individual nurses who demonstrate capacity both for outstanding practice and clinical leadership of a nursing team would be elevated to the position of clinical nurse.

With continuing experience and, likely, with advanced, formalized educational preparation, the clinical nurse would qualify as the master clinician. As such, she would have to maintain excellence in practice, serve as an outstanding role model, and participate in the tutorial and experiential development of the less-qualified, less-experienced nurse practitioners.

In such a conceptual scheme for professional development, the nurse grows

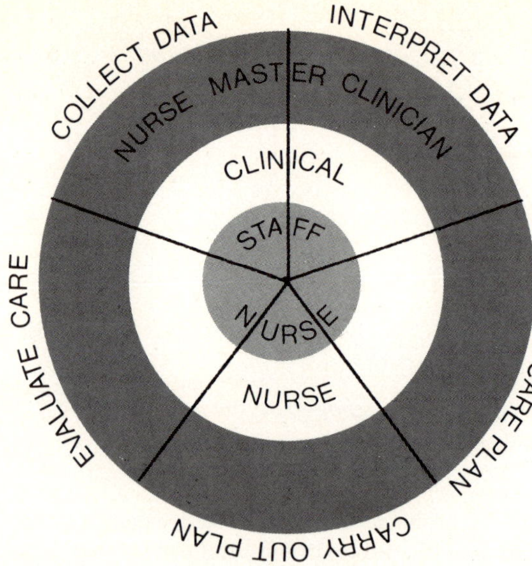

Figure 4-8. Professional development model for nursing practice.

around rather than *away from* client care. The system serves to expand and deepen the knowledge of the practitioner, and to call upon the nurse to evidence increasing ability at assessment, diagnosis, patient management, intervention, and evaluation.

There is a natural and rational progression from one level to another based on demonstrated excellence in clinical nursing performance. Rather than compelling one to become less involved in practice, promotion would provide an opportunity for greater professional challenge, accomplishment, and recognition.

Is such a concept truly possible? Can we implement such a plan for career development and enlargement? The National Commission has, over the period of the implementation phase, continued to examine and publicize documentary evidence that such approaches not only can, but do work.

> *Good Samaritan Hospital, Phoenix, Arizona.*[39] In late 1967, the decision was made to restructure the nursing service so as to make the nurse personally responsible for the quality of patient care. In order to carry out this determination, basic changes were required in terms of both nursing roles and the functions of related health occupations.
>
> Perhaps the most obvious shifts in terms of nursing practice were related to the restructuring of traditional levels and functions of nursing service. At the staff nurse level, clinical teams were organized under the leadership of experienced professional nurses. The team leaders were assigned patients, and the patient could identify and relate to "his" nurse. The team leaders obtained histories, developed care plans, and wrote nursing orders for the direction of the nurse team members. These individuals, in turn, carried out the plan, and assisted in evaluation. Specific procedures and treatments

were discussed with the patient and modified, if necessary, to ensure his understanding and cooperation. The staff nurses were encouraged to utilize each other as consultants while the team leaders made assignments in terms of patient requirements and an individual nurse's ability to perform care practices. The team leaders write progress notes, change orders as needed, and continuously review care plans.

At the next level of expertise, the one consistent with the model category of "clinical nurse," Good Samaritan replaced the traditional Head Nurse with nursing coordinators whose responsibilities are continuous (they do not work shift assignments, for example, but are on 24 hour call) and patient care centered. Their role is multifaceted, but devoid of the non-nursing functions that weigh so heavily on the head nurse in the customary setting. The nurse coordinator is responsible for the actual, direct practice of nursing care, and she is also the manager of the care provided by the nursing teams in her area of responsibility. She serves as a consultant to team leaders and to other coordinators, and has responsibility for teaching aspects of assessment, planning, execution, and evaluation of care.

At the level we have designated "master clinician," Good Samaritan appointed seven clinical supervisors, each responsible for several episodic nursing care units. These individuals differ significantly from the traditional behavior of the supervisory nurse. They are patient care oriented, and provide a role model for the entire nursing service in terms of knowledge and care provision. They are the clinical leaders who set the tone for qualitative advancement in nursing roles, and assume responsibility for overall direction of practice in the acute setting.

At all levels, entry requirements, formal educational expectations, and demonstrated competence are being developed and scrutinized so that the nurses can look toward a rational and planned career perspective centered on the enhancement of patient care. Authority is increased, responsibility is defined and accepted, and the entire thrust of nursing service has been redirected.

Other departments than nursing had to reexamine their functions and commitments. One of the major changes enacted in Good Samaritan was that support departments throughout the hospital were required to plan round-the-clock, seven-day-a-week provision of services in any way they desired *except by using nursing personnel and time.* This decision alone relieved nurses of a considerable portion of the "non-nursing" functions that have been traditionally performed by the service to the diminution of patient practice.

In addition, ward clerks and unit managers worked with the clinical supervisors to set up procedures and systems to relieve the team leaders and staff nurses of various housekeeping and maintenance tasks, as well as secretarial functions. The unit managers now assume responsibility for training ward clerks and for the *management of the units* twenty-four hours a day—leaving the nurse staff to manage patients full time.

Veterans Administration Hospital, Northport, Long Island.[40] In 1969, the VAH at Northport undertook an extensive revision of organization and functions in order to establish what it termed Nurse Administrator Units to provide for the treatment and care of patients.

The patients in these units are generally older individuals who are suffering from acute and chronic health problems. Their illnesses include psychiatric, medical, and surgical problems. For the most part, they have received maximum benefit from prior continuous treatment by the medical staff.

While the nursing service is not as differentiated as the model proposes, with staff and clinical nurses not firmly delineated, the assigned duties and responsibilities of the Nurse Administrator clearly are those associated with the concept of the nurse master clinician rather than those of supervisory nurse or director of service in the traditional institutional setting. For example, the Nurse Administrator is empowered to:

- Plan, implement, and evaluate the total care and treatment program of a group of patients.
- Function as the primary care provider for the group.
- Take initial and subsequent medical history of the patient.
- Order appropriate laboratory tests, x-rays, EKG, and other procedures on patients.
- Conduct daily rounds, observe and record observation about patient progress.
- Initiate, continue, or modify the patients' treatment regimens within published station policies.
- Within limits of station policy, order and adjust patients' medications on the basis of clinical observations, results of tests, etc.
- Discriminate between normal and abnormal findings on physical and psychosocial assessments.
- Make prospective decisions about treatment in collaboration with physicians.
- Initiate actions and treatments within protocols developed jointly by medical and nursing personnel—such as adjusting medication, ordering and interpreting laboratory tests, and prescribing certain rehabilitative and restorative measures.

Out of related planning, there emerged the concept of satellite clinics to be located in the community apart from the treatment center at the hospital. These clinics are under the direction of a clinical nurse practitioner, and are designed to provide therapeutic, social, and recreational programs for the veterans to assist them in reentering their community. Specifically, the clinics deal with the mental health problems of former clients while using referrals to the hospital for medical needs.

A single clinical nurse administrator (master clinician) floats among the seven satellite clinics, being directly responsible for the overall psychosocial program in the operation. To ensure, however, that there is still direct client involvement for all nursing staff, this nurse administrator spends approximately one-quarter time in patient examination, interviews, and therapy.

To provide for needed collaboration, each clinic has a physician on site for approximately three hours each week to see referrals and to prescribe drug changes. At the beginning of the program there were many hospital referrals from the clinic nurses due to client neglect of health regimens, but these have been markedly reduced. The reduction of neuro-psychological referrals has been even more significant through the institution of the localized therapy centers.

Role functions of the clinical nurses are quite varied, and include:

group therapy, individual therapy, crisis intervention, home visits, continuous evaluation and screening, and joint planning with the physicians.

Related to changes in individual roles and nursing service organization, however, must also come a basic reexamination of our health care facilities, their organization and structure. In order for professional nursing to extend its care features, it must have better understanding of, and greater participation in, the decisions which determine how care will be delivered and by whom. When we wish nursing to be a "clinical department" rather than "an arm of administration," then we must involve it in the decision making and planning for care.

Evanston Hospital in Illinois.[41] At this hospital, a pioneer attempt was made to develop a triad system which brought together in problem-solving committees the three essential determiners of care procedures (see Figure 4-9). At the patient care level, there were eight triads comprised of: a nursing coordinator, responsible to the Chairman of the Department of Nursing; an attending physician, responsible to the Chairman of Medicine, Surgery, or Obstetrics-Gynecology; and an administrator, Director of Patient Care Administration, responsible to the Vice President of Health Care Services. The triads met regularly to discuss patient care, to formulate joint plans for service and support, and to attack problems as they arose.

Within the care unit, the nursing staff closely paralleled the model proposed earlier. Most nurses were hired at the staff level, and after some six months of experience and in-service education, might move to the clinical nurse level. This second level was subdivided, and after a period of another six to twelve months, the clinical nurse might be appointed a senior nurse clinician. The nurse coordinator was to function as a role model and as an actual practitioner—roughly equivalent to the level designated as master clinician in the proposed career model.

At the management level of the hospital, an Advisory Council recapitulated the joint nature of the care committees. The council consisted of the Chairmen of Medicine, Surgery, Obstetrics and Gynecology, and Nursing, and the Executive Vice President of the Hospital.

In 1967, a study was made on the effects of such organizational restructuring in the orthopedic unit. Joint planning by the triad members resulted in a deliberate effort to increase the patient care aspects of the nursing role while non-nursing functions were assumed by a secretary and a unit administrator. The results are most interesting. Direct care provided by the head nurses jumped from less than 19 percent of their time to more than 33 percent. Time involved in patient care for all R.N.s increased from 28 to 43 percent of their time. Since the nurses were still attempting to examine roles, there still was a large percentage of time yet to be recovered. It was found, however, even in this preliminary period that duties adjudged to be inappropriate for nurses decreased from 15 to 9 percent even as patient care time increased. Idle time for nursing personnel dropped from 7 to 4 percent; Idle time for the ward secretary dropped from 14 to less than 1 percent. These figures surely indicate that the reorganization was beginning to move the system in the desired directions.

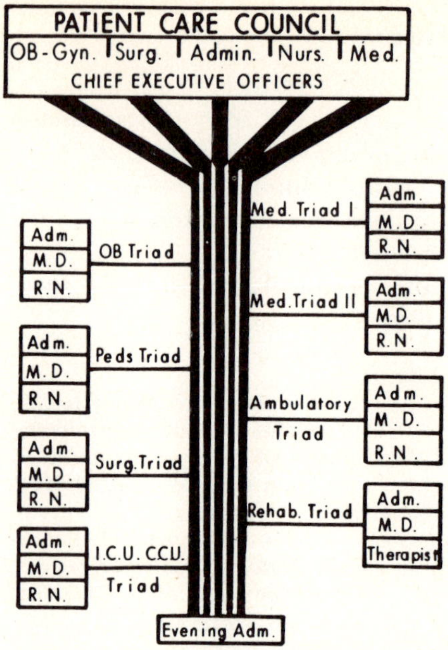

Figure 4-9. Extract from the Evanston Hospital organization chart.

Throughout the implementation phase, the National Commission has urged nursing, medicine, and health management to work in concert so that, "*Personnel policies in all health care facilities differentiate levels of responsibility in accord with the concepts of staff nurse, clinical nurse, and master nurse clinician . . . promotion should be based on demonstrated clinical competence . . . and non-nursing functions should be adequately and appropriately staffed.*"[42] With the help of the joint practice committees and the increased experimentation among health care facilities and maintenance organizations, the next few years should see progressive change toward extending the nurse practice role.

For too long, many of our health care institutions have pursued a policy of containment. We have attempted to add functions, occupational groups, and new services to our old skeletal frames without truly examining either the effectiveness of the basic structure or the impact of the additions. The National Commission emphasizes that, "*Planning, by definition, should be a projection, not a recapitulation. It is essential that planning facilitate change and improvement rather than serve as a report on the status quo.*" It is critical that structures and policies be examined in light of what nursing practice is becoming and ought to be. To ensure this, the Commission feels that nurses must " *. . . be appointed to, and hold full membership in, groups involved in health planning.*" Progress has been made over the past several years, but there is still much to do—and time becomes an ever more critical factor.

EXTENDING THE KNOWLEDGE BASE OF NURSING

While considerable progress has taken place in revitalizing the nursing commitment to excellence in practice, there must be a clear recognition that the final limitation to its extension, and its quality, lies in the body of knowledge by which it is guided. Underlying all the other recommendations made by the National Commission in the area of nursing roles and functions is this statement:

> The federal Division of Nursing, the National Center for Health Services Research and Development, other government agencies, and private foundations appropriate grant funds or research contracts to investigate the impact of nursing practice on the quality, effectiveness, and economy of care.[43]

Lack of research leaves us without a secure set of facts—or even perhaps a strong set of probabilities—to guide and assess the nursing care of a patient. In many situations, the clinical practice of nursing still consists largely of stereotyped techniques liberally sprinkled with personal idiosyncrasy. What a nurse does, and when, is frequently determined as much by the pressures in the external setting than by clear knowledge of resultant benefits to the patient. Without valid means for assessing differential care, it is almost impossible to define optimum practice.

In this respect, nursing faces the same challenges that confront all other professions. In 1900, for example, medical historians tell us that perhaps one out of every five cases presented to a physician was likely to be treated with procedures based on scientific knowledge. Eighty percent of the patients were approached through a combination of judgment, concern, and supportive care. Today, less than three-quarters of a century since American medicine began its impressive commitment to research, it is almost impossible to imagine the way things were.

Nursing stands today in much the same stance that medicine occupied earlier. It is still more an art than a science. Yet its best clinicians have already demonstrated that art is no longer sufficient, that patient care increasingly demands knowledge that can only come from scientific inquiry. At the same time, the aim of research should be to elevate the practice of nursing—not art *or* science, but art *and* science are needed to ensure the highest levels of humane and capable care.

What Research in Nursing Has Shown

No one would expect that scientific inquiry into nursing could duplicate the feat of medicine in creating a veritable knowledge explosion, but there are already strong indicators that increased investigation into nursing practice means significant contributions to the improvement of patient care.

- Separate studies at Cornell-New York and Kansas University document the effectiveness of expanded nursing care for the chronically ill ambulatory patient. Greater continuity of care, increased return to employment, and enhanced social adjustment were found to accompany the changed clinical nurse role.[44]

- Controlled study of survival and recovery rates in intensive cardiac care clearly shows that specially qualified nurse practitioners can be elemental in saving lives and preventing death.[45]
- An investigation of developmental behavior in premature infants provided a solid base for changing care procedures for nursing practice and enhanced the progressive development of the children.[46]
- Preliminary findings indicate that environmental stimuli (colors, noise, textures, odors) can be of vital importance in the nursing care of geriatric patients and their ensuing ability to cope with the activities of daily living.[47]

These are simply examples of the breadth of nursing inquiry. At the present time, nursing research is being pressed into many other areas including: family planning; evaluation of quality and conditions of delivery of nursing care in urban hospitals; bowel and bladder training for incontinent patients; therapeutic exercise for the stroke recovery patient; continuing care for children with *spina bifida;* and the long-term help of the diabetic patient.

From these efforts, and others, we shall learn how to improve the practice of nursing and, just as importantly, we may learn when our present or suggested interventions are not conducive to patient improvement. Even the negative findings are important since they can frequently point the way toward other, more salutary approaches.

Despite the measurable success of some of these beginnings, it is nevertheless true that their impact is still slight, and that we need to attain a far greater level of activity before we can begin to make substantial gains in terms of knowledge increments.

Support for Nursing Research

Clearly, one of the primary reasons for the slow growth of research into nursing practice lies in the lack of financial and institutional support of its study activities.

In 1950, the federal government's *total* expenditure for all nursing activities was $250,000. This figure climbed sharply over subsequent years, but most of the funds have been directed to construction grants, student loans, and traineeships.

In fiscal 1969 and 1970, the Division of Nursing of the Public Health Service received $3.8 millions per year broadly designated for research. On examination, however, this amount was intended to serve not only for support of actual investigations, but the training of researchers, the assisting of advanced graduate students, and the funding of other related activities. As an example of the effect, the Research Grants Branch of the Division of Nursing has received an average of only 54 grant applications per year between the fiscal years 1964-1970 and only 49 percent of these have been approved.

As a comparative benchmark, the federal government in fiscal 1969 and 1970 appropriated more than $350 millions *per annum* to medical research with additional sums for the teaching and training functions that might be related to these research activities.

Perhaps another illustration might serve to underline the problem. At the highest point of federal expenditure to support nursing research, our appropriations approximated $5 per year per active licensed professional nurse in these United States. As an investment in the long-term contribution of our nation's largest health practicing profession, this seems to be far below actual need.

Nursing research has generally found state and private support as difficult to obtain as federal moneys. Fewer than ten of the one hundred largest private foundations, for example, support nursing research on any form of regular or systematic basis. Very few states provide funds for research or related support in the appropriations they make toward nursing education.

Obviously, the first concomitant to the expansion of the corpus of nursing knowledge is for the profession to assume this responsibility and to support and encourage research themselves. This nursing has done to an extent through such means as the establishment and perpetuation of the American Nurses' Foundation, an organization designed to "conduct, support, and promote nursing research and disseminate research findings."[48] The ANF is supported by a dues contribution from members of the American Nurses' Association, contributions from individuals, and funds from business, industry, or other foundations.

In *An Abstract for Action*, the National Commission recommended that the federal government allocate $4 million to the support of nursing research in the next fiscal period, and that an additional $18 million be provided for the advanced training of graduate students and researchers, as well as related activities. This was a modest and seemingly realistic appraisal, not only of need, but of nursing's ability to "gear up" in order to use these funds wisely and well. The amounts suggested were more than those proposed by the administration and less than those authorized by Congress—and less than the American Nurses' Association would have liked the Commission to specify.[49]

The final appropriation for 1972 was $3.8 millions. The administration request for fiscal year 1973 was for $4.1 millions directed at nursing research grants and contracts, and that was the amount included by Congress in the two bills vetoed by the President in 1972. Thus, the Congress and the administration were both planning in terms close to the National Commission's proposals. In the request for fiscal year 1974, however, the administration has made *no* provision in its budget for support of nursing research.

At this point in time, no one can predict what the final appropriations will be. There would appear to be a number of actions, however, that should be taken in anticipation of the President's statements on budgetary requests. Nursing, through its organizations at the national and state levels, should attempt to gain relief in the form of transitional federal aid for the continuation of ongoing research and the progressive beginning of new efforts. At the same time, nursing must make every effort through state planning and joint practice committees, and through interdisciplinary informational activities to see that the funds provided through revenue sharing to the states do, indeed, go into the support of activities so vital to enhanced patient care and improved health delivery systems.

The National Commission has already provided the Congress and the administration with its fiscal estimates and has made available, at their request, additional materials which explain and expand upon many of the aspects of nursing practice, education, and research. The Commission will continue to support the need for, and the desirability of, increased support of nursing research through public funding. Whether this be done by federal or state agencies is less important than the accomplishment, but nursing and all our health agencies must weigh the short and long-term implications of the proposed adjustments.

Aside from the concerns over federal funding, the Commission staff in February, 1972 contacted approximately 140 foundations known to be interested in the health and welfare fields. These foundations were provided a pamphlet prepared by the Commission on the need for research into nursing practice,[50] as well as a two-page cover letter which asked for their increased consideration to any future requests for the support of investigations related to nursing practice and patient care. More than 85 of the foundations replied, and some indicated that they might in the future consider the possibility of support. The general tone of reaction is indicative, however, that much more needs to be done in terms of informing the public and the private sectors of our society about the worthwhileness of investigations into nursing practice.

Related to the Commission's recommendation on funding for research was the proposal that federal, state, and private funds be made available for:

> . . . a national clearinghouse for the collection and dissemination of information about research and innovations in nursing.[51]

Both the American Nurses' Foundation and the American Nurses' Association have developed proposals related to this recommendation. The ANF seeks to establish a clearinghouse; the ANA is asking support to develop a compilation and inventory of nursing research which could provide the nuclear data bank for such a clearinghouse.

By any standard of measurement, nursing research has many grave problems facing it in the years immediately ahead. Only through continuing and intensified efforts can we begin to catch up on the unfinished agenda that we now possess; and we must find new and better approaches to support that which should be done in the future.

OTHER RECOMMENDATIONS ON ROLES AND FUNCTIONS

Through the impact of the National Commission's efforts to achieve their priority goals, it was expected that those other aspects of the proposals for nursing roles and functions might be attained. A systematic look at progress on each of the seventeen recommendations is provided in Appendix B.

Perhaps one recommendation to be singled out is that which proposes the bringing together of nursing education and service through such activities as:

> *a*. Nurse practitioners and clinical directors of nursing service receiving significant appointments to (or relevant association with) institutions for nursing education; and
>
> *b*. Nursing faculty in institutions for nursing education be given responsibility for providing or organizing significant elements of care.

This concept was, of course, based on the growing number of institutions such as Case Western Reserve, Rochester, Vanderbilt, and others which encourage joint appointments and increased communications between nursing education and service. To some extent, this idea had been viewed by the Commission as being noncontroversial. It was with some surprise, then, that they received word that the Council of Diploma Schools of the NLN had voted its nonsupport of the recommendation.[52]

Perhaps a clue to this action might be found in the report of the NLN Task Force which reacted in these words:

> The Committee members believed that the education and service sectors must work more collaboratively, but they expressed deep concern about the concept of dual appointments for high administrative positions . . . If the Commission is indeed recommending *dual appointments*, the Committee could support this only at middle and lower levels. . . .[53]

The Commission is, of course, primarily concerned about bringing service and education together in nursing; it will remain for experience and evaluation to determine the limits, if any, to the organizational levels at which this should proceed.

SUMMARY

The National Commission proposed seventeen specific recommendations in the area of nursing roles and functions. Four areas, which embodied most of the specific recommendations were particularly emphasized as priorities while a fifth, the area related to research support, was given continuing, if less intensive, attention.

The first area was that of the establishment of the National Joint Practice Commission. While the NLN task force, and others, indicated their preference for including health administrators as well as licensed practical nurses on the NJPC from the beginning, it was the considered opinion of the National Commission and its advisory groups that it was necessary to begin, first, with the nurse and the physician and build from there, bringing others into the developmental work of the task forces which would be established to address particular problems and projects.

Out of greater wisdom and experience, the NJPC itself could later determine changes in membership. The National Joint Practice Commission is now established, enjoys the support of the AMA and the ANA and is presently entering a phase of increased organizational activity following its initial structural efforts.

The second area was that of the statewide joint practice committees. At the present time, more than half of the states have initiated such committees or reorganized existing liaison groups which conform to the characteristics of the NJPC. Progress has already been achieved in a number of states, particularly the designated target states, toward changes in nurse-physician roles and in state practice acts.

The third area involved the publication and encouragement of consideration by nursing, and significant others, of a new formulation of the nursing role. Through the development of episodic and distributive concentrations, practice can be extended over the full range of consumer needs for health care. Throughout the implementation phase, the National Commission and its staff sought to involve nursing service and education in the contemplation both of needs and of opportunities that lie in this area. The terms, themselves, seemed to bother many individuals and groups. Yet, in the opinion of the National Commission, it was necessary to construct a new terminology for practice apart from the traditional terms with all their familiar connotations and perceptual images. Other commentators have expressed the same concerns, and recently, terms used by the National Commission, such as *episodic* and *distributive* are coming into increasing currency. Apart from the words, however, a greater number of care institutions are beginning to study the interactive model of nursing practice and to consider client care in the light of its formulations.

The fourth area concerns an expanded pattern for nursing careers anchored in practice. Here, the Commission and its staff sought to inform nursing and the public of the dynamic changes that are occurring in both individual and group nursing roles. To the extent possible, the Commission has recommended and supported developmental processes that encourage nurses to stay in practice while eschewing non-nursing functions. Likewise the Commission has publicized and encouraged experimental approaches to organization and structure which emphasize the use of nurses for patient care and not as administrative extensions.

The fifth area, and certainly the most problematic at this point, is the concern for nursing research—its adequate support, and its expansion. At present, there is, simply, insufficient public or private funding for this vital activity, and the prospects for the short term are far from bright. In all likelihood, the innovative practices in role functioning and interdisciplinary care will enhance the prospects of increased aid for nursing research, but one would have to be sanguine indeed to feel that this could occur in the next two or three years. Undoubtedly, this area is one that must be taken up by others—not only nurses, but all those who share concern for a better health care system in this nation.

Of the seventeen recommendations in the field of nursing roles and functions, the NLN task force, in the only published organizational review of the Commission's work, endorsed nine as stated, six with some modification such as the suggestion to add other groups to the National Joint Practice Commission, and two with some indication of concern over the specific interpretation of the recommendation. Only the Council of Diploma Programs of the NLN indicated formal nonsupport or rejection of any of the recommendations. They voiced their opposition to four specific proposals—three were ones having to do with episodic and distributive care; the other involved joint appointment of individuals to nursing service and education. Among the many other organizations and associations involved, there was general concurrence and, in many cases, overt endorsement of the recommendations.

Much, of course, remains to be done in implementing recommendations in the area of roles and functions, but a great deal of work has been initiated and is underway. With continuing growth and activity, we can anticipate significant changes in the future practice of nursing.

FOOTNOTES

1. Garfield, Sidney R. "The Delivery of Medical Care." *Scientific American.* 222:4:15-23 (April) 1970.
2. "Extending the Scope of Nursing Practice." A Report of the Secretary's Committee to Study Extended Roles for Nurses. Washington, D.C.: U.S. Department of Health, Education, and Welfare. November, 1971. pp. vi-vii.
3. See, for example, "A Joint Statement of the American Nurses' Association, Division on Maternal and Child Health Nursing Practice and the American Academy of Pediatrics, Guidelines on Short-Term Continuing Education Programs for Pediatric Nurse Associates," January, 1971. Also, see "The American College of Obstetricians and Gynecologists and the Nurses Association of the American College of Obstetricians and Gynecologists, and the American College of Nurse-Midwives Joint Statement on Maternity care," January, 1971.
4. As one example, "An Act Relating to the Practice of Nursing; Amending Section 54-1413, Idaho Code, by Authorizing a Professional Nurse to Perform Acts Recognized as Appropriate According to the Rules and Regulations Promulgated by the Idaho State Board of Medicine and the Idaho Board of Nursing." March, 1971.
5. The National Commission for the Study of Nursing and Nursing Education. *An Abstract for Action.* Jerome P. Lysaught, Director. New York: McGraw-Hill Book Company, 1970, p. 89.
6. Memorandum from Jerome P. Lysaught, Director, NCSNNE, to members of ANA Congress for Nursing Practice and AMA Committee on Nursing entitled, "Notes on August 4, 1971 Joint Meeting with Summary of Agreements Reached," dated August 11, 1971.
7. "The National Joint Practice Commission: New Bottles, New Wine." Rochester, New York: The National Commission for the Study of Nursing and Nursing Education, 1972 (pamphlet).
8. "A Guide for Establishing Statewide Joint Practice Commissions." Rochester, New York: The National Commission for the Study of Nursing and Nursing Education, 1970 (pamphlet).
9. Memorandum from Robert A. Hoekelman, Chairman, and Shirley A. Smoyak, Vice Chairman, NJPC, to State Joint Practice Committees, Medical Societies, and Nurses' Associations, dated August 3, 1972.
10. "The Graduate Education of Physicians." The Report of the Citizens Commission on Graduate Medical Education. Chicago: The American Medical Association, 1966, p. 86.
11. Lysaught, Jerome P. "Distributive Health Care Needs and the Occupational Health Nurse." *Occupational Health Nursing.* 20:11:8-9 (November) 1972.
12. Data displayed in Figure 3 are obtained from *Statistical Abstract of the United States, 1970* and *Facts About Nursing, 1970-71.* All figures are rounded for simplicity.

13. The National Commission for the Study of Nursing and Nursing Education. *An Abstract for Action,* op. cit., pp. 91-92.
14. "Extending the Scope of Nursing Practice," op. cit., pp. 11-12.
15. Helmer, Joy. "Letters." *American Journal of Nursing.* 71:10:1922-23 (October) 1971.
16. The National Commission for the Study of Nursing and Nursing Education. *An Abstract for Action,* op. cit., pp. 64-69.
17. "Extending the Scope of Nursing Practice," op. cit., p v.
18. ibid.
19. Brown, Esther L. *Nursing Reconsidered: A Study of Change, Part I. The Professional Role in Institutional Nursing.* Philadelphia: J. B. Lippincott Co., 1970, p. 1.
20. "Trends in European Nursing Services." Report on a Working Group. World Health Organization, Regional Office for Europe. December, 1970, p i.
21. "Extending the Scope of Nursing Practice," op. cit., p. 16.
22. ibid.
23. Brown, Esther L., op. cit., p. 1.
24. See "Episodic Nursing Practice: Refinement and Expansion of the Roles." Rochester, New York: The National Commission for the Study of Nursing and Nursing Education, 1971 (Pamphlet).
25. Personal interview, March 2, 1971, between Gwen Marshman, R.N., and NCSNNE staff at Strong Memorial Hospital, Rochester, New York.
26. Personal interview, November 18, 1971, between Catherine Baldy, R.N., and NCSNNE staff at Henry Ford Hospital, Detroit, Michigan.
27. Personal interview, December 3, 1971, between Joan Templeton, R.N., and NCSNNE staff at St. Francis Memorial Hospital, San Francisco, California.
28. "Extending the Scope of Nursing Practice," op. cit., pp. 17-18.
29. "Distributive Nursing Practice: Development and Fusion of the Roles." Rochester, New York: The National Commission for the Study of Nursing and Nursing Education, 1971, p. 11. (Pamphlet).
30. ibid., *passim.*
31. David, Janis H. "Liaison Nurse." *American Journal of Nursing.* 69:9:2142 (September) 1969. Information and interpretation was also provided by site visit and interview by NCSNNE staff, October 20, 1969.
32. Rosner, Aria C. "The School Nurse Practitioner—A New Concept in School Health." October, 1971. (mimeo). See also: Flebbe, Ruth. "The School Nurse Practitioner—A New Approach to the Delivery of Health Care to Children." *School Nurse Practitioner Newsletter.* January, 1972, No. 2.
33. *The Dr. Martin Luther King Jr. Health Center Fourth Annual Report.* January-December, 1970. See especially pp. 1-78.
34. The National Commission for the Study of Nursing and Nursing Education. *An Abstract for Action,* op. cit., p. 92.
35. Treat, Margaret and Marlene Kramer. "The Question Behind the Question." *The Journal of Nursing Administration.* 2:1:20-27 (January-February) 1972.
36. Anderson, Odin W. *Toward an Unambiguous Profession? A Review of Nursing.* Chicago: University of Chicago Center for Health Administration, Pamphlet A6, 1968, p. 8.
37. Duff, R. S. and A. B. Hollingshead. *Sickness and Society.* New York: Harper and Row, 1968, p. 374.
38. The nursing practice model is adapted from: Hoekelman, Robert A. and Harriet Kitzman. "Introduction to the Pediatric Nurse Practitioner Training Program at the University of Rochester School of Medicine and Dentistry." February, 1972 (mimeo).
39. Gabrielson, Rosamond C. "New Approaches for Nursing Service." *New York State Nurse.* 41:4:46 (August-September) 1969.
40. Personal communications, April 10, 1972, with Barbara Eckert, R.N., and May 11, 1971, with Marguerite Burt, R. N., Chief Nurse, together with NCSNNE staff visit, VAH Northport, April 21, 1971.
41. NCSNNE staff visit and interviews, Evanston Hospital, June 5, 1969.
42. The National Commission for the Study of Nursing and Nursing Education. *An Abstract for Action,* op. cit., pp. 130-136.
43. ibid., p. 156.
44. Wang, Mamie K. "A Health Maintenance Service for Chronically Ill Patients." *American Journal of Public Health.* 60:4:713-721 (April) 1970. See also: Lewis, Charles E. and Barbara Resnik. "Nurse Clinics and Progressive Ambulatory Patient Care." *New England Journal of Medicine.* 277:23:1237-1241 (December 9) 1967.
45. Pinneo, Rose. "Nursing in a Coronary Care Unit." *American Journal of Nursing.* 65:2:76-79 (February) 1965.

46. Neal, Mary V. "The Relationship Between a Regimen of Vestibular Stimulation and the Developmental Behavior of the Premature Infant." Unpublished doctoral dissertation, School of Nursing, New York University, 1967.
47. Center for Nursing Research, Wayne State University. "Sensory Perception in the Aged with Implications for Institutional Environment." Unpublished paper prepared for the Institute of Gerontology, University of Michigan-Wayne State University, 1971.
48. *Facts About Nursing, 1970-71 Edition.* New York: American Nurses' Association, 1972. pp. 257-258.
49. "ANA Approves NCSNNE Report's Four Central Recommendations." *ANA in Action.* 3:3:14 (Fall) 1971.
50. "Professional Partnerhood in Health Care: The Need for Research into Nursing Practice." Rochester, New York: The National Commission for the Study of Nursing and Nursing Education, 1971 (pamphlet).
51. The National Commission for the Study of Nursing and Nursing Education. *An Abstract for Action,* op. cit., pp. 83-87.
52. Personal communication from Frances K. Peterson, Director, Department of Diploma Programs, NLN, to Jerome P. Lysaught, Director, NCSNNE, dated May 15, 1972.
53. "Report of the Task Force to Study the Implications of the Recommendations Presented in *An Abstract for action." Nursing Outlook.* 21:2:113 (February) 1973.

FIVE TOWARD CHANGE IN NURSING: EDUCATIONAL PATTERNS

Paralleling the ferment in nursing roles and functions, there has been, since mid-century, a significant shift in the institutional patterns of nursing education. Spurred by the rising demand for increased and extended health care delivery, the nursing profession has responded with a dramatic increase in numbers of students and educational programs. In 1955, for example, there were slightly more than 45,200 students admitted to the various preparatory programs for nursing. Eighteen years later, that figure more than doubled, with 94,150 students beginning their studies. This increase averages slightly more than six percent per annum, and was a vital factor, not only in the growth of the profession, but in the marshalling of personnel and resources which expanded the health care delivery system throughout the sixties and early seventies.

Just as the number of students and nurse practitioners has grown, so too has there been a related increase among the institutions involved in providing their instruction. In 1955, there were approximately 1,100 schools of nursing; eighteen years later, there are more than 1,350—an increase of almost twenty-three percent. These overall figures, however striking they may seem, mask the actual velocity of change and fail to suggest the wrenching experiences through which nursing education has passed. Over the fifteen-year period from 1958 to 1973, the number of hospital schools of nursing *decreased* from 940 to 540; in contrast, the number of associate degree programs *grew* from 40 to 540. This fundamental trade-off in institutional patterning, combined with an increase of some 100 baccalaureate programs, meant that the computed gain of 250 nursing programs since 1955 has actually involved the entrance or exit of no less than 1,000 institutions involved in nursing education. What might on the surface appear to be a smooth upward slope of institutional participation in nursing education becomes, on examination, a heavily serrated curve strewn with the skeletons of abandoned programs. Well over a third of the programs offering preparatory education in 1958 no longer exist. Their places have largely been taken by a number of junior and community colleges whose programs in nursing are not only new, but whose entire institutional existence dates back only a few years.

This change, rapid as it has been in coming and so profound in its effects, has not been the result of conscious national or regional planning. Frequently, at the local or institutional level, the decision to open or close a program in nursing education has been made, essentially, on institutional idiosyncrasy. Meanwhile, throughout this period, nursing students have frequently become the confused victims of institutional shifts and rearrangements. Graduates of some preparatory programs continue to find that their further progress is hazarded and sometimes prevented because of institutional impediments that they neither understand nor accept. Labels have been attached to programs—and to their graduates—which stereotype them in ways that seem to have little to do with the reality of observed performance. Faculty and educational administrators are also bemused by this state of flux. Fundamental questions have been raised about almost every traditional concept concerned with nursing education, its curriculum, its articulated patterning, and its very objectives since 1923. No true consensus has yet been reached on many of the answers.

Over the course of its investigation, the National Commission attempted to take a fresh and dispassionate look at the problems which nursing education faced. Some were quite clear, and their required resolution apparent. It is patently harmful, for example, to maintain a bifurcated system of education in which some of the institutions are positioned in the collegiate mainstream while others are located within the independent locus of the hospital schools of nursing. It is harmful for a variety of reasons, but most particularly for the detrimental effect it has had on students wishing to develop an extended career for themselves within the profession. It is harmful in a particularly wasteful way, too, for the divisive and destructive part it has played within the house of nursing. So much energy has been expended, and so much antipathy engendered, that continuing controversy must be ended. For these reasons, then, the Commission sought, as a first priority, the establishment of statewide master planning committees that could work on the ultimate resolution of this issue while paying proper attention to the need for transitional programming and long-term resource allocation.

Second only to the priority for severing the Gordian knot of the bifurcated educational system is the need to ensure that our emerging pattern of two- and four-year collegiate programs becomes involved in interinstitutional planning for articulated curricula. If there is one thing that our Commission, and society as a whole, would find intolerable in nursing education, it would be the spectacle of our having solved the dilemma posed by the collegiate-noncollegiate institutional impasse only to have it replaced by a gulf between the two collegiate components. Nursing and nurses need systematic, articulated educational opportunities as surely as they need role enlargement and extension. For this reason, the National Commission sought to encourage, publicize, and support efforts at curricular planning and articulation—particularly in the latter cases where there is multi-institutional involvement.

A third priority relates to the rapprochement between nursing practice and education in such ways as to hasten educational planning that will support and complement the changing roles and functions already seen in practice settings. This kind of planning, however, must be directed at the very point of entry into the educational sequence and, then, at each succeeding stage through upper-division and advanced curricula. Changing practice requirements should be the criteria for thorough academic reformulation; the diversity and depth of the new roles are such that simply appending "courses" or "clinical experiences" is insufficient to the task at hand. To this end, the National Commission sought out those experimental programs which attempted to increase in significant ways the joint involvement of education and practice in the development of new content, course arrangements, and clinical experiences. These, in turn, can become the catalysts for an emergent pattern of nursing education geared to new assumptions and realities.

Frequently lost among all the expressed concerns for preparatory programs is the fact that no clinical profession can afford to ignore, or even deemphasize, continuing education for personal mastery. When we deplore the complications of institutional rivalry and lack of program fit faced by recent graduates, we must certainly add regret that more has not been done for practitioners who need periodic updating and refresher courses. Whether these are presented on an ad hoc basis or as part of a formal graduate program leading to a degree, there are evident problems of availability, resources, support, and individual opportunity. The fourth priority, then, of the National Commission, throughout the implementation phase, was to determine and effect some incremental steps that would encourage and assist nursing in planning post-preparatory educational programs.

Apportioned throughout the implementation phase was a continuing concern for the support of all educational programs in nursing, particularly as these were determined and fashioned by statewide master planning committees working on the evaluated needs and resources of the profession. The effort to inform and elicit support was a constant included within each of the priority efforts to initiate change.

Altogether, the National Commission proposed twenty-two specific recommendations related to the emergent needs of nursing education. Most of these are subsumed in the four priority categories, along with the general concern for financial support. Within the descriptive accounts of implementation activities, a general focus is discernible; information or progress toward each individual recommendation is provided in Appendix B.

A COMPREHENSIVE PATTERN FOR NURSING EDUCATION

From the beginnings of formalized nursing education in this country, the hospital school has played a leading and, for a long time, dominant role. As late as 1969, these institutions still comprised a majority of all preparatory programs for nursing. Only the dramatic growth of the community colleges in the fifties and sixties effected the significant shift of programs into the collegiate pattern. Much of our present concern, however, must take into account that somewhere between eighty and ninety percent of all our current nurse practitioners received their induction into the profession through the medium of the hospital school-including most of these who now possess advanced graduate degrees.

This actuarial data must be seen in context. The preponderance of hospital nurse graduates might be viewed nostalgically, but it can also simply indicate the fact that there was little choice for entering students over much of the period reported. At one time, for example, a similar percentage of our professional elementary teachers would have been recorded as products of the normal schools which abounded across the country. As educational choice and change developed, however, that institution found it necessary, like the hospital school is today realizing, to transform itself or disappear.

Since 1923, a series of independent, national studies have stressed that nursing education should be brought together into one comprehensive pattern centered in the mainstream of the collegiate system for higher education. Goldmark,[1] Brown,[2] Ginzberg,[3] Bridgman,[4] and the National Commission[5] have all emphasized the fact that a bifurcated system is by nature an unequal and incompatible structure. Yet, fifty years after the first of these proposals for change, nursing, alone of our professions, still has almost forty-five percent of its preparatory institutions outside the collegiate system.

Such changes as have occurred, have frequently been marred by emotionalism, anger, and personal attack. And as the number of noncollegiate programs continues to diminish, the remainder begin to assert themselves ever more aggressively in predictable patterns of defensiveness and closure of the herd. In 1971, forty-eight years after the report of the Goldmark study which called for the phasing out of hospital training schools, the following resolution was adopted by a national organization of some 325 hospital schools of nursing:

> Be it resolved, That the Assembly of Hospital Schools of Nursing (Type VIII membership) of the American Hospital Association direct the Assembly's Governing Council to exert every possible influence to obtain from the American Hospital Association an official statement repudiating those groups and individuals who are alluding to the phasing out of diploma programs of nursing education.[6]

This proposition was allowed to die quietly. Not only were the governing council and the board likely indisposed to exhuming the former reports in order to carry out full retribution and repudiation, but they had already gone on record, in adopting the findings of the AHA advisory committee to study the report of the National Commission, as supporting "... the improvement academically and organizationally of all programs in nursing education ... and the establishment of new programs associated with systems of higher education. ..."[7]

To the detached observer, it might make good sense to avoid this issue, eschew confrontation, and let nature take its course. Attractive as such a solution might be from a personal standpoint, the National Commission observed:

> One might be willing to let the competing schools play out the game in a crescendo of social and economic clashes were it not for the fact that the problems are too critical to be left unresolved.[8]

The most critical single issue, of course—the one for whom solution and resolution is absolutely essential—is the student of nursing. While institutions may joust and administrators pronounce, it is the student whose future is being most intimately affected.

The Student in Crossfire

The National Commission, throughout its report, refused to discriminate among registered nurses by resorting to labels. Our investigation confirmed that diploma school graduates compared favorably with collegiate students at the point where both groups began their careers in practice. In fact, the differences within programs are at least as great as those between, and the similarities among all preparatory programs are greater than the distinctions.

It is because of the intrinsic worth of the individuals involved that the Commission sought to equalize the rewards and the opportunities extended to students coming out of the preparatory programs. Our recommendations were based not so much on what *is* but, rather, what *ought to be* the pathway provided for personal choices in nursing. Three very simple propositions summarized the conditions that should obtain for all nursing students:

> 1. Academic recognition and reward should be so arranged that nursing students are equitably recompensed in comparison with their peers in other fields. As the Carnegie Commission puts it, "... a degree (or other form of credit) [should] be made available to students at least every two years in their careers."[9]
> 2. Every nurse should be provided with continuing opportunities for career mobility, specifically including the right to extended, formal education, with a minimum of obstacles and a maximum of choice.
> 3. Each nurse should be encouraged, within the educational framework, through both experiential and environmental factors, to become as full, mature, and self-actualizing a personality as possible.

Our answer to "Why change?" is bound up in the consideration of these three conceptual givens and the present circumstances, in which many students find themselves caught in a crossfire of institutional imperatives.

Academic Recognition. Hospital schools of nursing began as institutions which frankly offered training in return for student service. This concept may have received acceptance at a time when society regarded lightly any post-secondary education for women, but it has little contemporary currency. This quid pro quo conception has been considerably reduced through the impact of changing customs and accreditation requirements, but it is nonetheless true that hospital schools have never fully adjusted to the insurance of equal compensation for equal investment by its students as compared to that enjoyed by their peers in other institutions.

Because of the traditional patterns, the student in a hospital school most frequently spends two-and-one-half to three years in course work. At the end of that time, however, no degree is presented. While one can claim that a school diploma is "another form of credit," the student quickly discovers that it is not a standard means of exchange. Students in two-year programs within the collegiate system spend less time in their program, sit for and pass the same licensure examination, receive the designation as Registered Nurse, and, in addition, acquire an Associate Degree which testifies to their successful completion of a universally recognized increment of advanced education. In short, the hospital school perpetuates unequal treatment and, in doing so, treats its students differently not only from other nursing students, but from all those other college students of varying disciplines whose temporal investment is similar.

Continuing Opportunity. If nursing students simply stopped at the completion of the preparatory period, it might at least be arguable whether the extraction of three versus two years is so great a social wrong as to demand institutional reconstruction. Unfortunately, it is precisely at this point that the problem is compounded. Increasingly, more nurses do *not* wish to terminate their education at the completion of the preparatory program. Then, for far too many, comes the sad recognition that their diploma isn't standard currency, and that they must resort to the barter system to accomplish any further advancement.

The students discover that their education—outside the collegiate mainstream with its standardized arrangement of courses, credits, and hours—now must be validated by equivalency examinations, placement tests, and a pervasive challenge to prove one's self again and again.

The enormity of this wastefulness in terms of time, expense, frustration, and human dignity cannot be measured. The extent of it in student numbers alone, however, is unconscionable. Approximately one out of every five baccalaureate students today has previously earned the RN license. This proportion bespeaks the shifted pattern to collegiate schools because in earlier periods, from 1958 through 1968 for example, these RNs comprised between sixty-five and eighty percent of all the so-called graduate students in American collegiate nursing programs.[10] If this many students survived the hazards, how many fell victim to the nonsystem we have perpetrated? How many have dropped by the wayside convinced that they have been callously used as pawns in an institutional game?

At base, the question is one of ethics as surely as it is one of education. Our rival institutional patterns must be reorganized into a comprehensive unity that will facilitate the student's progress and provide a rational system for the coming generations of graduates. No amount of institutional sophistry can justify neglecting a unification of the system.

Student Self-Actualization. Formal education inherently is an exercise in individual and societal values. It is no accident that our western culture has largely moved away from apprentice types of training toward broader, more liberal learning. There is, undeniably, a high degree of social efficiency in only teaching persons to "do things." For social effectiveness, and for mature citizenship, however, we need deeper understandings and attitudes which can direct and humanize the "doing" of those "things."

In the course of the investigation phase, the National Commission asked student nurses to assess their educational world in terms of its affective values. From their replies, it became readily apparent that there were significant differences between the environmental setting of the collegiate and hospital school settings that are deeper than the scientific content of the courses, the arrangement of the calendar, or the details of the curriculum. These distinctions are displayed in Figure 5-1.

Factor	Significantly Different Perceptions: Higher	Significantly Different Perceptions: Lower
General Esteem	BSN ADN	Dipl
Academic Enthusiasm	BSN ADN	Dipl
Breadth of Interest	BSN ADN	Dipl
Intrinsic Motivation	BSN ADN	Dipl
Extrinsic Motivation	ADN Dipl	BSN

Figure 5-1. Comparison of student reactions to the nursing school environment inventory.

TABLE 5-1 COMPARISON OF ACADEMIC PREPARATION AMONG NURSE FACULTY MEMBERS

Level of Preparation	Type of Institution		
	Hospital School	Two Year College	Four Year College
RN (non-degree)	21.0%	1.1%	.4%
BSN or equivalent	57.1%	35.3%	14.2%
MSN or equivalent	20.7%	62.3%	78.2%
DNS or equivalent	1.2%	1.3%	7.3%

It is obvious that students in both two- and four-year collegiate programs perceive their surroundings to be generally similar and, on the whole, quite different from the world viewed by the hospital school student. General esteem for the program, academic enthusiasm, breadth of interest, and intrinsic motivation are all seen as being more valued and stressed in the collegiate setting.[11]

To some extent, the differences distinguished by the students mirror distinctions to be found in their faculties. If a teacher is to broaden the horizons and perspectives of a student, then it stands to reason that the mentor must have had broadening experiences and appropriate education in preparation for the task. The comparative academic preparation of the nurse faculty in the collegiate and noncollegiate programs, however, bears out the observations of the students. As shown in Table 5-1, there are significant shadings toward greater preparation among those appointed to collegiate faculties.

One out of five faculty members in hospital schools of nursing has taken advanced formal preparation for her position. By the same measure, one out of five has never even completed a collegiate education.[12] This situation cannot help but affect student-faculty interaction and the environmental setting within the hospital school itself.

The point, of course, is what do we value in our nurse practitioners? What values do we want them to develop and nurture? Our society has largely shown its preference for the broader scope of education that fosters breadth of interest, intrinsic motivation, esteem, enthusiasm and other factors calculated to unleash the human potential of the student. Our Commission felt that the restructuring of the educational patterns of nursing would simply place that profession alongside all others that have been positioned in the mainstream of American education. In doing so, we equalize the rewards for accomplishment, enhance the opportunities for career mobility, and broaden the personal vistas of the nursing student. No institution that styles itself an educational facility can, in conscience, provide its students with less.

Progress Toward Implementation

A combination of economic and social pressures, combined with the active efforts of many leaders in nursing and higher education, has fashioned an evolutionary growth toward a collegiate system of nursing education—a growth, however, that has seldom been well planned or cooperatively executed. In part, this movement has reflected our growing acceptance of fourteen years of general education as a societal norm; in part, the institutional shift in nursing education is an example of economic determinism.[13] By whatever combination of factors, the trend is unmistakable. As indicated in Figure 5-2, there has been a steady swing toward the collegiate pattern.

As a first priority, the National Commission sought—through its informational contacts with nursing organizations, other health professions, higher education bodies, and the public—to explain and interpret the obvious developments in nursing education. In so doing, the Commission and staff emphasized the positive impact that such changes could have for the student, for the consumer of health care, and for the public who is, at one time or another, taxpayer, parent, student, or recipient of health care.

In their endorsement of the Commission's summary recommendations, the American Nurses' Association, the National League for Nursing,. the American Medical Association, and the American Public Health Association approved the proposition that we should move forward on placing all nursing education in the collegiate system. The American Hospital Association advisory committee did not comment directly on the point, but did propose that all new nursing programs be associated with the system of higher education. By these actions, or statements, the Commission felt free to move on to more detailed activities.

During the succeeding stages of the implementation effort, therefore, three specific areas were identified for continuing follow-up: organizational contact with the hospital schools; specific assistance to selected hospital schools; and an information campaign designed to foster acceptance of the changing patterns for nursing education.

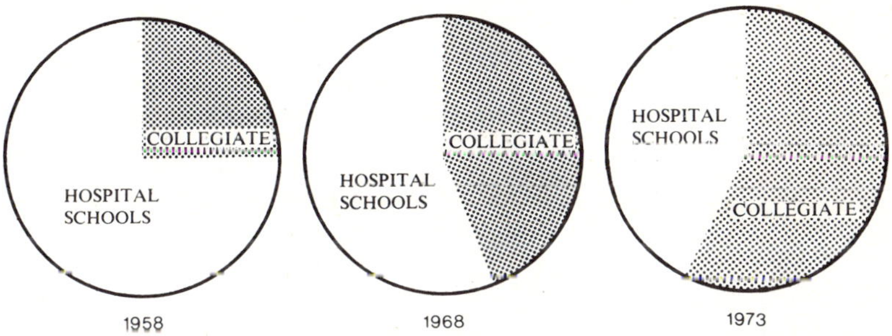

Figure 5-2. Changing patterns in nursing education: institutional shifts, 1958-1973.

Organizational Contacts. There are two large organizations of hospital schools of nursing: one is the Council of Diploma Programs of the National League for Nursing; the other is the Assembly of Hospital Schools of Nursing of the American Hospital Association. There is, of course, some overlap of membership and even a form of interlocking leadership since some individuals have held top positions in both organizations.

The swift action of the NLN Board of Directors in endorsing the summary report and recommendations of the National Commission in February, 1971[14] was not happily received by the membership of the Council of Diploma Programs. Their concern and dismay, particularly over the recommendations that would lead to the demise of the hospital schools, were vigorously brought to the attention of the board at the biennial convention of the league in 1971. This, in turn, led to the appointment of the NLN Task Force to Study the Implications of the Recommendations Presented in *An Abstract for Action.* This group, after airing a number of concerns about the transition of nursing education, endorsed the basic recommendation to place "... nursing education ... in the mainstream of American educational patterns with its preparatory programs located in collegiate institutions."[15] The task force did remove the word *deadlines* from the recommendation in its endorsed form because "... The implied threat of forcing institutions to close was rejected as unnecessary. . . ."[16]

Meanwhile, the staff of the National Commission had approached the executive committee of the Council of Diploma Programs with the proposal that an ad hoc committee be established to discuss areas of mutual concern and to consider whether or not there might be transitional projects that could be worked on jointly. In April of 1972, this was discussed with the Executive Committee and a formal request was tendered to them to establish an ad hoc planning committee. On May 15, 1972 the director of the Council of Diploma Programs conveyed the following:

> Your request that a joint ad hoc committee be established was given first consideration when the committee reconvened following the April 6-7th annual meeting of the Council of Diploma Programs. Actions of the membership assembled at the meeting included non-support of the following recommendations published in *An Abstract for Action*. . . .
>
> This expression of non-support and the existence of the NLN Task Force to Study the Implications of the Report of the National Commission for the Study of Nursing and Nursing Education led the committee members to conclude that collaboration at this time was not possible. . . .[17]

While the executive committee thus refused any organizational involvement, at least for some period of time, the National Commission did carry the matter to the council membership by supplying the hospital schools with copies of a position paper in pamphlet form—"The Diploma Nurse, the Hospital School, and the National Commission."[18] This document elaborated upon the rationale for the Commission's recommendations and subsequent efforts at implementation. It emphasized that their conclusions did not repudiate either nursing schools or their graduate products, but were aimed at the development of an improved comprehensive pattern of education that would be superior to anything we have had to this point.

The Assembly of Hospital Schools of Nursing of the American Hospital Association had, in 1971, resolved to take steps to "repudiate" those groups and individuals who suggested the phasing out of diploma programs. Despite this unpromising pronouncement, the Commission staff met with the governing council of the assembly in early 1972 and proposed the establishment of an ad hoc committee to examine and discuss mutual concerns. The governing council agreed to name such a group, and in March of that year, a joint announcement of the committee was made by that council and the National Commission. In the text of the release on the newly formed group, Joy Lynn Douglas, chairman of the governing council stated:

> There is much in the Commission's report that our members have long supported. In terms of educational patterns, the time has come for all of us to look at varying models and relationships. The hospital schools of nursing have long made an essential contribution to the nation's health care; it is important, therefore, that any changes made in educational patterns represent a real advance for both the public and the student.[19]

Ensuing discussions with the ad hoc committee led to some improved understanding, if not to any commitment to change. One direct outcome was an invitation to the director of the Commission to participate in the program of the annual meeting of the assembly in 1972. The changed atmosphere, resulting both from the discussions with the ad hoc committee and with the Commission's administrators' advisory committee, was clearly observable. While the assembly might not agree with the Commission's viewpoint, they recognized that there had been a significant effort on the part of that body to discuss and listen to spokesmen of the hospital schools.

In the words of an editorial staff member from *Hospitals*, the Journal of the American Hospital Association, if the director of the Commission

> . . . had appeared before the Assembly of Hospital Schools of Nursing last year, it's a good bet he would have been torn limb from limb—figuratively at least . . . Last year, the Assembly passed a resolution urging the American Hospital Association to publicly repudiate groups and individuals who alluded to the phasing out of diploma nursing education—a thinly veiled slap. . . . This year's Assembly, considerably subdued—or perhaps caught by surprise . . . listened politely, although discussion following . . . was lively.[20]

In the spring of 1973, the governing council discharged the ad hoc committee, but by this time it had served the useful functions of facilitating exchange of ideas, delimiting areas of agreement and disagreement, and fostering a recognition that change is coming in nursing education and that the real choice is the extent of one's own involvement in shaping the direction of that change.

Specific Assistance to Schools. In its recommendations concerning the development of a collegiate system for nursing education, the National Commission attempted to suggest a variety of alternatives. While a number of hospital schools might wish simply to close their institutional doors for a variety of reasons, others might want to continue some form of involvement in nursing education. Some might choose to provide clinical facilities for the instruction of collegiate students, thus ensuring that nursing education continue in the hospital—though in altered ways than before. Other hospital schools might look forward to a blending of institutional relationships with collegiate schools so that faculties could be joined and resources and facilities shared. There is even the possibility that a small number of hospital schools, endowed with greater financial assets, and possessing highly qualified faculty, combined with strong motivation, might conceivably become collegiate schools in their own right.

This last alternative, perhaps more than any other single recommendation of the National Commission, elicited a great deal of negative reaction. The NLN Council of Diploma Programs voiced their "nonsupport" of this proposal, and the NLN Task Force to study *An Abstract for Action* chose to delete this one recommendation out of all those proffered by the National Commission. Likewise the authors of the "Appraisal" of the report, published in the *American Journal of Nursing,* expressed concern for this recommendation and related it to what they perceived to be ". . . an apparent underlying bias in favor of hospital schools. . . ."[21] It is indeed interesting that the same recommendation has been seen both as a threat by hospital schools and as a subterfuge by collegiate spokesmen.

Rather than leave concerns such as these to theoretical disputation, the National Commission and its staff sought to help a number of hospital schools as they explored alternatives in response to the developing pattern of collegiate education. Consultation was offered to several schools which were planning a phased program of closure or cooperative realignment with collegiate schools. At the request of a number of institutions, particularly in the states of New York, Pennsylvania, and California, planning and assistance was given to the exploration of new educational arrangements, or consortia, in which a number of programs, including hospital schools of nursing, might be consolidated into a collegiate system.

Perhaps the most intriguing of these efforts to assist particular institutions in their planning for change was that which involved the highly controversial switch from a diploma school of nursing to a collegiate institution. Actually, this proposal had stemmed from the fact that a precedent already existed. In the investigatory phase of the Commission's work, we had become acquainted with St. Mary's Junior College of Minneapolis.[22] This institution had originally been the St. Mary's Hospital School of Nursing, but in 1962 the faculty initiated a number of activities designed to explore the possibility of attaining independent collegiate status. By 1964, St. Mary's had received an educational charter from the State of Minnesota designating it a nonprofit junior college institution; in 1966, the school made formal overtures to the North Central Association of Colleges and Secondary Schools for collegiate accreditation. The school subsequently moved through the lengthy and rigorous process of accreditation by the regional association and is today a fully accredited education institutional member. Currently, St. Mary's Junior College offers associate degree programs in seven areas: child development, inhalation therapy, medical laboratory, medical records, nursing, occupational therapy, and physical therapy.

During the final stages of the study, our staff had become acquainted with a planning group at the Catherine Laboure School of Nursing near Boston. After an exhaustive two-and-one-half-year study of trends and resources, the faculty and administration concluded, in April of 1970, that the school should shift from a diploma to a collegiate institution. Because the approximate date of that decision coincided with the promulgation of the National Commission's recommendation that some hospital schools explore the possibility of becoming a collegiate institution, there was an obvious mutuality of interest. Over the next several months, the Commission staff worked with the school-planning group to consider ways and means of effecting the desired changes and to find possible sources of support for such a development. One consequence was the publication by the National Commission of a documentary case study of the effort undertaken by Laboure to become a collegiate institution.[23] The decision was finalized in the spring of 1970, and steps were undertaken to secure an educational charter from the Commonwealth of Massachusetts and preliminary accreditation status from the New England Association of Colleges. Since that time, the institution has continued on its course and, today, Laboure Junior College and St. Mary's Junior College are living evidence that hospital schools can transform their programs if they choose. The way is costly and arduous, but far from impossible for a select number of diploma schools.

In 1969, just before the appearance of the National Commission's report, there were 695 diploma programs in nursing education. In 1973, almost three years following the publication of *An Abstract for Action* and its resultant discussion and airing, there are 540 hospital programs, a decrease of 155 from our base year, and a decline of over twenty-two percent. Certainly, many of these adjustments would have been made in the regular course of events; hopefully, through our contact with some of these institutions, there was a more considered transitional effort, and, in some cases, the emergence of stronger collegiate programs through joint planning and cooperative use of resources.

Informational Efforts. Over the course of the implementation phase, a series of pamphlets was prepared to assist nursing organizations and state planning groups in their exploration of institutional trends in nursing education. Some of these reported case examples of change in process, such as the accounts of the two hospital schools that have become junior colleges. Other materials treated such concerns as continuing education, institutional articulation, and the collegiate-noncollegiate controversy.[24]

While many of these were specifically intended to document and encourage institutional transition, it was also necessary to address some of the common misconceptions that have frequently been mentioned in discussions about nursing education. For example, many of the non-nursing groups and organizations had little idea of the difficulty encountered by graduates of hospital schools in their efforts to continue their formal education in collegiate programs. Similarly, nurses and non-nurses alike were surprised when comparative data on nursing education revealed that differences in costs among the various kinds of preparatory programs were not in the directions generally assumed.

In a Commission publication, "Costs of Nursing Education and a Case for its Greater Support,"[25] figures from a limited sample of recent studies in New York and Tennessee were reported which corroborated and updated earlier large-scale investigations conducted by the National League for Nursing. The results showed that the average costs per student per year were as indicated in Figure 5-3.

Because of the early custom of training in return for service that was utilized in hospital schools, and because these institutions have traditionally charged low tuitions, many people have assumed them to be inexpensive vehicles for nursing education. Furthermore, many of us still draw our ideas about college costs from the institutions that were far less egalitarian than those of today. These unsustained generalizations have led to some downright false conclusions about the actual and relative costs of nursing education.

Most of the hospital schools of nursing provide not only for the instruction of their students but, also, for a broad spectrum of noninstructional support including housing, meals, uniforms, etc. These expenses are borne by the school and dramatically affect the cost picture. In the data presented in Figure 5-3, all instructional and noninstructional costs reported by the institutions have been included in arriving at the average figure displayed. The comparative costs also undoubtedly reflect some of the economy realized by collegiate programs through the utilization

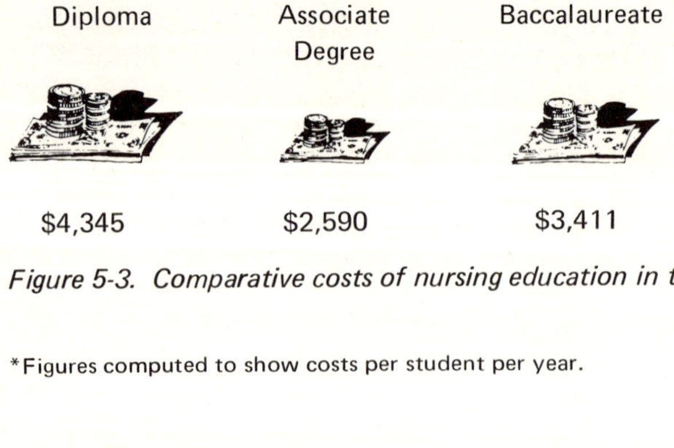

Figure 5-3. Comparative costs of nursing education in three kinds of institutions. *

*Figures computed to show costs per student per year.

of common arts and science courses for a variety of students in addition to those matriculated in nursing.

This is a simple illustration of the educational campaign necessarily conducted by the Commission in pursuance of the implementation effort. While the complete intricacies of institutional accounting are a field of study in themselves, it is essential that the health professions and the general public come face to face with the question of whether long-held assumptions—such as the "economy" of hospital education—can any longer be valid. In many cases, the answer is that our beliefs must be revised—or discarded.

The Prospects That Lie Ahead

One of the key points to be understood in terms of the resolution of the remaining problems in educational patterning is that *no action* is, most assuredly, activity of the most pernicious kind. While hundreds of institutions for nursing education have been involved in the tremendous effort to transform and revitalize the system, more than 125,000 diploma students have graduated over the six years of the National Commission's existence and have already begun to feel the effects of our present stupidities. We are continuing to admit students to the remaining diploma programs at a rate of almost 30,000 per year. And each one of these is a future victim of our "nonsystem."

In the long years of contest and debate, the surest outcome to date is that nursing students have generally paid the price of our intransigence and separatism. Each of our institutions for nursing education has contributed to the growth of our nation's delivery of health care. Yet, we still have a long way to go toward eliminating the flaws and the shortcomings of our present system. The National Commission's concern is that the future begins today, and that each delay permitted, each procrastination allowed, simply defers our appointed rendezvous with reality—to construct a comprehensive pattern for unified nursing education.

THE STATEWIDE MASTER PLANNING COMMITTEES

Because education is an area constitutionally reserved to the states, and because local conditions are important ingredients in the planning and timing of change, the National Commission proposed that the primary agency to effect the needed changes in educational patterns be formally designated, interdisciplinary committees knowledgable about the grassroots needs and resources of their area. To this end, *An Abstract for Action* proposed that:

> Each state have, or create, a master planning committee that will take nursing education under its purview, such committees to include representatives of nursing, education, other health professions, and the public, to recommend guidelines, means for implementation, and deadlines to ensure that nursing education is positioned in the mainstream of American educational patterns.[26]

The variability of nursing needs and resources from one state to another, the internal distribution of people and facilities, and the current status of educational patterning all dictate that local involvement and decision making is required to develop a plan and a timetable that have cogency and validity. It is also imperative that a multidisciplinary approach be initiated. In the truest sense of the word, many of the educational problems we have enumerated are ones that nursing, itself, did not create. It behooves all those who are involved to assist nursing in their resolution.

So strongly did the National Commission feel that participative planning and joint solution are needed to effect a new, comprehensive pattern for nursing education, that it urged all parties concerned:

> No hospital school should close and no collegiate program should open, until planning bodies have assured that an orderly transfer of functions and facilities has been developed. It is in the best interest of the whole country that this is carried out with speed and positive direction.[27]

With a spirit of cooperative concern replacing the emotionalism and partisanship of the past, it is possible in the last quarter of this twentieth century to end the divisiveness that has so long deflected nursing education from its primary aims.

Objectives of the SMPCs

In anticipation of the implementation operations, the first of the series of specialized pamphlets prepared by the National Commission was entitled, "A Guide for Establishing Statewide Master Planning Committees." In addition to reviewing briefly the needs and the historic disputes in American nursing education, the monograph propounded the purposes of the SMPCs as viewed by the Commission, subject, of course, to alteration at the state level on the basis of local concerns and priorities. In summary fashion, these are the tasks proposed:

1. The systematic reconstitution of nursing education within the patterns of higher education for the state.
2. Planning for emerging college programs so that they are developed in cooperation with existing health care facilities in such ways as to secure optimal clinical experience for the students.
3. Encouragement of joint planning between junior and senior collegiate institutions so that their curricula may be articulated and individual access and career enhancement for the student is maximized.
4. Provision of aid and direction to hospital schools in the exploration of alternative institutional response to the emergent patterns in nursing education—including the possibility in some cases of becoming collegiate schools in their own right.
5. Examination of statewide allocation of resources to both preparatory and advanced nursing education for the purpose of encouraging ex-

pansion or consolidation of programs to effect optimal utilization of faculty, facilities, and financial support.

6. Identification and encouragement of institutions to assume responsibility for continuing education on a state or regional basis to ensure that nurse practitioners are given greater opportunity to update and enlarge their skills.[28]

In approaching these objectives, the National Commission recognized that the statewide planning groups would find that, in bringing about an orderly transfer of educational programs, each of the existing kinds of institutions has characteristics and contributions that should be preserved in the emergent, comprehensive system that we wish to design—a system that could be better and stronger than any of our contemporary components.

The hospital schools of today, for example, have particular values embedded within their self-image that are surely to be encouraged within the new colleges for nursing education. These include: the close relationship so often found between faculty and students; the emphasis that is placed on student-patient involvement in care; the provision of early exposure to clinical care; and the identification of the curriculum with clinical excellence. These points are not the sole possession of the hospital school, but the best of these institutions have long exemplified their essentiality to student excellence.

The baccalaureate schools of nursing have outdistanced all others in the development of science related courses that extend the comprehension of nursing practice and provide a strong foundation for continued expansion of knowledge. These institutions, further, have worked to develop interdepartmental arrangements to bring the full resources of the collegiate institutions to bear on the support of nursing education. Faculty and students in nursing benefit from the combined knowledge and research activities of the college or university as they seek to determine better ways of meeting health care needs through nursing resources.

As the newest, and many would say the brashest, of our schools for nursing education, the community colleges have made their mark by taking leadership in instructional innovation—many of them have been pioneers in such fields as instructional technology and communication media. Likewise, many of these institutions have encouraged experimental curricula and innovative programs that are in sharp contrast to both tradition and the more staid advances of baccalaureate and hospital schools. While many of these experiments have not been successful, and the two year schools are the first to admit this, there is a healthy quality to their willingness to question many of the things that more settled institutions take as givens.

It is certainly one of the concerns of the statewide master planning committees that we distill out the best elements in our current patterns of nursing education and preserve them within the solution that will be our comprehensive system of tomorrow.

Establishment of the SMPCs

In its initial guidelines for the formation of state master planning committees, the National Commission emphasized that an official state body or other recognized authority must be involved in the legitimation of the group. The approach to securing this imprimatur was necessarily seen to vary from state to state. In some cases, the office of the governor might be the appropriate point of departure. In other states, existing offices for comprehensive health planning, higher education, or health might, by custom or by evinced interest, be the best vehicle. The parent agency would, in turn, likely become the appointing body for the committee using the suggestions for multidisciplinary involvement as well as the inclusion of concerned lay members.

As a preliminary step, the National Commission urged in 1970 that the state boards of nursing, the state nurses' associations, and the constituent leagues for nursing work in joint efforts to determine the best course for proceeding in each of the fifty states. Their attention was drawn to recently concluded studies on nursing needs and resources in Virginia,[29] Wisconsin,[30] North Dakota,[31] and South Dakota.[32] These four reports provided illustrative examples of the kinds of data that statewide master planning committees would require in order to assess nursing needs and resources, and contained suggestions for a revised educational pattern. In addition, the state groups were reminded of Lucile Leone's monograph on *Statewide Planning for Nursing Education,* prepared for the Southern Regional Education Board, which provides a detailed blueprint for the organization of a model state planning group.[33]

Out of the early experience gleaned from interaction with state nurses' organizations, the National Commission in April of 1971 designated the nine target states as ones in which planning and development efforts would be concentrated so that we could learn more, at first hand, on how to go about structuring the statewide master planning committees. Following their formal notification and acceptance, the Commission staff began to work with groups from these states to secure the official designation of a planning body. In Georgia, Governor Carter named the Georgia Educational Improvement Council to be the parent agency for such a committee; this function was later transferred to the Comprehensive Health Planning Office as a result of a complete reorganization of state offices and departments. In California, the Coordinating Council for Higher Education was recognized as the agency for development of a statewide master plan, and work had been begun on a comprehensive plan when the state legislators involved withdrew the charge from the Coordinating Council. At the present time, the work is inactive, but could be resumed on short notice. In North Carolina, the Joint Committee on Nursing Education of the State Board of Education and the State Board of Higher Education has been designated as the master planning committee. Still another variation is to be found in Kansas, where the planning committee was formed and designated by joint organizational action of the Kansas Nurses' Association, the Board of Nursing, the League for Nursing, the Medical Society, the Hospital

Association, and the Nursing Home Association. Thus, it went—each state finding its optimum way to develop a recognized and accepted planning body.

As anticipated, and as experienced in the case of the joint practice committees, the ripple effect from the target states soon involved a number of other states in the developmental steps of master planning. Some, of course, like Virginia, the Dakotas, and Wisconsin had only recently completed resource studies which involved multidisciplinary boards or committees. Other states had advanced to the stage of establishing an organization of nurse associations to plan strategy for the designation of a statewide master planning committee. Over the two-year span, from April 1, 1971 to April 1, 1973, a considerable effort has resulted in significant accomplishment. Through the support of state nursing organizations, medical societies, hospital associations, and interested consumers, there has been a nationwide pattern established. The results are shown in Table 5-2.[34]

As indicated in the table, approximately half the states have reached the operational stage of statewide master planning. Less than half a dozen are still largely unorganized; many have accomplished preliminary steps such as contacting other health organizations, initiating discussions with comprehensive health planners, etc. Those that have reached the operational stage are now beginning to program specific activities in line with their charges.

Georgia, in accordance with the governor's executive order, has developed a thirty-nine member SMPC whose offices are located within the state Office of Comprehensive Health Planning. A full-time project director is actively coordinating the work of this board and its subcommittees. To date, the SMPC has adopted and forwarded to the governor five major recommendations which include: the inclusion of nurses on all policy-making groups concerned with the state's health services; the establishment of specialized training programs for registered nurses to prepare them as primary care practitioners, particularly for rural areas of the state; the development of counseling and referral services for nursing school applicants previously rejected by education programs; the extension of comprehensive health services to school children through expanded nurse roles and adequate supporting personnel; and the formal recognition and support of the Georgia State Joint Practice Committee. Two subcommittees are now taking the general framework of

TABLE 5-2 STATUS OF IMPLEMENTATION: STATEWIDE MASTER PLANNING COMMITTEES

Category of Status	Number of States*
Operational master planning committee	26
Master planning committee in process of development	21
No organized body	4

*Total of 51 includes the District of Columbia.

nursing education and nursing practice under advisement to examine goals, establish priorities, make recommendations, and propose specific means and methods for implementation. In the near future, subcommittees are to be established to consider continuing education and legislation.

The Wyoming Commission on Nursing and Nursing Education was formed in 1970 as a multidisciplinary group with broad organizational support. It is now in the process of seeking independent, incorporative status in order that it can qualify as a not-for-profit agency, in accordance with internal revenue service regulations, so that it can seek outside funding for the studies and projects which it hopes to initiate. Meanwhile, subcommittees have been established to publicize the work of the Commission, to study and report on Wyoming's nursing needs and resources, and to investigate the educational patterns and career mobility opportunities for nurses in the state. Because the concerns of the Commission are even broader, perhaps, than the charge of the statewide master planning committees from the National Commission, there is consideration that an enlarged subcommittee known as the task force committee might be designated as the SMPC, while the entire commission would work on related projects and assist in implementation. A meeting with the governor has been proposed to obtain official sanction of the commission's activities.

In Kansas, where master planning is the product of interorganizational agreement, objectives have been identified and task forces have been at work in: continuing education, joint practice, articulation of nursing curricula, needs in nursing service, and levels of nursing practice. The task force on continuing education has already developed a set of guidelines which has been endorsed by the Kansas State Nurses' Association. Like the commission in Wyoming, the committee in Kansas has styled itself the Master Planning Committee for the Study of Nursing and Nursing Education. With task forces in education and joint practice, which serve as the state's SMPC and SJPC, the master committee assumes the role of an umbrella organization that coordinates and facilitates planning between the two sub groups along with aiding in implementing the recommendations of either or both.

As in the case of the state joint practice committees, what began in the target states soon spread into others. To cite one example, nursing organizations in Minnesota had long sought some link with a state agency that would have the charge to develop a coordinated plan for nursing education within the state. In 1972, the governor designated the Minnesota Higher Education Coordinating Commission as the group responsible for drawing up a statewide plan for nursing education. The commission, in turn, has established a multidisciplinary advisory committee along the lines of the proposed SMPC and is assisted by staff personnel from both state agencies and the professional health organizations. Through its designation and status, the commission is in a position, not only to plan, but to implement its recommendations throughout the state.

Maine and Arkansas have recently completed a first step toward statewide master planning with the completion of studies on nursing needs and resources.

Rhode Island has moved on to the demonstration model stage to effect changes in nurse utilization and practice patterns. Delaware has submitted the first half of a two-volume report on nursing to the governor, and Idaho has gone so far as to submit their master plan for nursing education to the State Board of Education and receive that body's approval for implementation. Many other states' master planning committees could be used as examples, but the general variety of activities has been indicated. Progress and pace of activity are varied; however the groundswell of involvement and planning for action is clearly observable.

ARTICULATION IN NURSING EDUCATION

Development of a comprehensive plan for nursing education implies more than simply shifting the responsibility for that education into the collegiate institutions of this country. There is a need to ensure that those institutions, in turn, provide reasonable linkage between two-year and four-year programs so that students see an educational ladder they might ascend. The collegiate schools are to be included in the indictment implied in the title, "You Can't Get There from Here: Articulation in Nursing Education."[35] The author of that paper, Bonnie Bullough, points out that the rigidities of our current educational patterns make articulation between two- and four-year collegiate programs as difficult as the historic lack of fit between hospital schools and colleges.

There are, of course, historic antecedents for the present state of affairs. The long, grinding effort to get nursing education into collegiate settings, plus the protracted internecine struggle over continuation of hospital schools, made collaboration between these institutions difficult at best. Students have paid the price for the lack of articulation. The beginning nursing programs in two-year colleges were envisaged as "terminal, vocational, and technical" sequences which were not designed for educational continuity. Again, students are paying the price for our systemic deficiencies. Whereas few students in the community colleges may have expressed interest in going on to baccalaureate programs in the fifties, perhaps as many as eighty percent of the graduates today say they would like to continue their education—particularly after some period of clinical experience.[36]

In a sense, the entire question of educational articulation falls into two somewhat separate considerations. There is the need to consider the immediate plight of students prepared in our current system. And there is the need to plan for an improved, more rational patterning that will facilitate future mobility among nursing students as well as cooperation among the institutions engaged in their instruction.

Remedying the Short Term Defects

Most students who apply to a school of law or medicine present a fairly consistent pattern of prior educational experience. They usually possess a college degree in arts or science, frequently with a pre-professional sequence or major, but without any clinical experience in the discipline which they wish to pursue.

In nursing, the situation is vastly different. Many students come to baccalaureate institutions as registered nurses graduated from either hospital schools or associate degree programs. A goodly number of students are also attracted into nursing from the auxiliary health fields so that licensed practical nurses, aides, and orderlies see registered nursing as a career process, and they bring to their educational experience a background of experience and on-the-job instruction that includes a good deal of the content of the preparatory nursing program. There are also the vast training programs in the military and in some civilian agencies that produce corpsmen and health workers. Many of these persons come to registered nursing programs equipped with a combination of knowledges and skills relevant to the profession. The extent of this overlap is epitomized by the results of a study conducted by the Allied Health Professions Project at the University of California at Los Angeles. This group identified some 300 nursing tasks, sixty percent of which were performed by all levels of personnel from aide to RN.[37] Thus, work experience and prior education do involve many procedures and tasks that are commonly taught in nursing programs.

Examination and Placement. In the past, nursing educators have agonized over many of the problems presented by these applicants. At one extreme, some have proposed blanket acceptance of various groups; at the opposite pole, others have argued that all such students start afresh. The first viewpoint reflects a primary concern not to penalize the student; the other emphasizes the desirability of a lock-step system of nurse preparation. Most faculties and institutions have gone to the middle ground of assessing student transcripts, providing challenge examinations, and, occasionally, evaluating individual clinical competence.

Few, however, would argue either the problems or the vagaries of such an approach. Not only may one institution be more demanding, but some individual faculty members may significantly skew the situation through the development of teacher-made tests that have high levels of difficulty. A much more objective and standardized approach is needed.

Faced with a similar situation, the National Committee for Careers in the Medical Laboratory secured funding for a test development project from the U.S. Department of Labor. With the help of major organizations, including the American Society of Clinical Pathologists and the College of American Pathologists, plus psychometric consultation of the Educational Testing Service, four standardized tests in medical laboratory proficiency were developed and first administered in 1971. The program has been continued and is a vital force in determining advanced placement or recognition.[38]

Nursing has no comparable development at the national level. Individual schools, like Mesa College in Grand Junction, Colorado, have embarked on sophisticated development projects employing both paper-and-pencil and videotape techniques to test knowledge and clinical skill.[39] Perhaps the most ambitious project, however, is that begun by the University of the State of New York. At the direction of the Regents, the State Department of Education has developed a series of professional examinations in: nursing fundamentals, medicine-surgery, psychiatric nursing, and maternal-child.[40]

The promise—and the disappointments—of this approach became very clear in the first three years of administration. No less than eighty-five percent of the applicants who took the Fundamentals of Nursing made a passing grade. As a result, 211 credit requests were made to fifty-five nursing programs in New York State. Only seventy-seven of those requests were granted, whereas 134 were rejected. Only twenty-four of the nursing programs approved even one request; thirty-one approved no requests. Of the approved requests, eighty-three percent were granted by associate degree institutions.

In the face of such evidence the National Commission concluded that nursing, through its national organizations, must develop clearer policies and better tools to ensure that students caught in the nonsystem of today are given reasonable opportunity to demonstrate their competence—and then are afforded proper placement and credit. Until this is done, students will continue to be unfairly and unjustifiably restricted. Only the moral suasion of nursing itself can correct the picture presented by the experience of the New York State testing program.

Accessibility of Programs. Despite the fact that there are more than 1,300 preparatory programs in nursing, many of the baccalaureate programs are well removed from the residences and work places of the nurse practitioners who desire to advance their formal education. In addition, residency requirements and other traditional academic restrictions have hampered the extension of educational opportunities to the graduate registered nurse. More recently, however, there has been a profitable reexamination of these policies and provisions.

The Michigan State University School of Nursing is establishing an extension program that will permit registered nurses in one locality to complete their baccalaureate degree by taking all courses, both lecture and clinical, in their own community through the combined utilization of university and local resources. If the model trial is successful, it will be extended throughout the state.[41]

Even more revolutionary is the announced plan of the New York State Regents to offer an *external* degree in nursing by which an individual conceivably could receive an earned degree through demonstrated competence without any of the customary residence requirements or formal course recognition.[42] Funded by an educational grant from the W. K. Kellogg Foundation, this project may well point the way to solving the backlog of individual problems caused by our present ill-fitting system for nursing education.

In addressing these problems, the National Commission has attempted to inform, publicize, and encourage those people and activities that are working to solve, or at least ameliorate, the short-run defects of our system. In terms of effecting basic change, however, it must be recognized that the various statewide master planning committees are in a more strategic position to ensure that those successful approaches to educational problems are implemented at the grassroots level.

Planning Long-Term Articulation

From the standpoint of the student—and the general public—placement tests and challenge examinations are better than nothing as a help to educational mobility. We should strive, however, for a resolution of the basic ills that beset the system for nursing education while continuing to meet the needs of those who presently need help. The ultimate solution to the problems of educational patterning requires coming to grips with the relationship between two- and four-year collegiate programs in nursing.

Altman has predicted that by 1980, between sixty-two and sixty-six percent of all admissions to preparatory programs in nursing will be through the associate degree institutions.[43] Paradoxically, Bullough points out that, today, the National League for Nursing is still encouraging a concentration of nursing courses in the upper division of baccalaureate programs—and that this factor alone militates against easy articulation of institutional curricula.[44]

So long as one views two-year programs as technical and terminal, and four-year programs as professional, there will remain a semantic and perceptual bar to the examination of what is really going on in both kinds of programs. In its examination of objective data provided by licensure examinations, the National Commission found that there were differences between the graduates of the two programs, but not to the degree imagined.[45] There was considerable overlap of scores, and the best two-year programs compared favorably with four-year institutions. If one takes into account the relative newness of the programs, the age differences commonly found among the students, and other environmental aspects, much of the observed difference can be explained in ways that have little to do with the nursing curriculum itself.

In the responses to the Nursing School Environment Inventory, the collegiate programs closely resembled each other, and both showed significant deviation from the responses of hospital schools of nursing.[46] Likewise, observed performance of beginning practitioners indicates that individual differences are more significant in demonstrated skill than is institutional background.[47]

For all these reasons, we must discard the outdated notion that the two- and four-year programs should be intrinsically different, and recognize two quite evident points:

1. Increasingly, the two-year institutions will become feeder schools to the baccalaureate programs. Students will enter upper division courses possessed of formidable amounts of knowledge and skill, and already licensed to practice as a registered nurse.

2. Four-year institutions must not only reorganize themselves to admit these students, but must cope with the fact that what they have been doing in "upper division" courses must be sharply altered to provide a true continuation of education with expanded electives and deepened scientific and clinical content.

These emerging trends will largely remake the face of baccalaureate nursing education. Some institutions are already emerging as upper division "schools" which are designed to admit students from preparatory nursing programs and provide them with an expanded curriculum. Other four-year colleges are now planning to push their traditional nursing courses down into the first two years of the academic calendar so that their own students, as well as transfers, will have completed basic preparation and be ready for true "upper division" courses by the beginning of the third year. Both these developments recognize that the customary offering of nursing courses only in the third and fourth years of a baccalaureate program does not make them, in fact, upper division courses. While the realization is not new, its acceptance is far from complete. Davis[48] pointed out in 1966, "There is not much to distinguish the baccalaureate graduate . . ." and, somewhat later, Reinkemeyer[49] observed that baccalaureate preparation ". . . has not differed ostensibly from that of the diploma or associate degree programs."

These criticisms, of course, are not intended to castigate the baccalaureate program, but to urge a basic reexamination and reformation. If four-year institutions are today doing much that is, or can be, done in a two-year school, then we are missing great opportunities for doing more—and doing it better. In the course of the implementation phase, the National Commission sought to investigate new departures in educational articulation, publicize them, and, in particular, call them to the attention of the statewide master planning committees which could be their advocates and proponents. Examples of these innovations include:

Georgia State University in Atlanta has developed a two plus two nursing curriculum that is designed to offer an associate degree in nursing, and then accept graduates of that program, plus degree students from other two-year programs, into the third year of a baccalaureate program. The curriculum includes lower division nursing courses in the first two years, and upper division, advanced courses appropriate to students who have demonstrated mastery of the preparatory sequence. The University has also experimented with enrolling diploma school graduates in the junior year of the upper division program with good results.[50]

The Purdue University Department of Nursing is linked in an articulated system of education with technical colleges at Calumet and Lafayette. Students at these two-year colleges complete a lower division program in nursing and then are permitted to transfer to the Purdue campus. The university program admits only RNs and presents only upper division courses which are planned to build on the structured base developed in the associate degree programs. The linkage is maintained through joint planning and discussion among the school faculties involved.[51]

> The State College of Arkansas has extended its concept of articulation to permit even more variation in the lower division. Using a core curriculum approach, with a spiral of concepts and skills that permits students to refine and deepen their understanding, the program is designed so that first-year students are prepared to practice as licensed practical nurses and to pass the regulatory examination. The students are encouraged, however, to move directly into the second year of studies. At the end of that year, the students are prepared to take the RN license examination and receive their Associate degree. They are encouraged, however, to move right into the upper division of the program leading to the baccalaureate degree. Transfer students from other associate degree programs are welcomed into the upper division course of study.[52]

A continuing series of institutional variations could be cited. Governors State University has embarked on an upper division baccalaureate program in nursing, and is working cooperatively with associate degree programs in its locality to assure an articulated, interlocking program. The University of Health Related Sciences and Rush-Presbyterian-St. Luke's, both of Chicago, have upper division programs in the late planning stages that will represent new departures in articulated patterning. So, too, has the University of Nebraska School of Nursing.

If all change were to take place school by school, however, it would be years before all 1,350 institutions for nursing education might adjust their sights appropriately. Recognizing this, the National Commission proposed:

> No less than three regional or interinstitutional committees be funded for the study and development of the nursing curriculum to develop educational objectives, universals, alternatives, and sequences for instruction. These committees should seek to specify appropriate levels of general and specialized learning for the different types of educational institutions.[53]

This recommendation never intended to establish a "Super Board" or inject greater rigidity into the nursing curriculum. By the very proposition that there should be *no less than three* examinations conducted by interinstitutional collaboration, there is little likelihood that autocracy could develop or orthodoxy be established. Hopefully, some consensus and a great deal of variety might be found in the attainment of an articulated, comprehensive pattern of collegiate nursing education.

Throughout the implementation phase, the Commission and its staff worked with institutions and groups interested in pursuing this recommendation for interinstitutional curriculum planning. To date, two projects have been funded by the W. K. Kellogg Foundation that are capable of meeting the expectations of the proposal. The Southern Regional Education Board began in 1972 a three-year project to relate educational competencies and skills to future roles of nurses. Specifically, the investigation focuses on two related concerns:

1. The development of a blueprint for education programs of sufficient flexibility to train nurses in the South for their different roles—present and future.

2. The evaluation of the importance of advanced and continuing education, the better coordination between the different levels of nursing education (associate degree, baccalaureate and advanced degree programs), and the effect of these on flexibility in the nursing curriculum.[54]

As the main working body of the project, a thirty-six member seminar has been constituted composed of nurses and non-nurses. The results of their deliberations will be tested over the last months of the study through the selection of institutions to serve as demonstration models of changed curricular patterns.

Also in 1972, an articulated nursing education program for Orange County, California was instituted. The development of this program was sparked by an earlier survey of institutional facilities for nursing education which revealed, among a large number of findings, that it could take approximately six years of college study for a licensed vocational nurse to obtain a baccalaureate degree in nursing—some two years longer than if she had entered a program fresh from high school. This situation arose because there simply was little or no communication, let alone articulation, between and among the educational programs.

Three community colleges—Fullerton, Golden West and Santa Ana—have come together with California State University at Fullerton and the University of California at Irvine to effect joint planning and curricular compatibility so that the "individual interested in nursing may begin in one of the two-year colleges and earn an associate degree, continue at CSUF through a bachelor of science degree in nursing, and progress into the postgraduate program at UCI without losing academic credits through these transfers."[55]

Planning has already begun on the development of the curricular modules, and the first innovations will be instituted in 1973. The principal features of the projected system will include: all nursing levels to be incorporated within the educational system; at the end of one semester a student could receive an aide certificate; at the end of one year the student could write the LVN examination; at the end of two years the student would receive an associate degree and write the RN examination; there would be a common core curriculum at the lower division levels among all the participating institutions; there would be liberal use of qualifying and challenge examinations at all levels; and the upper division college would admit only graduates of lower division programs.[56]

Hopefully such fresh breezes in nursing education are catching. In 1972, the Colorado Planning Committee announced that it was working on "a proposal for a career ladder program for nursing education involving all the schools in the state."[57] This, of course, is the only logical response to the need for providing all citizens of the state access to improved nursing care while providing all nurses with access to enhanced career development.

DEVELOPING CURRICULAR CONCENTRATIONS

An unintended consequence of the similarity among preparatory nursing programs, coupled with the historic relationship of nursing to hospital practice, is that almost all of our institutions are now committed, consciously or not, to the development of practitioners for episodic care. So pervasive has this been that we refer to our educational programs, with their concentration of clinical experience in acute settings, as "generalist" preparation. It is this acceptance of tradition that prompts Davis to link baccalaureate and hospital nursing programs and conclude, "During the course of their professional schooling, each has been exposed to much of the same round of clinical experience in the hospital."[58]

If we can begin to accept that there has not been much difference among our programs—certainly not all that has been implied or believed, then we may be able to take the next step toward critical assessment and recognize that the chief distinction between nursing content in baccalaureate programs and all others is the inclusion of a learning sequence devoted to community or public health nursing. The point, in fact, is that this comes as too little, too late in terms of the expressed needs for developing functional nursing competence over the full range of episodic and distributive client care requirements.

In this country, we have become increasingly aware that our health care system has been cure oriented and that we need to develop a companion concern for health maintenance and disease prevention—a commitment to wellness that at least accompanies our involvement with illness. The documentation of this, discussed at length in Chapter Four, is too detailed to require repeating. There is, however, an absolute necessity to relate these changing role requirements to our educational system so that it, in turn, can reflect them in both students' curricula and clinical preparation.

In an almost prophetic way, Peplau several years ago stated, "When the attention of the public focuses on areas of public need which hitherto have received scant attention from the available professions, new areas of specialization tend to be formulated."[59] From the viewpoint of Millis, this is precisely what is occurring in health care today, through the concurrence, in time, of the *articulated* cry for expansion of traditional health care service into areas where it has not been traditionally available—slums, isolated rural settings, and impoverished pockets of society—and the *unarticulated* demand of a whole new proportion, "Don't only save my life, but keep me well!"[60]

Nurse practitioners have already begun to respond to this expressed need. Now nursing education must move swiftly to provide them the backup and the replacements that will be required. It may be some satisfaction to note that, even if there were not cries from the field for differentiated practice, nursing itself, impelled by the research findings it has already begun to accumulate, would have found it necessary to reorganize its "generalist" curriculum. As Peplau notes, "Any large increase in knowledge about phenomena germane to a particular field tends to lead toward specialization. In the professions, such increased knowledge places a new and major burden on the generic programs which cannot teach all that is new, nor can they quickly revise curricula. . . ."[61] Especially since the generic programs have been an unrecognized form of specialty preparation, we are faced with problems. Because the crisis is already upon us, we cannot indulge in the luxury of slowly revising curricula.

Opening the Curriculum

Perhaps the first thing that a school of nursing can do to begin curricular adjustment is to develop elective courses in nursing science that permit a student to make meaningful choices along lines of personal interest. This has been near impossible in the past because there was little difference in the content of the standard nursing courses regardless of the institutional level at which they were presented—and even less in the way of elective courses. Articulated programs necessitate upper division courses with differentiated and intensive content. As one observer, Thurston, views it:

> In almost every health care setting, nursing roles are gradually changing and expanding. In any setting, however, the present professional nurse has three primary functions or roles: dependent, independent, and collaborative. The nurse seems to have little difficulty functioning in a dependent role, but the independent and collaborative areas of practice seem neglected. Why does this occur? Do our curriculums contain some "hidden agenda"? That is, do we assume that the majority of nurses will function *primarily* in acute care settings? Do we assume that the most important learnings are related to the dependent role? Thus, do we focus student learning and clinical experience in settings which foster the dependent role?[62]

Whether the emphasis on episodic care and the acute setting is conscious or simply accepted, the outcome is the same. The answer must lie in our effort to do things differently. As Thurston sees it, the answer would lie in new concentrations and curricular differentiation:

> The proliferation of knowledge and the expansion of needed skills make it unrealistic to try to prepare professional nurses to care for *all* individuals at *all* levels of health and illness and wherever they may be . . . One possibility is to develop tracks for specialization at the baccalaureate level whereby students could gain additional knowledge and skill in *either* distributive or episodic care environments consistent with their own career goals and interests.[63]

At the University of Kansas, nursing students take four core courses taught by teams of nurses with expertise in varying clinical areas. The first two of these courses are intended to develop a conceptual model around which the individual student can organize concepts of wellness, health care, and the various stages of the nursing process. The second two core courses are designed to extend the students' concepts and skills, together with an acquaintance with nursing functions in *both* episodic and distributive practice. As soon as students have completed the second core course, they may enroll in various electives in nursing science, including upper level courses in distributive and/or episodic care. Among the electives in episodic care are: Nursing Care in Physical Illness Crises; Nursing Care of the High Risk Mother; and Nursing Intervention in Specialized Care Units. Electives available in distributive care include: Nursing Intervention in the School Age Child; Perspectives in Aging Related to Nursing; Nursing Care of the Person with Addictive Behavior Patterns; and Nursing Care of the Handicapped Child. In addition to the formalized course electives, students are encouraged to engage in independent individual and group projects related to their own practice interests. These projects have varied from the development of a joint physical diagnosis seminar with medical students to the provision of staffing for a community hospital in a rural area of the state.[64]

The University of Wisconsin School of Nursing has been laboring since 1967 to develop, evaluate, and revise a new curricular model similar to, but even more extensive perhaps than, that at Kansas University. One of the major characteristics of the new program is that each student can choose, at the end of the second year, to concentrate in either distributive or episodic nursing. Through the use of concurrent tracking and elective learning opportunities, the students are developed as individuals prepared to serve "specialized professional functions."[65]

The faculty is agreed that there are knowledges and skills basic to all nursing practice; this core content is taught in the first two years of the baccalaureate program, thus enabling the ready transfer of students from other preparatory programs. There is agreement that it is no longer feasible to prepare nurses to care for all patients in all types of settings; the students are encouraged to concentrate and specialize in reasonably defined areas of practice.

The curriculum differs from the traditional in several ways: students enroll in nursing courses from their first year on; students take core courses which are interrelated with other health care programs; students progress at their individual rate through the program; and a considerable portion of the clinical experience is built around group practice, both in nursing teams and in interdisciplinary teams organized for delivery of care.

Still another variation of curricular concentration is to be found in the proposed pattern for Sonoma State College in California.[66] This is planned as a two-year upper-division program which is directly articulated with two-year associate degree programs. The lower-division courses will represent the preparatory core; the upper-division courses will provide for specialty concentrations.

In the first year of the upper division program, all students will focus upon community health inasmuch as the traditional lower division programs will have stressed episodic and acute care. Two other courses, one in combined sciences, the second in change processes, are general requirements. The students, however, choose between preceptorships in episodic or distributive nursing which include: field studies, clinical practice, surveys, and investigatory studies.

Selection of supporting courses and electives will be determined by the choice of preceptorship and prior educational and experiential background. The student in episodic nursing, for example, might choose more chemistry, physiology, or biochemistry. The distributive nursing student might elect to take additional courses in psychology, sociology, anthropology, or ethnic studies.

A recent proposal for curricular change in nursing education at Stanford proposed a three-level design to develop specialized nurse practitioners who possess extended skills in either episodic or distributive practice as well as an advanced consumer's knowledge of research related to that field and experience in collaborative delivery of care together with other health professionals.[67]

At the first level, all nurses would complete core seminars and laboratories while already selecting arts and science electives related to their intended areas of practice. A decision on the field of concentration would be required at the second level when the students would begin seminar and laboratory work in either episodic or distributive care. This would be supplemented by continued electives in related fields. At the third level, students would be involved in advanced case and field work and in clinically directed research. Electives would be geared to their individual projects and to the field of concentration.

Kathryn Smith, the developer of the proposal, has suggested examples (see Table 5-3) of the related electives that might be appropriate to the defined areas of practice.[68]

While these course listings are partial and tentative, they suggest the varied resources existing within the university setting that can be brought to bear on the enhancement of the nursing curriculum.

There is much to be done, both by the institutions housing nursing education programs and by the regional curriculum study groups, in assessing the needs and directions for the future of the upper-division program. With the support and assistance of the statewide master planning committees, we should be able to facilitate the pace of revision throughout the country. The impact of the National Commission's challenge is already evident, but these recorded efforts at the cutting edge of change must be multiplied. As Longway suggests, there is need to address change:

> The areas in which change will most likely be accommodated may be in a redefinition of nursing or in early specialization in the educational process. Perhaps the day of the general practitioner in nursing will go the way of the general practitioner in medicine. The recommendation for a two-track system of nursing preparation—episodic and distributive—may well indicate the direction of change for the future.[69]

Too many in nursing education have long voiced the opinion that specialization in nursing could only occur at the post-baccalaureate level. This betrays a lack of understanding both of the emergent two-year, four-year collegiate relationship and of the fact that much of our generalist education has truly been specialized

TABLE 5-3 COMPARATIVE SAMPLE OF ELECTIVE COURSES OUTSIDE NURSING SCIENCE FOR EPISODIC AND DISTRIBUTIVE PRACTICE CONCENTRATIONS

Episodic Majors	Distributive Majors
Level One	Level One
Principles of Biology	Community Medicine
Vertebrate Biology	The Environment of Man: Health Resources and Physical Environment
Physiological Basis of Behavior	Infectious Diseases of Man
Principles of Pharmacology	Human Nutrition
General Biochemistry	
Level Two	Level Two
The Family in a Hospital	Health Care Organization
Trauma and Emergencies	Personality Development in Childhood
Fetal and Neonatal Physiology	Methodology in Social Science
Abnormal Human Development	Family and Kinship
Medical Genetics	Comparative Social Systems
Level Three	Level Three
Statistical Methodology	Introduction to Sociological Research
Analysis of Data	Medical Anthropology
Methodology and Research Techniques	Field Methods in the Study of Organizations

education for episodic or acute practice. Shibboleths must give way to societal requirements and to common sense. The development of a true, deepened, and open upper division curriculum is one idea whose time has arrived and whose success is demonstrable. Its application and extension must become a priority for all collegiate nursing.

Lower Division Concentrations

When the programs in associate degree nursing were being developed, in addition to some common conceptions about technical and terminal programs, there was a general acceptance of preparing nurses for episodic practice. Like the hospital school and baccalaureate programs before them, the associate degree curriculum emphasized clinical experience in the medical service units of the hospital. And like the other programs, the ubiquitous title of "general nursing" was applied to the sequence and to its products. The most obvious distinction between the community college and the two older institutional forms has been the length of its curriculum rather than the difference in its experiential content.

Educational leaders at the community or junior college level have begun to raise significant questions about this replication of effort and about whether, indeed, their programs are general preparation for nursing. As DeChow puts it:

> It is time to move away from the concept that this program prepares a generalist. . . . I believe a registered nurse prepared at the associate degree level has a role in all clinical areas—in both episodic and distributive settings. But if she is to be an effective beginning practitioner in these settings, the education for her role must be different from what it is today.[70]

After pointing out that nursing teams will be required to deliver optimum care in both episodic and distributive settings, DeChow points out that it is critical, then, to ensure that beginning staff practitioners, prepared at the associate degree level, are ready to work in concert with advanced nurse clinicians in a variety of settings and with whatever patients need care. This logic leads inexorably to her point of decision:

> Would it be wiser for students, after having a broad basic core of nursing experiences which would allow for horizontal mobility in the field, to select a particular area of focus or concentration for the last quarter or semester of their basic nursing program—even at the AD level of preparation? I believe the answer to these questions is yes, and is not in contradiction to the purpose of the associate degree nursing program as originally envisioned.[71]

Similar awareness has already come to an increasing number of associate degree programs. Perhaps the most advanced of these, currently, is that planned by the faculty of Bakersfield College in California. The increasing demand from the community for beginning nurses prepared to serve in "family health nursing" has prompted the development of a parallel track system at the associate degree level for nurses who can now select a concentration in either episodic or distributive practice.[72] The decision has been reinforced by the positive reactions of physicians, administrators, and nursing students to the idea of developing these kinds of practitioners—and offering students an elective choice.

The faculty of the department of nursing was convinced that merely inserting some community health nursing into the established associate degree curriculum with its heavy concentration in episodic care would only dilute the quality of the latter. Rather, it was agreed that both types of practitioners are needed, and that both could be prepared in the same institution through the use of elective courses and a variety of clinical experiences.

The family health nurse program is now designed to prepare nurses for beginning practice in nonacute settings. The graduates should be capable of providing a level of primary care to individuals in the community, of coordinating the work of auxiliary health personnel, and of teaching health instruction in community settings. The nurse is also prepared to serve as a team member, under the guidance of a clinical nurse or master nurse clinician in the community or public health setting.

In the first year of the collegiate program, students from the two areas attend the same nursing science courses and clinical experiences. These in combination represent the core of the curriculum. In the second year, however, the elective concentrations come into play. While the episodic student major is involved in the traditional courses and clinical settings, the family health major will be working in health departments, neighborhood treatment centers, and mental health clinics. The last semester of the second year includes extended work in: local agencies, epidemiology, health teaching, and comprehensive health service.

Developments, like those at Bakersfield, are beginning to reach the implementation stage in Florida, Missouri, Indiana, and Illinois. With more than forty percent of our nursing students now being admitted to associate degree programs, and with the affinity that these institutions have for innovation and experimentation, it is conceivable that rapid change might be engendered. This would, in the opinion of the National Commission, be very positive, but would be even more effective if it is jointly planned and articulated with emergent trends in upper division programs in nursing education.

The indications seem quite clear. There is a place for concentrated study in nursing at the associate degree level which is positively related to both societal requirements and the steady encroachment of specialization throughout the entire nursing profession. Recognizing that our traditional programs and curricula have involved concentration in episodic practice, we can now balance the picture and begin to provide practitioners for the full range of the health care system. In doing so, interinstitutional planning can make for effective programming and close articulation. That, in turn, will ensure not only better health care but improved career mobility for the students involved.

GRADUATE EDUCATION IN NURSING[73]

Almost lost sometimes in the emphasis on preparatory nursing education, with its bifurcated patterns and unarticulated ladders, is a recognition of the need for graduate nursing education. In *An Abstract for Action,* the National Commission sought to address this concern and restore it to perspective. There are critical needs for nurses who have advanced, formal preparation, in at least four areas:

1. Clinical nurses or master nurse clinicians capable of providing excellent direct care while serving as a role model and preceptor for nursing students and less experienced practitioners.
2. Instructors and professors for educational positions in the emergent collegiate pattern.
3. Specialists in the organization and delivery of nursing services in both episodic and distributive care settings.
4. Researchers prepared to investigate and enlarge the *corpus* of nursing knowledge.

In 1972, there were approximately eighty graduate programs in nursing education. In total, these enrolled approximately 4,100 full-time and 1,600 part-time students. In terms of our identified areas of critical need, there were almost 1,700 full-time students in programs leading to advanced clinical practice, 1,400 enrolled in teacher preparation, 700 in health delivery organization, and 300 in advanced research. Both the number of programs and students have shown small, but steady, incremental growth since 1958. The total number of students, however, is far below our needs in any area, and the support for these programs has been largely, and in some cases almost entirely, from federal appropriations under the Health Manpower and Nurse Training Acts. State governments and private foundations, with few exceptions, have remained uninvolved in graduate nursing education, and the general public is largely unaware of the proposition however attuned it might be to problems in preparatory institutions.

Because we have been laggard in our provision of opportunities and support for advanced education, the National Commission was concerned that careful stock be taken of needs and resources in order to determine how best to "catch up." There is no question that we need to attack all four areas of indicated need; we cannot, however, do an effective job, simultaneously, across the board without large amounts of aid. Moreover, there are variations in levels of need from one area to another, and there are also differences in the capacity of the various states to respond to the several requirements. Obviously, a state without a graduate program in nursing is not likely to start—nor should it—by establishing a doctoral program. To ensure local participation in the planning and ranking of priorities, the Commission therefore proposed:

> The state master planning committee . . . be particularly concerned that the number of graduate programs in nursing be consistent with human and economic resources, and that the inauguration or expansion of weak programs not be permitted.[74]

To provide the wherewithal for carrying out this plan of controlled expansion, the Commission suggested that federal, state, and private funds support the development of programs and personnel that could meet the identified needs. Thus, early progress from 1970 through 1972 in the development of federal support for nursing education was encouraging. In fiscal 1972, the actual funds supplied nursing for all educational and support programs amounted to $144.9 million. Almost $31 million of this was assigned to scholarships and traineeships that were related to specific student aid. The total administration request for fiscal 1974, however, is less than $53 million, with substantial reductions in both scholarships and traineeships.

The long and short of this is that state funds, particularly those realized through revenue sharing, and private support must be expected to play a larger part in advanced nursing education than ever before. There are, of course, possibilities that budgetary compromises and adjustments will be worked out between the legislative and executive branches of our federal government. There is little likelihood, however, that funds for graduate nursing education would be more than maintained in categories and amounts similar to those of fiscal 1973. And this is not conducive to meeting the needs of our health care system.

The Commission and its staff have undertaken informational activities related to these concerns; however, it seems clear that the statewide master planning and joint practice committees will be in a much more salient position in the immediate future to influence decisions and allocations. It is fortuitous that so much progress has been made in multidisciplinary planning, because now, more than ever before, we need to have cooperative assessment and joint presentation of needs and proposals. Meanwhile, we can briefly inventory some of the needs of graduate education in nursing.

Two general observations should be made before we look into the four personnel areas. The first is that eighty graduate programs in nursing are quite few in comparison with 1,350 preparatory programs. That same number of graduate programs, however, looms larger when we consider the fact that there are only 4,100 full-time graduate students across the nation—an average of little more than fifty students per graduate nursing program. State master planning committees must look closely at the mass of these graduate programs, and severely question the inauguration of any new programs until established ones can demonstrate their lack of capacity. The resources of faculty and facilities, as well as finance, can be overextended. We do not need more graduate programs in nursing if they reduce the quality of the ones we have or if they simply redistribute the same general numbers of students among a few more programs—thus reducing the student-program ratio.

The second general observation, noted in the investigation phase and reconfirmed frequently throughout the implementation phase, is that nurse educators and state master planning committees, as well as the regional curriculum planning groups, must question the length and the academic requirements associated with graduate education in nursing. Many of the master's degree programs in nursing require up to seventy semester credit hours and two years, or more, for completion. In contrast, many academic disciplines require thirty to thirty-six hours and one academic or calendar year for the master's degree. This is particularly true when, as in the case of nursing, the undergraduate major is in the same field. The National Commission's staff has suggested two factors that, taken together, tend to explain the lengthy graduate programs in nursing:

1. The traditional curriculum of the generic baccalaureate program in nursing meant that these students did not, in truth, receive upper division nursing courses prior to entering graduate school. In their junior and senior years, they received courses similar to those taught in the associate degree institutions.
2. Nurse educators, having fought so long and hard for academic acceptance and respectability, now approach graduate education with a zeal to be "purer than Caesar's wife." In doing so, they seek to produce graduates who need fear comparison to no one—and they create requirements second to none.

These statements are made with only a touch of hyperbole. It will become apparent, as collegiate institutions are articulated and true lower- and upper-division curricula emerge, that graduate programs, particularly for the master's degree, may be reduced in length and demands with no diminution in quality or output. This is an important consideration both in institutional and statewide master planning because the present system operates to increase costs significantly and to reduce the numbers of applicants. A shorter program with high standards, but fewer academic "hurdles," would lower per capita costs of graduate nursing education by a considerable factor.

Advanced Clinical Practitioners

The fastest growing area of concentration in graduate nursing education is that of advanced clinical practice. By 1970, the clinical programs had enrolled more students than any of the other graduate majors, and many of the newer institutional programs had just begun to accept students. There are programs of choice in four general areas (medical-surgical, maternal-child, psychiatric-mental, and public health nursing) with a number of specialties and divisions within them. These programs and their graduates are the nucleus from which we must recruit the advanced nurse clinicians and master clinicians required to man the developmental model of the emerging health care delivery system.

The sheer poverty of our efforts to date is staggering. From 1966 to 1970, for example, we graduated 2,000 advanced clinical practitioners from all of our graduate programs combined. If we consider for just a moment the fact that there are approximately 7,000 hospitals in the United States, not to mention all the other kinds of existent and emerging health care facilities, plus the growing demand for community practitioners, then the enormity of the situation is appalling.

Strides have been made, nonetheless, toward improving the situation. More than one-third of the graduates cited above completed their work in 1970. In 1971, there were almost 1,600 students enrolled in master's programs, and this figure went up again slightly in 1972. The deficit, however, in terms of needed practitioners, particularly in distributive care, has likely widened.

Decisions made over the next two years will be critical in determining whether or not we produce the clinical practitioners required. A combination of improved support, increased enrollment, and shortened academic programs could go a long way toward matching supply with demand. Without each of those ingredients, however, the prospects are dim, to say the least.

Qualified Nurse Faculty

As real as the shortage of advanced practitioners is the shortage of qualified faculty for the some 1,350 educational institutions in nursing, and for the increasing number of continuing and in-service educational programs. In the period from 1966 through 1970, approximately 3,300 nurses received master's degrees in educational specialties. In contrast to the clinical practice majors, however, there has been some indication of a slight drop in enrollments in these teacher preparation sequences.

In the face of the progressive transition of nursing education from a dual system into a single, collegiate pattern, there must be an accompanying shift of faculty members from the closing to the emerging institutions. This poses a unique problem in nursing education. As indicated previously in Table 5-1, more than seventy-five percent of the faculty in hospital schools of nursing hold either no degree or that of the baccalaureate. Thus, there is a pool of some six to seven thousand individuals who will need to pursue advanced preparation to increase their capacity for teaching and, at the same time, enhance their opportunities for future advancement in academic rank and recognition. Unless means are provided, these individuals cannot make the shift to the collegiate institution.

This problem is of such significance to the re-patterning of education that the National Commission has urged collegiate schools to appoint faculty members from the hospital schools on the basis of their ability and experience, while, at the same time, providing opportunities for extending formal academic study. The Commission has also urged that:

> Congress provide earmarked funds for faculty members of schools of nursing to enable them to obtain additional formal academic preparation equal to that required for regular appointment to faculty posts in collegiate institutions. These funds should have forgiveness features based on years of continuing service.[75]

A developmental program such as this, encouraged by the statewide master planning committees on the basis of their analyses of area needs and resources, could provide a shorter, more efficient, less expensive approach to meeting the shortage of nurse faculty. In the long run, however, we must nurture institutional support, increased enrollment, and attractive programs to produce the numbers we need.

Leadership in Care Delivery

As surely as changing patterns are affecting our needs for clinical expertise and faculty preparedness, so the growing complexity of health care delivery demands more skilled and qualified nurses in positions of administrative leadership. Not only is there the demand to provide more care to all people, but there is an insistence that it be delivered through new kinds of institutional and organizational structures. At the heart of the problem for nursing administration is a growing recognition that many traditional functions and tasks need to be reexamined, and a new role set established. In the Commission publication, "New Patterns in Nursing Administration: The Vanishing Supervisor," there is clear documentation of two interrelated trends.[76] The first is the divestment of more and more non-nursing functions by nursing service and administration. The second is a resumption of care functions, both episodic and distributive, by senior nurses who formerly devoted almost all their time to systems maintenance.

These trends, of course, are only reported by the Commission; they were set in motion by nurses, and nurse administrators particularly. In terms of educational preparation, these developments mean that the individuals involved must not only develop organizational and leadership skills, but they must maintain greater currency with clinical practice than we have formerly thought necessary. To provide this leadership, nursing graduated some 1,600 individuals from advanced programs in administration in the period from 1966 to 1970. These figures would seem to be in better balance with expressed need than most other areas of advanced preparation except that the functional reexamination of the administrative role began in this same period and only now, perhaps, are we getting changed input into the curricular programs of graduate schools. Thus, even our more recent graduates have likely been prepared for a traditional role that is rapidly being altered.

We need, then, to maintain support levels for graduate education in nursing administration while, at the same time, encouraging program changes that can facilitate the restructuring of health care institutions.

Fostering Research Capability

In Chapter Four, we discussed the National Commission's concern for enlarging the scope of nursing practice through research into the basic aspects of intervention and care. Support and funding of nursing research have always been problematic, but intimately related to the matter of funding is the fact that we have a great need to develop more qualified nurses capable of conducting rigorous inquiry into the clinical practice of their profession.

In the United States, today, there are between 600 and 700 nurses who have completed doctoral programs which involve research training and significant original investigatory work. (It is not so much the advanced degree that is important as the fact that this is the level at which true research competency is developed.) This small number of people, dispersed among the nation's educational and care facilities, is simply inadequate to the task of developing a corpus of knowledge to direct improved nursing practice. The situation is not likely to better itself very rapidly. As indicated in Figure 5-4, the total number of nursing students enrolled in doctoral programs has risen slowly over the years, ranging from 100 to 300 students at any one time.

Enrollment is not a sure measure of completion. Over the entire period, 1957 through 1972, approximately 250 students received the doctoral degree—a figure far below the number of students in course. In concrete terms, the net effect of the situation is to depress the number and quality of research projects in nursing practice—over and beyond the limitations imposed by inadequate funding.

The announced reduction in federal requests for support of nursing trainee-

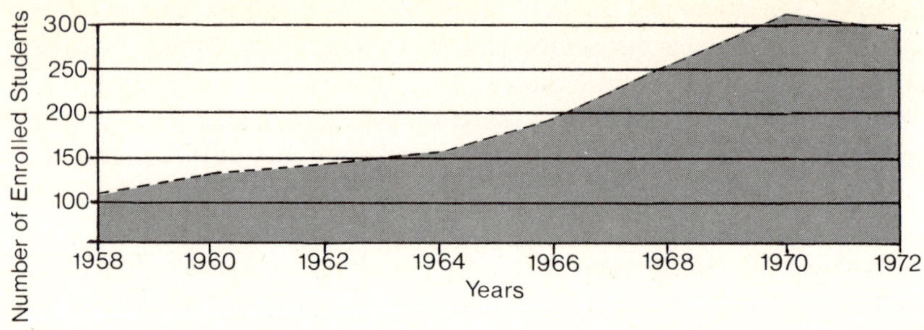

Figure 5-4. Enrollment of nursing students in doctoral programs, 1958-1972.

ships and scholarships comes at an acute time for nursing research. We need time and support for developing capable individuals, and we need time and support to capitalize on their ensuing discoveries. The statewide master planning and joint practice committees will find the areas of research and research training among the thorniest problems they will deal with.

CONTINUING EDUCATION IN NURSING

In the course of the investigation phase, the National Commission found that one area of universal concern and almost uncommon agreement was that of continuing education. A survey of medical societies, hospital associations, state departments of health, health insurance groups, planning representatives, and a wide variety of nursing groups found more than ninety percent agreement to the proposition that "social change and technological advances will increase the emphasis on continuing education in nursing." Similar consensus was apparent in the matter of in-service nursing education.

For purposes of distinguishing these two kinds of educational programs, the National Commission used the following definitions:[77]

> *Continuing Education.* Formalized learning experiences or sequences designed to enlarge the knowledge or skills of practitioners. As distinct from graduate education, continuing education courses tend to be more specific, of generally shorter duration, and may result in certificates of completion or specialization, but not in formal academic degrees.
>
> *Inservice Education.* Programs administered by an employer designed to upgrade the knowledge or skills of persons functioning within that agency.

These definitions are not sacrosanct, but they help to emphasize differences in specificity and control that are important in planning the extended education of the practitioner. From the standpoint of the Commission's involvement, we were most concerned with continuing education, but recognized its interrelationship with inservice education and the need for interagency planning at all levels.

Evolving care delivery, and changed nursing roles, have mandated some form of continuing education for all practitioners. The intensive care nurse in 1973, faced with immediate decision making for a cardiac patient, must have more specialized knowledge about patient response to respiratory support measures, electronic monitoring hazards, and onset of physical malfunction than would be required of a general medical practitioner. And, this is only an indicative example of changes in both distributive and episodic care. Continuing education, then, is far more than a one-time-only brush-up of information and skills. It is of equal importance with preparatory education and may be an even more integral part of excellence in clinical practice.

For continuing education to be soundly planned and efficiently conducted, there must be some more systematic approach than the laissez-faire operation we have employed. It is extremely expensive, for example, to have every institution that educates or employs nurses attempt to provide all the courses, workshops, or internships that might be required for the evolving practice specialties. As a matter of fact, this is so impossible that its attempt would likely have a disheartening effect on programming. Furthermore, letting each institution do only what it prefers may not meet the overall needs of patient care.

The best alternative seems to reside with the statewide master planning committees. These groups are in a unique position to assess the needs and resources of large planning areas for continuing education in nursing, and then to apply those findings to a matrix of institutional and geographic givens. In *An Abstract for Action*, the National Commission recommended:

> The state master planning committee for nursing education identify one or more institutions to be responsible for regional coverage of continuing education programs for nurses within that area.[78]

In addition, the Commission suggested those committees consider regional planning for many aspects of continuing education through such vehicles as the interstate compacts on higher education, and the development of increased interdisciplinary approaches to continuing education that reflect the growth of team delivery of health care.

It is significant that many of the statewide master planning committees have taken an early interest in continuing education; Kansas, one of the nine target states, has developed and proposed a master plan for continuing education throughout the state and Colorado is presently engaged in a similar developmental project.

During the course of implementation, the Commission and its staff worked with state groups and the interstate compacts to encourage the growth of planning and cooperative action for continuing education. In doing so, we made particular efforts to work with the National Conferences on Continuing Education for Nurses, the organizing group from those sessions, and the emergent organizations specifically directed at continuing education concerns such as Midwest Continuing Professional Education for Nurses. As the leadership group that had promoted the

National Conferences became more convinced of the desirability of formal organization, an ad hoc committee was formed to work in liaison with the National Commission staff to further our joint interests in continuing education. One result of this cooperation was the publication of the Commission pamphlet on "Continuing Education in Nursing: Necessity and Opportunity."[79] The beginnings generated by the ad hoc committee continued even after the new ANA Council on Continuing Education was established as the outcome of the search, by the original National Conference group, for an "organized home".

One of the initiators of both the conferences and the Council on Continuing Education, Betty Gwaltney, discussed the joint work, in a letter to the NCSNNE Director:

> You undoubtedly know the ANA Council on Continuing Education has finally been launched. . . . I will honestly say that the support . . . your staff have given to the National Conference meetings on Continuing Education in Nursing and the Organizing Group for the promotion of the Council has helped immeasurably to move all of us concerned with continuing education towards our now accomplished goals in record time.[80]

Appreciated as these comments are, the fact of the matter is that the various groups in continuing education have been instrumental in focusing attention on the needs of the practitioner for continuous professional involvement in the enhancement of care. Through the interaction between these groups and the Commission, there is evidence that planning and institutional commitment have increased, ensuring that the nurses' needs will be met.

Few would disagree with the necessity for the practitioner to keep skills and knowledge current. However, while emphasizing the importance of gearing up a plan and a system for continuing education, the National Commission has agreed with the many nursing organizations that have looked with dismay at recent efforts to connect relicensure of nurses with evidence of continuing education. The concerns that the nursing organizations, and the Commission, share include: the necessity for providing means before one demands compliance; and the entire question of recording and accounting for the varied educational experiences of hundreds of thousands of individuals. These very practical matters need further thought and planning.

The ANA Council on Continuing Education has already issued an "Interim Statement on Continuing Education," and there has been interorganizational agreement in nursing on basic approaches to be taken.[81] This encouraging progress should not be short circuited by a rush to enact legislation that will be at best difficult to implement and at worst unworkable.

OTHER EDUCATIONAL CONCERNS

Throughout *An Abstract for Action* there runs the thread of interdisciplinary education both in preparatory programs and in continuing work experiences. It seems so simple that we should prepare health practitioners together in order for them to work together later. However, like many another simple idea, the complexity of putting it into effect is enormous. There are approximately 100 schools of medicine and 1,350 schools of nursing. Most beginning students in nursing are female undergraduates whereas most medical students are older, more academically experienced, and male. A litany therefore could be composed of all the obstacles to joint education. Nonetheless, an increasing number of institutions, student associations, and practitioners are attempting to do something about the situation. At the Universities of Kansas and Rochester, for example, medical and nursing students are learning basic diagnostic procedures together and faculty members from the University of California recently reported on teaching strategies developed out of collaborative experience.[82] Likewise, a number of the regional medical programs have sponsored joint practitioner learning sessions. And an increasing number of collegiate programs in nursing are using medical school courses which bring students of the two professions together in the classroom. Perhaps the single most significant step to date, however, has been the selection of interprofessional education for joint practice[83] as one of the three beginning task forces of the National Joint Practice Commission. The emphasis thus placed on the interdependence and collaborative learning of the major health practicing professions may serve to overturn the forces of inertia and parochialism.

A second consideration in the general development of nursing education is that of widened access for students from a variety of backgrounds and socioeconomic levels. American nursing has long distinguished itself by its concerns for the care and recruitment of the disadvantaged. It is obvious, however, that more than concern is needed to overcome the obstacles that impede occupational mobility. The National Student Nurses' Association, supported by a $100,000 federal grant, is now engaged in a systematic effort in five target areas to recruit, "Black, Spanish-speaking, and Indian Americans, including men," into a nursing career.[84] This commendable approach adds planning and follow-through that is not often present in efforts to effect social change.

Nursing, now, must squarely face the fact that it remains a predominately white, middle class, female institution. It must strive to diversify itself by widening its doors to applicants from the many other groups within our society. Among the obvious groups to be approached are: men, particularly those with a demonstrated interest in the health care occupations; racial and ethnic minorities; college graduates without settled occupational plans; mature women returning to the occupational labor force after marriage and family; and the great numbers of aides, practical nurses and other health workers who naturally look to nursing as an avenue for advancement.

There are merits in almost any plan to increase career opportunities; the National Commission emphasizes, however, that its recommendations concerning recruitment of the disadvantaged and the under represented into nursing is not primarily for the purpose of social amelioration. Rather, it is to increase the quality of input into the nursing profession through tapping the best individuals wherever they may be found. The ultimate goal that nursing might seek to achieve is the development of a practicing profession that generally mirrors the population to be served. That objective should be tempered by the determination to maintain quality as the first priority in any recruitment efforts.

Still another area for development is that directed at bringing nursing education and practice back into a more unified relationship. In the general development of collegiate nursing, there has been an unfortunate separation of service and education that must be healed through a deliberate campaign of rapprochement. The National Commission has urged a variety of approaches to this end, including the use of joint appointments and the organizational reestablishment of combined departments.[85] While a number of institutions have initiated efforts in these directions, the NLN Council of Diploma Programs[86] and the task force[87] to study the Commission's report both expressed reservations about the proposal. The latter group indicated that its concerns were primarily directed at the problem of involving the top echelons from education and practice in these arrangements because of the workload now involved in these positions. The specifics of the arrangements can be worked out in the crucible of experience, but the general proposition of closer relationships is one that the Commission feels is essential. The combined activity of the statewide groups in educational planning and joint practice should produce impetus from both ends toward the reconstruction of a broadly based middle ground in which service and education are intimately involved in developmental activities jointly arrived at and mutually conducted. Only then will the two arms of professional nursing be rejoined in a common mission.

COSTS OF NURSING EDUCATION

In the early months of the implementation phase, the National Commission received a number of inquiries concerning the mounting costs of nursing education. Many of these were directly related to the transitional movement from hospital schools into collegiate institutions. Of the more than 200 preparatory programs closed in the period from 1958 to 1968, many reported costs to be an important, if not necessarily determinative, factor in their decision. On the other hand, many of the emergent programs found themselves under budgetary limitations which severely restricted the number of students they could accept. Overall, many preparatory programs reported that their costs were being scrutinized carefully in comparison with other kinds of academic departments.

In order to provide some assistance to the schools of nursing, the Commission staff reviewed two earlier major studies of educational costs produced by the National League for Nursing[88] and compared their results with two recently completed statewide studies in New York[89] and Tennessee.[90] These latter investigations demonstrated consistency with the national surveys, but provided us with dollar amounts more attuned to the seventies. The report of the Commission's analysis noted two significant generalizations:[91]

> 1. The costs for the professional nursing portion of a student's program ran between three and four times the costs of the related general academic portion, although the student time was roughly divided equally between the two areas.
>
> 2. In all programs reviewed, there was a considerable and widening gap between "income" from sources such as tuition, and "expense" in terms of academic salaries, costs of instruction, overhead, etc.

In Tennessee, for example, the average cost of a baccalaureate nursing program for a single student was a little more than $12,000 for the entire four years. The professional sequence constituted more than $9,000 of the total while the related arts and science courses comprised less than $3,000. In large part this is explained by the greater costs of any program which involves clinical practice. Professional education, with its supervised student teaching, has higher costs than liberal arts programs. Nursing, however, tends to be more expensive than professional education due to its lengthier periods of close supervision in practice settings, low faculty-student ratios, and concomitant increases in indirect expense related to these factors. While few would argue for reduced clinical supervision in nursing education, there is some indication that costs related to faculty-student ratios might be alleviated. In a comparison of "small" and "large" programs, there was consistent evidence of reduced per capita costs among those programs with more than 200 students as contrasted to those with fewer than 100.

On the basis of this finding, plus the related experience of working with a number of schools exploring various forms of consolidation or joint operation, the National Commission recommended that:

> Small programs be terminated or consolidated into larger programs in order to reduce the per unit costs of education and in order to make better allocation of qualified faculty.[92]

While the state planning committees can review and recommend the rearrangement of nursing programs throughout their areas in order to arrive at more effective numbers and sizes of institutions, the reduction of per unit cost will not solve the entire problem of nursing education costs.

In both New York and Tennessee, there was a sharp disparity between student tuition and institutional costs—even among those schools with lower per capita expense. In Tennessee, baccalaureate students met approximately twenty-seven percent of their costs through tuition while junior collegiate students paid for about nineteen percent of their total educational expense. Most educational administrators—and parents—would agree that tuition has a practical ceiling and that it is not reasonable to increase tuition to the point where it could cover all costs. This is particularly true when there is a commitment to recruit students from disadvantaged socio-economic groups.

If tuition does not cover costs, then obviously, support is coming from somewhere else. The "somewhere else" in the case of nursing education is the harboring institution, public agencies, and private philanthropy.

Historically, the primary source of support has been the educational institution that houses the nursing program. The schools themselves have made up the considerable difference between income and actual expense through endowments, contributions, and other sources of income. It must be recognized, however, that when an institution supports nursing education in this manner, it is, in effect, requiring other people and other departments to subsidize the program through the redistribution of funds in a manner disproportionate to generated income. As in the case of student tuition, there is a practical limit to how much an individual institution can do and how willing other departments and schools may be to support nursing.

Public agencies, in recent years, have played a larger role in the provision of financial support to nursing education. The growth of the community college system has had a considerable effect on the support structure of nursing education. Whereas over eighty percent of the hospital school programs are located in private institutions, more than ninety percent of the community college programs are found in public institutions. This means that the general tax base of the area and/or the state is used to subsidize the difference between tuition and educational costs. In addition to the support of public colleges, a number of states have provided scholarship funds, institutional grants, and incentive programs to encourage an increase in class size.

Federal support of nursing education showed a dramatic expansion over the sixties and into the seventies. Millions of dollars were provided in student assistance through loans, scholarships, and traineeships.

These student assistance programs, however, did not meet the critical need of the institution to make up the difference between tuition and expense. For this purpose, the federal government supplied additional money for construction, institutional financial distress, and capitation grants for program enlargement. (It is in precisely this area that the greatest effects of President Nixon's proposed budget for 1974 will be felt.) While student loans and scholarships are to be retained, even if somewhat reduced, the entire area of institutional support will be removed except for the carry-over of limited funds for projects already authorized and underway.

This development, along with the promise of revenue sharing among the states, makes the task of the statewide master planning committees more crucial than originally thought. All nursing programs, wherever located, have commonly experienced an institutional deficit between income and expense. State funds have helped to reduce these losses, particularly through the extension of the public sector of higher education. The anticipated loss of federal funds, however, must be considered a severe economic threat to many educational institutions. The National Commission—as well as related health professions—has moved to alert the state planning groups to this situation. At this point in time, no one knows what the precise results of the budgetary proposals will be, but it is evident that nursing education must continue to receive broad help from public agencies and governing levels if we are to maintain viable institutional programs.

It is likely that private philanthropy and foundations can continue to make their greatest contribution to nursing education through the support of specific research and innovation. This support, however, should be directed at those areas for which public funds are not available and should encourage experimentation and demonstration rather than long-term support.

Given the opportunity through improved statewide master planning, nursing can generate a convincing case for needed support; it is essential that the profession and the public recognize the mutuality of the problem and the necessity for prompt resolution.

SUMMARY

In *An Abstract for Action,* the National Commission proposed twenty-two specific recommendations dealing with nursing education, its institutional patterns, articulation, advanced programs, and financial support.

Its first priority was to seek consensus on, and accelerated movement toward, a comprehensive collegiate pattern of nursing education. This concept is not new, but the intensive effort to publicize its necessity and to propose alternative measures for accomplishing it has been unique. In the past three years, there has been, for a variety of reasons, steady progress toward resolution of the traditional stand-off between collegiate and noncollegiate nursing programs. For the first time in American history, we have seen a majority of nursing students in collegiate schools and a majority of institutional programs housed in the colleges. Since 1970, there has been a reduction of twenty-two percent in the number of hospital schools; a clear trend seems to have been set in motion.

The establishment of a collegiate pattern for nursing education is not an end in itself. It is simply the first step toward a reformation of all nursing education so that a clear plan of curricular anticipation can be generated between two- and four-year institutions. The National Commission has publicized, encouraged and assisted a number of experimental programs designed to show that the junior and senior colleges can have jointly planned, interlocking programs that facilitate career mobility and enhance depth of learning. This is particularly critical for nursing in the face of accumulated evidence that sixty percent of all nurses will, in the next ten years, be graduating from associate degree programs. These schools and their graduates will look to the senior colleges to provide upper division programs that mesh with an extend the educational pattern.

With the articulation of these two kinds of collegiate programs, we can move toward the resolution of educational concentrations in nursing. A growing body of data testifies to the fact that nurses cannot be prepared to practice effectively over the full range of human care needs, in all settings, and in all cases. If we accept the concept that some degree of concentration, or specialization, will be required, then it is necessary to reexamine our present curricular structure to see what elements of specialty are already incorporated in what we have traditionally regarded as our generalist preparatory program. If, as the Commission contends, these programs are essentially aimed at the development of nurse practitioners to function in episodic care, then we must look to the development of alternative sequences that prepare qualified clinicians for distributive care. Again, the Commission has encouraged and publicized experimental programs of concentration in both upper and lower division levels and has published reports on the outcomes of a number of demonstration projects.

Related to all this has been cooperative planning with two large scale curriculum projects—one by the Southern Regional Education Board and the other by an Orange County educational consortium—to develop planned articulation, curricular interlocking, and practice concentrations which will provide impetus to a strengthened collegiate pattern for nursing education.

Over and beyond the concerns of preparatory nursing, the Commission has worked with institutions and organizations involved in graduate and continuing education for nursing. These areas of professional development are essential to the qualitative growth of practice and education and deserve comparable attention and assistance. Our present inability to produce advanced clinicians and qualified faculty is a limiting factor to the overall progress of nursing and its contribution of health care delivery. Therefore, we must expend post-preparatory educational opportunities.

In order to bring about this reorientation and reformation, the Commission has not only worked with the nursing organizations at national and state levels, but has helped in the establishment of structures that can facilitate needed changes—the statewide master planning committees. To date, approximately half the states have moved to the operational stage of development in master planning, and very few have not made at least some progress toward that end. These multidisciplinary groups composed of nurses, other health professionals, educators, and consumer representatives are charged with examining educational needs and resources and with effecting those changes required to produce a comprehensive and articulated system of nursing education throughout the states. Many of these groups have already made substantial progress and their recommendations have begun to make impact among educational and health planning agencies.

Some progress has been made in related concerns for interdisciplinary educational programs between medicine and nursing, the widening of recruitment efforts, and the rapprochement of nursing education and service in joint efforts to improve health care and teaching. In these efforts, the further work of the state master planning and joint practice committees can provide continuing encouragement and a communications network to disseminate information on successful projects and approaches.

The overriding problem in nursing education, and one that may be heightened by the President's budgetary recommendations, is that of financial support. Tuition charges have never borne the full expense of educational costs in nursing—and it is unlikely that they ever can. The growth of the public sector in nursing education has meant that more institutions are receiving help from state and local tax proceeds and this has been of help. Several of the states have institutional support programs for nursing education in addition to the general funding provided state and community colleges.

It must be emphasized, however, that state and federal funds provided for student support and scholarships do not go to the critical area of deficit between tuition and expense. As a matter of fact, adding students who are induced through receipt of scholarships merely lengthens the dollar gap that the institution experiences. For this reason, federal programs of institutional support, including construction grants, capitation funds, and financial distress payments have been a vital element in program planning. Elimination or redirection of these funds through revenue sharing poses, therefore, an awesome problem that nursing and the statewide master planning committees must address. The solutions produced will determine the constraints on nursing education for some time to come.

In pursuance of the implementation of its educational recommendations, the National Commission anticipated and found some organizational opposition. The NLN Council of Diploma Programs voted nonsupport of seven of the twenty-two recommendations including all those which related to changing the institutional patterns in preparatory nursing education. The AHA Assembly of Hospital Schools of Nursing adopted a resolution calling for the repudiation of all those alluding to the phasing out of diploma programs. The NLN Task Force to study *An Abstract for Action* accepted eighteen of the twenty-two recommendations as stated, proposed minor word modifications in three, and deleted one recommendation posed minor word modifications in three, and deleted one recommendation—that dealing with the transformation of a hospital school into a collegiate institution.

On the whole, however, the degree of controversy was less than had been expected, largely because the general trend of institutional patterning is now set. Some individuals have called for a last ditch stand to preserve hospital schools of nursing, but it is not likely that many institutions will follow that lead in the face of mounting economic and social pressures.

The greatest area of concern left to the Commission, aside from the ever-present problem of financial support, is the development of improved articulation between the two levels of collegiate programs. Experimentation and demonstration have taken place in both kinds of institutions and the general outcomes have been impressive and encouraging to the concept that true interinstitutional planning and programming can take place. The overall inertia is still considerable, however, and it will remain to the nursing organizations and the statewide master planning committees to continue the movements that have begun in this direction. The interinstitutional curriculum study groups and higher education planning bodies will also have significant effects on the articulation of nursing education. In the last analysis, however, nurses themselves must exert the initiative for change.

FOOTNOTES

1. Goldmark, Josephine. *Nursing and Nursing Education in the United States.* New York: The Macmillan Co., 1923.
2. Brown, Esther L. *Nursing for the Future.* New York: Russell Sage Foundation, 1948.
3. Committee on the Function of Nursing. *A Program for the Nursing Profession.* Eli Ginzberg, Chairman. New York: The Macmillan Co., 1948.
4. Bridgman, Margaret. *Collegiate Education for Nursing.* New York: Russell Sage Foundation, 1953.
5. The National Commission for the Study of Nursing and Nursing Education. *An Abstract for Action.* Jerome P. Lysaught, Director. New York: McGraw-Hill Book Co., 1970.
6. Resolution adopted by the Annual Assembly of Hospital Schools of Nursing, Type VIII Membership of the American Hospital Association, dated October, 1971.
7. "Statement on Report of National Commission for the Study of Nursing and Nursing Education." *Hospitals.* 45:10:131 (May) 1971.
8. *An Abstract for Action,* op. cit., pp. 156-157.
9. "Less Time, More Options: Education Beyond High School." The Carnegie Commission on Higher Education, June, 1971, p. 15.
10. *Facts About Nursing,* 1970-71 Edition. New York: American Nurses' Association, 1971, pp. 106-107.
11. The National Commission for the Study of Nursing and Nursing Education. *An Abstract for Action: Appendices.* Jerome P. Lysaught, Director. New York: McGraw-Hill Book Co., 1971, pp. 287-327.
12. *Facts About Nursing,* op. cit., pp. 37-42.
13. Altman, Stuart H. *Present & Future Supply of Registered Nurses.* Washington, D.C.: U.S. Department of Health, Education, and Welfare, DHEW Publication No. NIH 72-134, 1971, pp. 65-95.
14. Personal communication from Margaret E. Walsh, Secretary and General Director, NLN, to Jerome P. Lysaught, Director, NCSNNE, dated February 23, 1971.
15. "Report of the Task Force to Study the Implications of the Recommendations Presented in *An Abstract for Action.*" *Nursing Outlook.* 21:2:115 (February) 1973.
16. ibid., p. 114.
17. Personal communication from Frances K. Peterson, Director, Department of Diploma Programs, NLN, to Jerome P. Lysaught, Director, NCSNNE, dated May 15, 1972.
18. "The Diploma Nurse. the Hospital School, and the National Commission." Rochester, N.Y.: The National Commission for the Study of Nursing and Nursing Education, 1972 (pamphlet).
19. "National Commission and Governing Council of Diploma Schools Seek Mutual Aims in Education." News release of the National Commission for the Study of Nursing and Nursing Education, dated March, 1972.
20. "Type VIII Members Meet." *Hospitals.* 47:1:94-95 (January) 1973.
21. Christy, Teresa E., Poulin, Muriel A., and Julie Hover. "An Appraisal of *An Abstract for Action.*" *American Journal of Nursing.* 71:8:1581 (August) 1971.
22. "From Diploma School to College: Two Case Studies on Changing Patterns Within Institutions for Nursing Education." Rochester, N.Y.: The National Commission for the Study of Nursing and Nursing Education, 1970 (pamphlet).
23. ibid.
24. See Appendix A, "Publications Related to *An Abstract for Action.*"
25. "Costs of Nursing Education and A Case for its Greater Support." Rochester, N.Y.: The National Commission for the Study of Nursing and Nursing Education, 1970 (pamphlet).
26. *An Abstract for Action,* op. cit., p. 107.
27. ibid., p. 158.
28. "A Guide for Establishing Statewide Master Planning Committees." Rochester, N.Y.: The National Commission for the Study of Nursing and Nursing Education, 1970 (pamphlet).
29. *Nursing in Virginia.* Report of the Governor's Committee on Nursing, 1969. Available from the State Council for Higher Education in Virginia.
30. *Nurses for Wisconsin's Future.* Report of the Commission on Statewide Planning for Nursing Education, 1970. Available from the Wisconsin Nurses' Association.
31. *The Need to Know.* Report of the North Dakota Joint Committee on Nursing Needs and Resources, 1969. Available from the North Dakota Hospital Association, the Nurses' Association, or the League for Nursing.
32. *Pulse of the Community.* Report of the South Dakota Planning Council, 1970. Available from the South Dakota Nurses' Association, Board of Nursing, and Comprehensive Health Planning.

33. Leone, Lucile P. *Statewide Planning for Nursing Education.* Atlanta, Ga.: Southern Regional Education Board, 1967.
34. See Appendix C, "Summary of Progress within the States."
35. Bullough, Bonnie. "You Can't Get There from Here: Articulation in Nursing Education." *The Journal of Nursing Education.* 11:4:4-10 (November) 1972.
36. "Purdue University Department of Nursing Baccalaureate Degree Program," First Annual Report to the W. K. Kellogg Foundation, April 1, 1970 to March 31, 1971.
37. UCLA Allied Health Professions Projects, *Summary Report,* Los Angeles, California, April, 1970, p. 24.
38. National Committee for Careers in the Medical Laboratory. "Proficiency Examination for Clinical Laboratory Personnel, Progress Report XI, October 31, 1972 (mimeo).
39. Johnson, D. A. "Mesa College's Project to Develop Proficiency Examinations in Nursing." Paper presented at the American Vocational Association Convention, Portland, Oregon, December, 1971.
40. Nolan, D. J. "College Proficiency Examinations in Nursing." Paper presented at the Annual Meeting of the New York State Council of Licensed Practical Nurses, April, 1971.
41. "Off-Campus Degree Program for Nurses Being Tried." *American Journal of Nursing.* 72:2:220 (February) 1972.
42. Schmidt, Mildred S. "Statewide Planning for Educational Transition and Articulation." Unpublished report to the National Advisory Committee, NCSNNE, Chicago, Illinois, December 8, 1971.
43. Altman, Stuart H. op. cit., p. 4.
44. Bullough, Bonnie, op. cit., p. 7.
45. *An Abstract for Action,* op. cit., pp. 105-108.
46. ibid.
47. Wilson, Fay O. and Marion Greiner. "The Role of the Registered Nurse as a Beginning Practitioner." Unpublished paper transmitted to NCSNNE by letter dated March 13, 1973.
48. Davis, Fred. (ed) *The Nursing Profession.* New York: John Wiley & Sons, 1966, p. 172.
49. Reinkemeyer, Sister A. M. "A Curriculum Plan to Prepare the Professional Nurse at the Graduate Level." Unpublished paper transmitted to NCSNNE, by letter dated May 3, 1971.
50. "Rationale." A statement sent to NCSNNE staff by Evangeline B. Lane, Chairman, Department of Nursing, Georgia State University dated June 11, 1971.
51. "Purdue University Department of Nursing Baccalaureate Degree Program." op. cit.
52. "Career Option Program in Nursing." Report on experimental program materials sent to NCSNNE staff by M. Armour, Chairman, Department of Nursing, State College of Arkansas, dated October 5, 1971.
53. *An Abstract for Action,* op. cit., p. 116.
54. "News Release." Southern Regional Education Board, Atlanta, Georgia dated October 4, 1972.
55. "News Release." University Relations Office, University of California, Irvine dated July 28, 1972.
56. "Articulated Nursing Education Program in Orange County." Grant application to Division of Nursing, Bureau of Health Manpower Education, NIH, submitted by University of California, Irvine for Orange County Consortium for Nursing Education, dated September, 1971.
57. Personal communication from V. S. Ward, Executive Director, Colorado State Nurses' Association to Jerome P. Lysaught, Director, NCSNNE, dated January 28, 1972.
58. Davis, Fred., op. cit., p. 172.
59. Peplau, Hildegard. "Specialization in Professional Nursing." *Nursing Science.* 3:4:268 (August) 1965.
60. "AHME Panel Cites Need for Future Changes in Medical Education." Continuing Medical Education Newsletter. 3:11:7 (May) 1972.
61. Peplau, Hildegard., op. cit., p. 268.
62. Thurston, Hester I. "Education for Episodic and Distributive Care." *Nursing Outlook.* 20:8:520 (August) 1972.
63. ibid.
64. ibid., pp. 521-522.
65. Chioni, Rosemary M. and E. Schoen. "Preparing Tomorrow's Nurse Practitioner." *Nursing Outlook.* 18:10:50 (October) 1970. See also, "Baccalaureate Curriculum Project to Plan New Curriculum." Faculty of the University of Wisconsin School of Nursing, August, 1970.
66. "Tentative Proposal for New Department of Nursing." Memorandum to NCSNNE staff

from Mary W. Searight, Chairman, Department of Nursing, Sonoma State College, dated December, 1971.

67. "Planning for the Future of Nursing Education, 1971-1981, A Ten-Year Plan." A Report to the Executive Committee of the Stanford Medical School, dated July 30, 1971.
68. Smith, Kathryn M. "Episodic and Distributive Nursing in an Emergent Curricular Plan." *The Journal of Nursing Education.* 11:4:11-20 (November) 1972.
69. Longway, Ina M. "Curriculum Concepts–An Historical Analysis." *Nursing Outlook.* 20:2:116 (February) 1972.
70. DeChow, Georgeen H. "Future Directions for the AD Nurse." *Nursing Outlook.* 21:2:109 (February) 1973.
71. ibid.
72. "Development of Associate Degree Program in Family Health Nursing." Proposal submitted to the Division of Nursing by Bakersfield College, dated January 14, 1972.
73. All data in this section are derived from: *Facts About Nursing,* op. cit., passim.; and a memorandum from Constance Holleran, ANA Washington Office, to Jerome P. Lysaught, Director, NCSNNE, dated January 29, 1973 together with enclosures on past and present federal budgets for nursing.
74. *An Abstract for Action.*, op. cit., p. 117.
75. ibid., p. 118.
76. "New Patterns in Nursing Administration: The Vanishing Supervisor." Rochester, N. Y.: The National Commission for the Study of Nursing and Nursing Education, 1972 (pamphlet).
77. "Continuing Education in Nursing: Necessity and Opportunity." Rochester, N.Y.: The National Commission for the Study of Nursing and Nursing Education, 1971 (pamphlet).
78. *An Abstract for Action.*, op cit., p. 122.
79. "Continuing Education in Nursing: Necessity and Opportunity." op. cit.
80. Personal communication from Betty H. Gwaltney, Director, Continuing Education Program, School of Nursing, Virginia Commonwealth University to Jerome P. Lysaught, Director, NCSNNE, dated March 22, 1973.
81. Zschoche, Donna A. "Report on the National Nurses' Congress." *Heart and Lung.* 2:2:168-174 (March-April) 1973.
82. Rosenaur, Janet A. and Dorothy J. Fuller. "Teaching Strategies for Interdisciplinary Education." *Nursing Outlook.* 21:3:159-162 (March) 1973.
83. "The National Joint Practice Commission: New Bottles, New Wine," Rochester, N.Y.: The National Commission for the Study of Nursing and Nursing Education, 1972 (pamphlet).
84. "Breakthrough: Right On!" *Imprint.* 19:1:7 (January) 1972.
85. *An Abstract for Action,* op. cit., pp. 94-96.
86. Personal Communication from Frances K. Peterson, Director, Department of Diploma Programs, NLN, to Jerome P. Lysaught, Director, NCSNNE, dated May 15, 1972.
87. "Report of the Task Force to Study the Implications of the Recommendations Presented in *An Abstract for Action.*" op. cit., p. 113.
88. Rowe, Harold R. and Hessel H. Flitter. *Study on Cost of Nursing Education. Part I, Cost of Basic Diploma Programs.* New York: National League for Nursing, 1964. Also, Rowe, Harold R. and Hessel H. Flitter. *Study of Cost of Nursing Education, Part II, Cost of Baccalaureate and Associate Degree Programs.* New York: National League for Nursing, 1965.
89. Unpublished financial data collected and supplied by the Division of Professional Education, The State Education Department, The University of the State of New York, 1969.
90. Rust, J. H., Jr. *The Cost of Collegiate Nursing in Tennessee.* Nashville: The Tennessee Higher Education Commission and Tennessee Mid-South Regional Medical Program, 1969.
91. "Costs of Nursing Education and A Case for its Greater Support." op. cit.
92. *An Abstract for Action.*, op. cit., p. 111.

SIX TOWARD CHANGE IN NURSING: CAREER PERSPECTIVES

Throughout the investigatory phase of its work, the National Commission was constantly reminded of the circularity of concerns in nursing. To improve the delivery of health care through developments in nursing, one must consider the roles and functions of the nurse practitioner, the educational system and curriculum related to her preparation and continued growth, and, quite as importantly, the means and patterns that ensure a long career of professional service. All of these are interrelated. Just as one should not change an educational program without regard for emerging nurse roles, so one cannot omit the career attractiveness of the profession in planning for the numbers and kinds of nurses needed in the coming months and years.

Nursing is a troubled profession. From its hundreds of preparatory programs, we have turned out students by the thousands each year. Yet, we find that reports of chronic shortages persist. Fifty percent of all our American nurses are professionally inactive and so we have begun, as in medicine, to recruit foreign practitioners.[1] Ironically, some of these individuals come from countries where the United States and its citizens helped found and support nursing education programs to extend care to badly impoverished areas. The removal of these nurses to our nation is a severe loss to their own country and a sad commentary on the American situation.

Withdrawal from professional practice is not the only sign of unrest; turnover rates in American nursing are extremely high. Seventy percent of the staff nursing positions in American hospitals, for example, experience personnel turnover in a one-year period.[2] In metropolitan areas, where the concentration of institutions is heaviest, this turnover rate sometimes climbs to 200 percent per annum. Compare this to elementary and secondary teaching, where the practitioners are also largely females from the same socio-economic backgrounds as nurses, and we find that the turnover rate of teachers in our public schools is approximately 20 percent per annum.

There are other manifestations of malaise. The confrontation of the collegiate and noncollegiate schools, the unarticulated relationship between two- and four-year colleges, the growing controversy over aspects of continuing education, and the insecurity of institutional financial support are educational factors that impinge on careers in professional nursing. Likewise, the limitations on both horizontal and vertical mobility in practice, the confusion of roles, the misutilization of nurses in care settings, and the lack of joint role development between nurses and other health practitioners materially affect professional careers. These are all reflected in nursing literature which mirrors the problems of identifications and goals. There is, in fact, anger, frustration, and a mounting disenchantment with the status quo.

In seeking to enhance career development in nursing, the National Commission acted to include such considerations in all those recommendations specifically pertaining to roles and functions, and education. A third area of activity both in investigation and implementation, was aimed directly at career concerns, however, because of their critical importance to the reconstruction of our health care system. Within this particular parameter, the Commission looked at such elements as:

1. The economic and social satisfactions of nursing.
2. New approaches and configurations that could extend the horizons of nursing careers.
3. The impact of organizations and associations on retention of qualified practitioners.
4. The effect of licensure, certification, and practice acts on career perspectives.

Based on its findings and conclusions, the National Commission proposed nineteen recommendations that dealt with nursing careers per se. For purposes of implementation activities, however, four priority areas were recognized. The first dealt with the motivational factors that impinge on nursing; these include both the economic returns from nursing careers and the noneconomic satisfactions that nurses commonly experience.

Because nursing is so predominately a female profession, it has long experienced the depressed levels of compensation common to all occupations largely staffed by women. This is even more evident in the case of nursing because the entire health field is affected by the eleemosynary aura that surrounds its institutions and facilities. Within the "female" occupations—elementary and secondary teaching, secretarial and stenographic workers, and the like—there can be found distinctions in salaries that indicate strong divergencies in our handling of the health sector. The Commission's concern, however, is that economic aspects of career satisfaction are only one part of the entire picture. If we resolved problems related to salary and compensation, we would still only be started on the agenda that must be taken up.

The human and social satisfactions derived from feeling valued, from contributing and accomplishing, and from realizing one's own complete potential, are of even more significance to the concept of a career. That we have not provided adequately for these satisfactions in the past is evident in the face of nursing's present problems. When many observers tend to agree that the level of commitment "... among those who aspire to nursing would appear to be relatively low as measured by both men and women in college teaching, medicine, law, engineering, and the ministry ... ,"[3] we must reflect on whether the flaws are within these individuals or within the system in which they find themselves placed. Through its investigation, the Commission determined that our career patterns for nursing do, indeed, militate in some important ways against intrinsic satisfactions that should be derived. Our first effort in implementation was to air these problems, suggest new arrangements and improved patterns, and publicize the positive results of experiments aimed at increasing satisfaction and reducing social dissonance.

A second priority was to seek greater harmony and organizational cooperation among the many groups that comprise the "house of nursing." In recent years, dramatic growth has occurred among the specialty practice groups in nursing. More than a dozen of these bodies have been established to date, and plans have been proposed for structuring additional ones in the near future. These groups count thousands of American nurses on their membership rolls, and have taken an active part in planning for continuing education, developing standards of practice, and seeking to provide a locus for the enhancement of care. Unfortunately, these same groups have often stood apart from each other and from the older organizations that draw their memberships from nursing. Thus, predictable problems have arisen in communications and relationships. The National Commission sought, as a definite implementation goal, to break down this psychological distance and to bring these groups into meaningful dialogue.

The third priority dealt with the concerns of individual involvement by nurses in their professional organizations. If we are to improve the delivery of health care, we need to have all nurses develop a commitment to professional excellence. Just as the organizations cannot function effectively in individual orbits, without concern for the paths of others, so the individual nurse practitioner cannot function effectively without interaction and communication with her peers, advanced clinicians, and the change agents functioning in her field. This, of course, is basic to the purpose for having professional organizations—to ensure the offering of opportunities for individual growth among the members. In this light, it is most distressing to note that only about one-third of the active nurses in this country belong to *any* professional or related organization or association.[4] Throughout the implementation phase, the commissioners and staff have addressed hundreds of informational meetings, emphasizing the need to involve *all* nurses in professional activities. Articles and monographs have been designed to appeal to nurses in a variety of roles and settings. In one sense, this approximates a missionary approach for our hope was first to arouse interest, then involvement among the targeted audiences.

The fourth priority in implementing recommendations for career enhancement lay in actions related to licensure, relicensure, certification, and health practice acts. During the course of the implementation phase, what had for some time been a rather prosaic area, suddenly blossomed with activity—much of it heated. Proposals to license new health occupations ran head-on into pleas for a moratorium on any such action. Relicensure in nursing, which has been widely viewed as a pro forma exercise, was suddenly related, through legislative proposals, to mandated requirements for continuing education. The emergence of clinical nurse practitioners, functioning in expanded roles and more independent settings, raised whole new issues in professional certification and responsibility. Finally, the health practice acts of a number of states became the focal point of the new "boundaries" of medical and nursing foundations. During most of the investigative period, these movements were in low key; during the implementation period, however, they moved toward crescendo. In this particular area, the National Commission sought to inform nurses, physicians, and relevant others, including members of the state boards, about the rationale of recommendations in *An Abstract for Action*, and to provide an objective analysis of the probable impact of some of the proposals on the delivery of health care. Through the establishment of the National Joint Practice Commission, and the subsequent work of its task forces, it was felt that there would be, in the near future, better data developed on which to base decisions in all these items of controversy. Whereas, in almost all other instances, the National Commission and its staff were assaying change, in this priority area, we frequently found ourselves urging groups to "go slow" until more facts were available.

Generally, the recommendations in the area of nursing careers were broad-gauge and long-term; some of the priorities were essentially related to advocacy and urging. In the other two general areas, nursing roles and nursing education, we could count the number of state practice and planning committees, observe curricular change, or view clinical nurses in new functional settings. In the area of career perspectives, however, there was less that was tangible. Even so, the commissioners and staff sought to develop a comprehensive approach to gaining public understanding and concern over issues which must be resolved if we are to develop strong career patterns in American nursing.

A summarized report on progress attained in each of the nineteen recommendations is provided in Appendix B. Emphasis in this chapter will be on the four priority areas selected for major implementation concerns.

MOTIVATION IN NURSING

In attempting to analyze and explain some of the phenomena in nursing related to career performance, it is useful to provide a general frame of reference. An increasing amount of research into human and organizational behavior has provided new insights into the understanding of motivation. In particular, the holistic approach of Abraham Maslow[5] displays a model from which hypotheses, generalizations, and probabilities may be drawn. As refined by the later contributions of Frederick Herzberg and his associates,[6] this model can be profitably applied to nursing careers.

Maslow proposes a sequence or continuum of needs that ranges from the most basic physiological requirements for survival through various psychosocial needs—for example, to be loved, to be esteemed, to reach that point of self-actualization or realization where one feels he has become what he *must* be. This theory can be illustrated diagrammatically as shown in Figure 6-1.

Certain generalizations proceed from this conception. The first is that there is a general priority of needs, from left to right, on the continuum. *Survival* has greater priority than *security* which, in turn, is more basic than *belongingness.* One usually needs to be sure of one's safety before seeking other requisites. A second generalization is that, while the general priority system seems universal, the need level in each specific area is different for each individual. Some of us have greater needs for security than do others. A third generalization is that an individual will strive to satisfy unmet needs in a given area until his own personal level of satiety is reached. An unfulfilled category becomes the focus of our current priority of activities. The fourth generalization, actually a corollary of the third, is that once an individual has attained his personal need level in a given area, he is no longer motivated by added satisfactions supplied at that level. Rather he seeks to begin obtaining minimum satisfaction at the next area of need. A final generalization is that a sudden threat to a prior level of satisfied need can cause regression along the continuum and focus the individual's attention on the restoration of former stability.

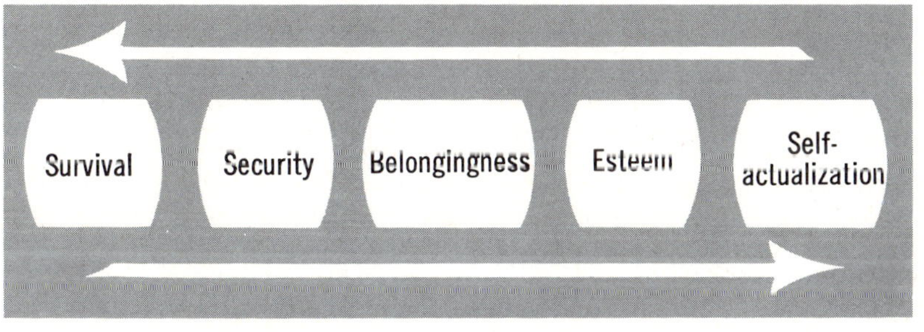

Figure 6-1. A representation of human need priorities.

The particular contribution of Herzberg to such a dynamic theory of motivation lies in his discovery of the distinction between factors that are satisfiers and those that are dissatisfiers in terms of reaching individual need levels. His research indicated that factors which surround the job, including salary and working conditions, are important, but are essentially hygiene matters which tend to prevent dissatisfaction—they do not necessarily lead to satisfaction. On the other hand, factors related to the work itself—peer recognition or increased responsibility, for example—can contribute significantly to heightened satisfaction and increased motivation.

Using this conceptual approach that Maslow, Herzberg, and others have fashioned for explaining human motivation and behavior, we can apply it as a measuring rod for examining American nursing. From the results of that analysis, we might obtain a better understanding of our present problems, emerging trends, and ultimate solutions.

Security Needs in Nursing

If we assert, as a starting point, that few American nurses are actually involved in a fight for physiological survival as a result of their career choice, we can then examine the current relationship between needs and satisfactions in the area of security. While economics is not the sole measure of security, it is certainly a common and useful tool for expressing certain levels and relationships. Table 6-1 shows a comparison between median full-time earnings of selected females in 1959 and 1969, together with a computation of the percentage of growth over the ten-year period.[7]

As indicated by these figures, earnings for all females and for all occupations rose sharply over this period. Nursing made steep gains exceeding those for all female workers and barely surpassing those for all professional and technical

TABLE 6-1 MEDIAN FULL-TIME EARNINGS FOR FEMALES IN SELECTED OCCUPATIONS, 1959 AND 1969

Occupation	Median Earnings 1959	Median Earnings 1969	Percent of Growth
All female workers	$3,161	$5,146	62.8
All professional or technical	4,209	7,291	73.2
Secondary school teachers	5,091	7,780	52.8
Elementary school teachers	4,546	7,380	62.3
Professional nurses	3,819	6,632	73.4
Clerical and kindred	3,544	5,384	51.9
Secretaries	3,807	5,777	51.7

workers. At the same time, however, because of its low starting point, nursing's median earning figure was still below that of teachers and other female professionals. While the gap has been narrowed somewhat in these cases, and while nursing has pulled away from clerical workers and secretaries, there still are salary indicators that nursing is not viewed on a plane with most other professional female occupations.

Much of the impetus for the gain in nursing salaries likely has stemmed from the formal decision, reached by the American Nurses' Association in 1966, to press for a starting salary goal of $6,500. By 1969, the median full-time earnings of younger nurses had reached $6,483 indicating that the ANA objective had largely been reached and, in many parts of the country, exceeded. As shown in Table 6-2, however, when we compare nurses with other professional female occupation groups having generally similar levels of preparation and responsibility, the results are clearly uneven.[8]

Table 6-2, though admittedly selective in terms of the occupations compared, illustrates the relative earnings of nurses to other professional groups outside the health field and to certain other professional groups encompassed within the health occupations. Note that all the latter, clustered at the lower end of the earnings scale, have relatively less difference between and among them.

To appreciate fully, however, the relative economic status of nursing, it should be viewed in comparison with male salaries in the health field. Table 6-3 displays selected male occupational incomes.[9]

TABLE 6-2 MEAN FULL-TIME EARNINGS FOR FEMALES IN SELECTED PROFESSIONAL AND TECHNICAL OCCUPATIONS, 1969

Occupation	Mean Earnings
Social scientists	$9,956
Computer specialists	9,609
Life and physical scientists	9,327
College and university teachers	9,170
Mathematicians	8,884
Social and recreation specialists	7,483
Librarians	7,469
Laboratory technicians	6,823
Dental hygienists	6,726
Registered nurses	6,632
Health technologists and technicians	6,427
Radiologic technologists	6,224

TABLE 6-3 MEAN FULL-TIME EARNINGS FOR MALES IN SELECTED HEALTH OCCUPATIONS, 1969

Occupation	Mean Earnings
Physicians	$30,521
Dentists	24,781
Dental hygienists	16,084
Radiologic technologists	10,441
Health technologists and technicians	9,657
Laboratory technicians	8,992

Not only is there, generally, a considerable difference in male and female earning levels, but in those cases of closest comparison (radiologic and health technologists, and laboratory technicians), the men are paid significantly more than their female colleagues and counterparts.

The briefest comment that can be made about these data is this: nursing salaries are depressed in comparison with certain female occupations, even more depressed in comparison with other female professional workers, and severely depressed in comparison with male earnings in the health field. At a time when we have been through, and are still experiencing, high costs of living, extreme inflation, and even such drastic actions as wage and price freezes, it is disturbing to find our largest body of health practitioners so hard-pressed to satisfy security needs.

Obviously the reasons for these conditions must be fully understood in order to be remedied. It is unarguable that women in our country have been economically deprived. The fact that ninety-nine percent of our nurse practitioners are women, while most of the decisions concerning compensation have been made by men, is eloquently enunciated in the foregoing tables. The sex linkage of nursing has undoubtedly affected the general view of the profession; to most men, such a preponderance of women would indicate that nursing ranks high in maternal caring, low in hard-core sciences, and is likely to be treated as an interim job, preceding marriage and a family. We must recognize, however, that this can be a self-fulfilling prophecy. The expectations and perceptions of parents, teachers, counselors, and friends may very well condition those entering nursing to "recognize and accept" these generalizations—if not to embody them.

A second factor that affects the entire milieu of nursing is a combination of attitudes about health and service occupations. Most men and women assume that there is some reasonable relationship between the importance of a job and the amount of salary that is attached thereto. While economists could readily find support, in general, for such a proposition, they have long recognized that, in our society, female roles, "mainly directed at serving a person and his situation . . . are low status . . ." and consequently undervalued and underpaid.[10] In such a generalized attitudinal pattern, nursing could be perceived as being closely linked with waitressing or household cleaning because all of these occupations have some elements of service on demand. Nursing has added to this, along with the other altruistic professions, by emphasizing an aura of an almost utopian concept of need and service. As Anderson points out, ". . . the non-profit and eleemosynary nature of health care and the dedication presumed to be expressed by the workers in being willing to care for the sick and disabled . . ." has affected our entire health care system.[11] Stress on research, scientific knowledge, and clinical excellence are relatively muted in the discussions on nursing that reach the public ear. The traditional view of the surrogate-mother with a lamp, at the bedside of the patient, fits more comfortably with the image of service and spiritual dedication. The inter-relatedness of these perceptions and attitudes probably accounts for Altman's finding that: ". . . nursing possesses work characteristics that give it 'status' above that related to . . . its monetary earnings."[12] Expressed in another way:

> This perceptual attitude does have positive as well as negative components. In the social sense, most people truly value and admire nurses. In the more mundane concerns it would appear that some people believe these "angels of mercy" subsist on manna and other blessings of heaven.[13]

The most pervasive factor of all, however, that has regulated and depressed nursing salaries is the interplay of supply and demand. Along with other professions dedicated to individual and social amelioration, nursing has aims that are essentially Edenic and limitless. Unlike "self-interested occupations [which] fear surpluses and prefer shortages . . . [the] occupations devoted to the public service . . . usually seek more recruits and complain about shortages."[14] The net effect is to continue to emphasize the problems of supply, manpower, recruiting, and preparatory training even in the face of evidence that "the nursing shortage is an illusion from the economist's point of view."[15]

The constant emphasis on *supply* in nursing has consistently overwhelmed any consideration of *demand*, and as a result we have tended to equate erroneous concepts of need with some real sort of social and economic demand. The history of American nursing is replete with efforts to produce large numbers of bodies to match projections "based upon generally unspecified criteria regarding adequate staffing [and with] practically no evidence . . . available concerning how any of these figures were arrived at. . . ."[16] From an economist's point of view, this approach can have a serious negative impact on the security level satisfactions in nursing. As Yett puts it so plainly:

> Without a program to translate the nation's "needs" into *effective* demand, the proposal to increase the *supply* of nurses could cause large relative salary declines. Under such circumstances, nursing will become an even less attractive career than at present.[17]

In economic terms, we have already produced sufficient numbers of registered nurses to equal or exceed almost every manpower estimate, however developed and however wisely conceived. We have, indeed, produced a nurse supply that exceeds the market demand at existing salary levels.

The paradox of having large numbers of inactive nurses coupled with "budgeted and unfilled" positions is explained when it is recognized that we are not dealing with a free market situation in which *salaries* (demand) could rise to a point where *nurses* (supply) would be attracted into the active work force. Yett argues that most nurses work in hospital settings and that these hospitals, through associations and cooperative approaches, often become, in fact, monopsonies or oligopsonies in terms of salary profferment.[18] So long as demand is artificially limited, we cannot truly speak of a supply shortage.

As another economist, Altman, views it, however, there is significant change in progress. In his opinion, ". . . the public is increasingly aware of the need to pay nurses a competitive wage so as to eliminate the often publicized shortages of hospital nurses."[19] He notes that public pressure, exerted on hospital administrators within the last few years, has resulted in sharp increases, such as those noted in Table 6-1. At the same time, however, he points out that, "Within the usual scope of general duty nursing, advancement and commensurate salary increases were small."[20] Clearly, there must be attention paid to increasing levels of pay for nurse practitioners and also to providing some form of career compensation pattern that will effectively meet security needs for the individuals involved.

Yett, for one, has argued that we need a national policy which will ". . . initiate a coordinated program to support demand [for nursing]."[21] This would require a sharp redirection of our historic emphasis. Most of the federal monies for nursing over the past years have been directed at increasing the supply of nurses through recruitment and preparatory programs. What effect might a switch of these amounts have had on the retention of qualified practitioners if the monies had been used to offer a more satisfactory level of financial security? As the Commission staff, in the course of the implementation, phrased the issue,

> It might be a most interesting and salutary experiment to increase the economic return of nurse practitioners, thereby increasing the personal needs satisfaction at the security level on the motivational continuum, rather than continuing to place our subsidies on the supply dimension only.[22]

Certainly our depressed salary levels of the past have bred reactions that are clearly not in the best interests of nursing or the public. The heightened emphasis on economic and general welfare, particularly since 1966, has brought new militancy to play. Over that period of time there has been a rise in nurses' unions, confrontations, charges and countercharges, and on occasion, strikes and work stoppages. Perhaps a switch in support emphasis from supply to demand might be the cure for the root problem.

Over the past three years, the Commission and its staff have emphasized that we should "... build on current improvements in starting salaries to create a strong reward system for remaining in clinical practice."[23] As in all the recommendations, this is not solely for the enhancement of nursing. Rather, it is aimed at *a long-term solution to nurses' security needs which, in turn, can enhance the delivery of care and limit or reduce the per capita costs to the consumer.* For the purpose of publicizing this effect, the Commission staff studied and reported on such innovative approaches as the Loeb Center for Nursing and Rehabilitation,[24] Metropolitan Hospital in Detroit,[25] and the Northport Veterans Administration Hospital.[26] In these and other instances, it has been demonstrated that improved salary levels, coupled with better utilization of nursing personnel, can produce lower care costs through reduced turnover, extended personal responsibility, and provision of professional care which hastens recovery and rehabilitation.

Solid progress has been made in the area of economic compensation for nursing, but much remains to be done. We cannot expect nurses to respond to higher levels of motivation so long as great numbers of them have their attention fixed on unmet needs in the area of financial remuneration. It is essential, therefore, that nursing and health management, together with the consumer, work toward continuing improvement in the area of security needs satisfaction.

Despite the complexity of solving these economic problems, it should be recognized that the machinery of our capitalist system is geared toward overcoming precisely these kinds of difficulties—once they are recognized and identified. Irregularities in supply and demand, adequate compensation for functions performed, and better ordering of our priorities and organization are the brick and mortar of our enterprise system. There is no reason to believe that the problems in nursing are any more incapable of solution than those of any other portion of society. It is primarily a matter of getting on with the job. And that the Commission has vigorously urged.

Psychosocial Needs in Nursing

As we continue to move forward on the solution of security needs, we must consider the range of psychosocial needs that nurses seek to satisfy. Studies have been conducted to determine why individuals choose nursing as a career and one reason has been preeminent—students have gone into nursing because they "want to help people."[27] This personal desire becomes a potent conditioner of perceived satisfaction at each area along the human needs continuum.[28] It suggests that in nursing, practice is the key to intrinsic motivational forces. In terms of the Maslow formulation, we might hypothesize the following need-satisfaction levels:

1. Basic personal competence in meeting routine client needs would represent psychosocial *security*.
2. Acceptance into collaborative team relationships that would expand both quality and quantity of care provided would satisfy *belongingness* needs.

3. Assumption of leadership and responsibility for care, accompanied by the recognition and respect of peers and associates, would fulfill *esteem* needs.

4. Perceived attainment of full professional competence and exhibition of role model characteristics in client care would represent *self-actualization* in nursing.

In this model of motivational levels, satisfactions are expressed in terms of *practice* related to the articulated pre-potency of feelings among nurses, both student and graduate. It is when we compare this model with the reality of present nursing careers that we recognize how much change is needed to ensure better congruency between human desires and work requirements.

An increasing number of nurses are becoming distinctly uncomfortable with the status quo. They perceive deeper problems than can be solved by rhetoric or surface change. They sense a malaise which involves fundamental flaws that must be corrected before the profession can progress. And they experience an increasing concern over goals, directions, and means. This phenomena is expressed by Davis in these words:

> Not long ago, my colleagues and I fell unwittingly into a sometimes tedious, sometimes oddly intriguing game of no known name. . . . Perhaps, it can be described as "find a one word name for the thing." The "thing" under scrutiny was a mass of diverse, seemingly irreconcilable and, we feared, hopelessly unmanageable findings and impressions from our four-year study of the professional socialization of student nurses. . . . The name we settled on finally . . . was "paradox."
>
> In retrospect, I believe this name was not only more appropriate to our research findings than it seemed at the time, but is equally fitting for contemporary nursing as a whole. For in bringing together the papers that make up this book, I am struck anew by the proliferation of paradoxes that characterizes nursing.[29]

Foremost among the paradoxes with which we must grapple is this: *nursing which exists to meet human needs has not yet evolved a career pattern which is linked to the needs of its practitioners.*[30] There is little argument over the primary motivation people bring to nursing, but there is clear evidence that length of service, increased responsibility, and promotion tend, inevitably, to draw the nurse away from direct client-centered activity. The inverse ratio is indicated schematically in Figure 6-2.[31]

Because present utilization patterns in nursing are familiar, the absurdity does not strike us, perhaps, until we realize that a nursing student in her clinical training will spend more of her time in direct patient care than she is likely ever again to be permitted in the system we have devised for using her skills. And, as a corollary, the better a nurse demonstrates capability for client care, the more likely she will be raised to a position farther removed from the dynamics of that care. In terms of the

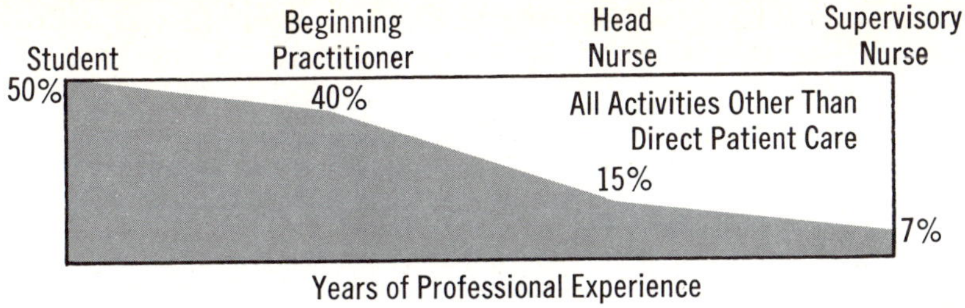

Figure 6-2. Comparative proportions of time spent in direct patient care activities by nurses.

motivational continuum, we can infer other consequences. Some good practitioners, failing to find psychosocial satisfaction in this career pattern, will drop out of the system altogether. Other capable practitioners might sublimate and attempt to find secondary satisfactions in administration or teaching and accept loss of client contact. The quality of patient services cannot help but be adversely affected by this disfunctional arrangement.

In documenting this problem, the Commission staff prepared two pamphlets over the course of the implementation period for distribution to nurses, health administrators, and concerned consumers. In "No Carrots, No Sticks: Motivation in Nursing,"[32] the basic conflict was presented. In "New Patterns in Nursing Administration: The Vanishing Supervisor,"[33] specific examples were drawn from research on the present system. It was found, for instance:

1. Promotional patterns in nursing do lead inexorably away from direct patient care and into the management of tasks.[34]
2. Nurse supervisors frequently find communication problems increasing because their concerns for personnel and systems maintenance are not congruent with staff and patient concerns for care.[35]
3. As a result of increasing discontinuity between the goals of the system and patient care, the traditional hierarchical structure has either forced nurses to conform or to become frustrated and leave.[36]

A number of experimental arrangements were examined to determine whether the traditional structure and functions of nursing service could be altered; results from these innovations were publicized as part of the implementation information effort. The Veterans Administration Hospital at Brockton, Massachusetts, eliminated the supervisory nurse position altogether and expanded the clinical requirements of the nursing staff. Satisfaction among the nurses was significantly increased.[37] At the Veterans Administration Hospital in Brockville, Ohio, head nurses were reassigned as care team leaders with authority and responsibility for making patient care decisions. Satisfaction and economic savings resulted.[38] Other examples were provided, as well, to emphasize that continuing attention must be paid to the interrelationship of our systems for nurse utilization and the resultant impact on psychosocial needs of the nurse.

Beyond the point of advocacy, the National Commission has encouraged both statewide master planning and joint practice committees to examine the concerns of career satisfactions in nursing and to emphasize the importance of clinical practice in realizing the psychosocial need requirements. These bodies, in turn, can recommend to the individual institutions and facilities that traditional systems of utilization and patterning be scrutinized in the light of emergent findings. As the Commission views it, the underlying motivational problems in nursing will be largely eliminated when:

> Personnel policies in all health care facilities are so designed that they:
> a. Differentiate levels of responsibility . . . according to the content of the position and the clinical proficiency required for competent performance.
> b. Provide for promotion granted on the basis of acquisition of the knowledge and demonstrated competence to perform in a given position.[39]

It has been ironic that in nursing one could find recognizable career paths in administration or education, but not in the practice of client care itself. It must be made possible for a nurse to satisy felt needs for belongingness, esteem, and self-actualization within the realm of patient care. To do so requires continuing and systematic efforts to separate out the non-nursing tasks and build up the care functions of the practitioner. There must be a basic reconstruction of leadership roles around patient care with the emergent concepts of clinical nurse and master nurse clinician replacing the traditional arrangement of head nurse, supervisor, and director with their diminishing involvement in client care.[40] From all of these changes, we may anticipate a functional system that satisfies the career expectations of those nurses with the strongest commitments to care and practice. Furthermore, we can realize the elimination of the paradoxical "fatal flaw" that has so long hampered American nursing—the career pattern that runs counter to the primary motivational urge to provide direct patient care.

REUNITING THE "HOUSE OF NURSING"

Second only to the concern of the Commission for the development of a functional career position for nursing has been the commitment to work for greater unity and organizational solidarity within the nursing profession. For as long as memory serves, American nurses have been at odds over educational patterns, institutional relationships, and organizational claims. Many of the earlier national studies of nursing had been victims of the internecine struggles within nursing leadership and between the nursing organizations. To an outside observer, it was evident that:

> . . . in the struggle to rearray itself and enhance the health care system of the nation, American nursing has sometimes evidenced suspicion, mistrust, and even paranoia. . . . When it was impossible to attack the real opponents and the real problems, nurses sometimes attacked each other.[41]

In the months after the appearance of *An Abstract for Action*, there began to emerge some of the anticipated complaints. Voices were raised to say "there is need for more study" or "the procedure for change is not clear" or "nursing is not yet ready for such a step."[42] To counteract these appeals to retain the status quo, a concerted effort was mounted to contact the various nursing organizations and enlist their aid in a common cause to implement the recommendations of the National Commission. Much of this activity has been reported in detail in Chapter Three.

The Commission's interest in unity went far deeper than securing the endorsement of its report by these nursing organizations. Our desire was to see those groups working together to address the many problems faced by the profession today so that there would be a pattern of relationships established by which tomorrow's problems might be resolved. Out of the experience of the first eighteen months of the implementation effort, during which we had talked to a great number of the organizations separately, the Commission staff sought to develop a common meeting point about which the various groups could rally. The rapid changes in nursing practice, the new and congruent roles with medicine, and general concern for expanded functions suggested that the issue, "the nurse as practitioner," might be the starting place. In an article for one of the specialty journals, the Commission commented:

> Never was there a time of greater need for American nursing to unify and present a combined front in the effort to improve total patient care. This need not be monolithic; there must be room for, and acceptance of, diversity. But there should be no mistake about the necessity. . . .[43]

To this end, the Commission proposed that ". . . representatives of all the nurse specialty bodies, as well as those divisions or sections of other specialty organizations which are essentially composed of nurses, meet at an early date. . . ."[44] The NCSNNE staff then began preliminary planning for such a meeting, but events soon obviated the necessity for this work.

The National Nurses' Congress

Early in the spring of 1972, the American Association of Critical-Care Nurses (AACN) proposed that a "National Nurses' Conference" be called that would include representatives from the many nursing organizations and associations. Preliminary reactions were generally quite favorable so the AACN set about determining dates, sites, and arrangements for such a meeting. In August of 1972, formal letters of invitation were sent to those nursing organizations, including the Nurse Corps of the three United States military services, asking them to designate delegates to attend a conference in January of 1973 at the Western White House in San Clemente, California.

This action was so complementary to the concepts of the Commission that, in September of 1972, a letter was sent from the NCSNNE to the same invited organizations saying, in part:

> . . . we are convinced that this meeting could be a beginning to the kind of unifying effort that is so badly needed within the profession. Accordingly, we have indicated to AACN our complete support for the call of this Congress and we urge each of the nursing organizations that has been invited to participate. . . .[45]

An unanticipated intervening activity then occurred. Acting independently, the American Nurses' Association invited many of the same organizations to a one-day meeting in Kansas City, scheduled for November 17, 1972. There was a time when such an action might have been viewed as the opening round in a game of organizational "one-upmanship," but all the principals involved displayed coolness and constraint. The ANA sponsored meeting was held as planned; the AACN went on with its plans for a lengthier conference in 1973.

Of the seventeen "civilian" nursing organizations invited to the congress, only one, the Council of Cardiovascular Nursing of the American Heart Association, failed to designate and send a representative. Of the "military" invitees, only the Air Force Nurse Corps indicated its intent to send a representative; the Army and Navy Nurse Corps declined to participate. In addition to the organizational representatives from nursing, the United States Public Health Service Division of Nursing and the National Commission were invited to attend as observers and discussants. Nursing organizations which took part in the January meeting are listed in Table 6-4.

In the fall of 1972, each of the organizations planning to attend the congress was asked to suggest items for discussion as well as priorities in terms of concern. From these individual listings, a composite was prepared by the AACN and the organizations were then asked to examine and react to the various proposals. On the basis of the replies, a final agenda was produced for consideration and adoption by the assemblage.

At the opening of the congress on January 25, 1973, Donna Zschoche, Executive Director of AACN, immediately emphasized the purpose and the shared responsibilities for the meeting:

> The burden of accomplishing our goals lies within each of us. AACN did not call the Congress to dictate or present a completed manifesto. . . . AACN called the Congress to ask each professional nursing organization to lend its thinking, expertise and strengths to determine its focus and method-

TABLE 6-4 ORGANIZATIONS PARTICIPATING IN THE NATIONAL NURSES' CONGRESS, JANUARY 25-26, 1973

Organization	Conference Status
1. American Association of Critical-Care Nurses	Participant
2. American Association of Industrial Nurses	Participant
3. American Association of Nephrology Nurses and Technicians	Participant
4. American Association of Neurosurgical Nurses	Participant
5. American Association of Nurse Anesthetists	Participant
6. American College of Nurse Midwives	Participant
7. American Nurses' Association	Participant
8. American Public Health Association—Public Health Nursing Section	Participant
9. American Urological Association	Participant
10. Association of Operating Room Nurses	Participant
11. Emergency Department Nurses' Association	Participant
12. National Commission for the Study of Nursing and Nursing Education	Discussant
13. National Education Association—Department of School Nurses	Participant
14. National League for Nursing	Participant
15. National Student Nurses' Association	Participant
16. Nurses Association of the American College of Obstetricians and Gynecologists	Participant
17. United States Air Force Nurse Corps	Participant
18. United States Public Health Service—Division of Nursing	Discussant
19. United States Veterans Administration Nursing Service	Participant

> ology in meeting those challenges which face us. . . . We will do all in our power to assist in whatever way we can to lay the groundwork for effective cooperation and harmonious relationships in our joint endeavors.[46]

This theme was repeated in the keynote address presented by the Director of the National Commission. Paraphrasing the text of Paul's first letter to the Corinthians, he commented:

> Now I beseech you, people . . . that you all say the same thing; and that there be no dissensions among you, but that you be perfectly united in one mind and in one judgment. For I have been informed about you, my people,

> by those of the house of Liberty that there are strifes among you. Now this is what I mean: each of you says, I am of ANA, I am of NLN, I am of the specialty organizations, or I am of the true realm of Nursing. Has Nursing been divided up?[47]

In the discussions which followed, it became evident that concern for greater cooperation and organizational harmony was widely shared. From this point of common departure, the participants moved to substantive matters on which action might be taken.

The first decision, arrived at unanimously, was that there should be no formal title at this time for designating the assembled group. The term *congress* seemed too formal and rigid for the present purposes, and there was a shared feeling that structure, organization, and therefore an appropriate title would evolve more suitably out of continuing interaction. It was agreed, however, that meetings should be planned on a continuing basis with sites and arrangements being determined among the participating agencies on a rotating basis. As an expression of their desire for better understanding and joint purposiveness, the group adopted the following statement of principle:

> We, as representatives of the several nursing organizations, will convene periodically and be mutually supportive in discussion of issues which face nurses and nursing in influencing constructive changes in health care.
>
> We have committed ourselves to the proposition that practice is the basic purpose of the nursing profession and that all organizations, all educational institutions, and all systems in which nurses practice should exist to enhance that primary goal.[48]

Out of ensuing discussion, four specific statements on current concerns were adopted by the group, subject to approval by the several parent organizations. These initial areas of common agreement were:[49]

> 1. The associations endorsed the position statements of the American Nurses' Association and the National League for Nursing which registered opposition to the application of institutional licensure to nursing personnel.
> 2. The associations encouraged the concept of continuing education, but disapproved of coupling this with relicensure at least until current studies on the issue are completed. The necessity of interorganizational discussion and planning was emphasized.
> 3. The continuing education unit for standardizing continuing education programs was endorsed as was the interim report of the ANA task force studying these matters.
> 4. The associations agreed to make universal, cooperative efforts to recruit all professional nurses into at least one of the professional organizations represented in order to foster greater understanding and solidarity.

The second meeting of these associations has been set for June of 1973 with the Association of Operating Room Nurses assuming the role of arranger and host.

At that time, the associations will have taken up the interrelationships in certification of advanced specialists, concerns in relicensure, and the enlarging field of continuing education. On these and a number of other topics, the ground seems to have been prepared for cooperative and constructive progress. As one indication of the understandings developed in the first sessions, four specialty practice groups took immediate steps to go on record as endorsing the implementation of *An Abstract for Action.* These organizations include: the American Association of Critical-Care Nurses,[50] the American Association of Neurosurgical Nurses,[51] the Emergency Department Nurses' Association,[52] and the Nurses' Association of the American College of Obstetricians and Gynecologists.[53] The actions of these groups following earlier statements by other nurse associations have placed the overwhelming majority of organized nursing behind the effort to establish an "unambiguous profession" within a unified "House of Nursing."

The Academy of Nursing

In the first volume of its report, the National Commission gave warm encouragement to the concept of an Academy of Nursing which could recognize and emphasize excellence in practice, as well as engage in other activities designed to promote professional growth. It was particularly gratifying, then, to receive notification that the American Nurses' Association officially launched a national Academy of Nursing in January, 1973, by designating thirty-six Charter Fellows of the Academy to organize and develop regulations and procedures for the new organization.

The majority of the charter fellows are highly expert clinical practitioners from a wide variety of specialty areas. In addition, there are some academicians, administrators, and researchers. The general guidelines in which they will operate are directed at, but not limited to, these primary concerns:[54]

1. Identification and exploration of issues in health, the professions, and society as they affect and are affected by nurses and nursing.
2. Development of new and innovative roles for nurses seeking to fill gaps in the health care system.
3. Application of research findings to the improvement of patient care services.
4. Elucidation of knowledge and skills needed to meet contemporary health care requirements.

Funding and support of the Academy of Nursing will be provided by the ANA, but detailed planning and functioning will be determined solely by the academy members to ensure a maximum freedom of inquiry and activities.

This development, in conjunction with the collaborative establishment of the "no name" association of nursing organizations, would seem to indicate that nursing is well on its way to overcoming the parochial problems of partisanship that have divided its members for so long. Moreover, the new academy reaffirms the dynamic concept of the role of practice within the profession. If the nursing congress participants agreed on "practice as the basic purpose" of nursing, the academy is the expression of "recognition for excellence in practice" and, thus, confirms the emphasis on career perspectives built around patient care.

RECOGNITION OF NURSING COMPETENCE

In *An Abstract for Action*, the National Commission reviewed the background and purposes of nurse licensure. Because any such regulatory power has both positive and negative aspects, the Commission considered a number of alternatives and proposals for change. Implicit in their discussions, and in the ensuing recommendations, were two key points: the maintenance of some form of surety as to competency for quality practice; and the inclusion of flexibility in the language of licensing regulations so as to foster rather than impede new practice roles and functions.[55] On these two principles, the Commission staff sought to develop, during the implementation stage, a continuing dialogue on licensure.

Basically, the concept of licensure is to protect the consumer. In the case of nursing, this should mean that a licensed registered nurse is competent to provide safe care for the normal demands of the patient. Traditionally, this has been established by passage of a state licensure examination—a paper and pencil test on matters related to nursing practice. All fifty states and the District of Columbia possess legal codes relating to licensure and relicensure, and, with few exceptions, these are administered and applied by state boards of nursing.

Currently, most state boards require periodic license renewal—generally on a one- or two-year basis. This renewal usually has not, however, involved reexamination or any other test of continued competency. Likewise, most states endorse licensees from other states without reexamination or other requirement. Therefore it is possible, in nursing, for an individual to obtain a license and maintain it for a lifetime without evidencing continuing capacity to practice at a safe and competent level.

This situation may have been acceptable for health care practice in less dynamic times. With changed demands on nursing service, including whole new technologies, drugs, and interprofessional roles, however, there is increasing awareness that evidence must be adduced to indicate that the nurse practitioner remains competent to render elemental "safe" practice. Without specifying exactly what means might be employed, the National Commission did recommend:

> All state licensure laws for nursing be revised to require periodic review of the individual's qualifications for practice as a condition for license renewal.[56]

While there is increasing agreement among nurses and the nursing organizations that some mechanism must be developed, and soon, to ensure continuing competency, few people anticipated that such procedures might become a polar issue in the course of the implementation phase. This became a controversy through the sudden appearance of legislation designed to mandate continuing education as a requisite for relicensure of nurses.

Continuing Education and Relicensure

As early as 1967, the National Advisory Commission on Health Manpower had recommended that "professional societies and state governments explore the possibility of periodic relicensing of physicians and other health professionals,"[57] and coupled this proposal with a commentary on the necessity of continuing education for quality practice. Four years later, the 1971 *Report on Licensure and Related Health Personnel Credentialing* urged the "specific requirement" of a continued level of practice competence as one condition of relicensure or recredentialing.[58] Both of these documents were clearly aimed at redirecting the traditional approaches to automatic extensions of health licenses and thereby substituting an "activist" role for the controlling boards in order to ensure consumer protection.

What seemed to be a theoretic concern turned into a very practical matter when, in 1972, the California legislature enacted a law mandating continuing education for nursing as a condition of relicensure. A number of other states (including Colorado, New York, Washington, and Indiana) have legislation proposed or pending that would specify similar requirements. While discussion of such regulations had taken place over a five-year period in generally temperate tones, the confrontation with reality elicited strong reaction. As an editorial in *RN* magazine saw it:

> We believe that nursing is drifting into a crisis. . . . At the heart of the problem is the move to make continuing education for nurses *mandatory* for relicensure. Such action at this time could result in confusion and chaos. It could drive thousands of nurses out of the profession, causing national problems in staffing of hospitals and other health agencies.[59]

When this editorial was transmitted to the Commission staff with a request for reaction, the director attempted to reduce the anxiety that had been occasioned by the tone of the magazine article, stating:

> By what rationale do you deduce that continuing education, required for licensure, would drive "thousands of nurses out of the profession?" I think our Commission and staff have seen a great number of nurses over the past five years. The vast majority of them are involved in continuing education, formal and informal, academic and inservice. They see this as their professional commitment.[60]

While rejecting the strident tones of the editorial, it is nevertheless true that there are very practical problems related to mandating continuing education for relicensure that cannot be dismissed with the wave of a hand.

Signe Cooper, one of the nationally recognized figures in continuing education for nursing, rejects the concept of mandatory learning for relicensure on the basis, in part, that we probably could not provide sufficient opportunities at present for compliance with such legislation. As she puts it:

> . . . it seems urgent to provide more continuing opportunities for nurses, upgrade the quality of the offerings, and prepare faculty for positions in continuing education.[61]

Given these conditions, Cooper believes that nurses would voluntarily engage in continuing education, obviating the necessity for compulsory requirements which could breed hostility and resentment toward advanced learning.

A second negative reaction to the possibility of mandated continuing education is focused on the need for some kind of national directing policy that would avoid the vagaries and compartmentalization that might be embedded in fifty-one sets of jurisdictional requirements. Speaking of continuing education in pharmacy, Clifton Latiolais, President of the American Pharmaceutical Association, stated:

> In the absence of a clearly defined program with specific objectives and appropriate criteria for evaluation, I believe that a national policy of mandatory continuing education for pharmacy is grossly premature and ill advised. With such ill-defined objectives, legal requirements for relicensure can only breed mediocrity at best and will inevitably lead professional "competency" to its lowest possible common denominator.[62]

The parallels to nursing, of course, are quite clear. If state requirements are couched in terms of "completed courses," "credit hours," or some other form of bookkeeping, there is every likelihood that decisions for compliance, by nurses, may be made on the basis of expediency or convenience without any form of planning and conceptual direction. Incompatibility of state requirements might only add to the complexity of the system and multiply the hazards faced by the individual nurse.

Still a third expressed concern with the present legislation revolves around the concept of control. There is some sentiment in favor of having the nursing profession, through its organizations, plan and provide the continuing educational curricula and, then, certify successful completion of courses or other types of experience. The nursing organizations would then endorse or attest to an individual's meeting of statutory requirements at the time that application for relicensure is made. This would maintain board control over the reissuance of the license, but provide professional control over the actual educational experiences and curricular design.

In the face of such controversy and confusion, organized nursing is beginning to shape definitive action. The American Nurses' Association has established a task force to study continuing education and its relationship to relicensure, meanwhile endorsing a moratorium on all new licensure changes until an opportunity has been afforded to look at both the pros and the cons of proposed legislation. At the

National Nurses' Congress in January, the assembled groups took specific action both to endorse the concepts of continuing education and to discourage mandatory programs for relicensure pending the results of the ANA inquiry. They further stated:

> . . . we deem it *essential* that the American Nurses' Association seek participation of all specialty nursing groups in their deliberations and ultimate decisions regarding continuing education as criteria for relicensure of registered nurses.[63]

Whatever the outcomes of the ANA study in terms of specific proposals, it is inevitable that greater emphasis will be placed on continuing, demonstrated competency in practice and that automatic license renewal on the basis of a single examination score sometime in the past, is not likely to continue. Since the mandatory features of the California legislation do not go into effect until 1975, there is still time for some concerted national policy to emerge; but the pressure is intense for the nursing organizations to cooperate and produce viable plans and policies that will protect the consumer, expand the professional capacities of the individual practitioner and, at the same time, do both effectively with a minimum of red tape and bureaucratization.

Institutional Licensure

In the 1971 *Report on Licensure and Related Health Personnel Credentialing*, in addition to the recommendation which urged the requirement of continued competency as a criterion for relicensure, there was a proposal for the study of a wholly different approach to licensure–one in which the institution, rather than the individual, would be licensed to comply with standards of safety and competency. In the words of that report:

> The concept of extending institutional licensure–to include the regulation of health personnel beyond the traditional facility licensure–has important potential as a supplement or alternative to existing forms of individual licensure. Demonstration projects should be initiated as soon as possible.[64]

Simply put, institutional licensure would replace the individual licensing of various health occupations and professions with a single authorization extended to a health agency under state regulation. As Hershey and Wheeler see it:

> Institutional licensure is a process by which a state government regulates health institutions by requiring the operator of such an institution to obtain legal authority (a license) to establish a health care facility, and to comply with certain standards in order to retain the license to operate his institution.[65]

The licensed institution could then establish job specifications, standards, and other criteria and appoint competent individuals to the various positions within the facility without regard to their possession of an individual license. The individual regulatory boards would be replaced by a single state board which oversees the compliance of the health care institutions.

There is, without doubt, a certain logical neatness to the concept of institutional licensure. From the standpoint of the state, there is the prospect of a single licensing board to replace the multiplicity of agencies now overseeing physicians, nurses, licensed practical nurses, and other health occupations. From the standpoint of the institution, there is the possibility of hiring qualified individuals without regard for "paper credentials." From the standpoint of the employee, there is the promise of increased ease of mobility and transfer. From the standpoint of the consumer, there is some indication that total overhead costs might be reduced.

In the face of all these indications, one might wonder why institutional licensure has become an issue. The reasons are several.

The first concern lies in the proclivity of the health field to begin studies and then embark on full-blown implementation of an activity prior to the conclusion of these investigations. At the urging of the 1971 licensure report, there are a few studies underway to determine what effects are to be found in the application of institutional licensing. None of these investigations is completed, but there is already proposed legislation in Massachusetts that would implement the concept statewide, and recent publications tend to sound as though all the results are in and that institutional licensure is proven to be a sound and positive concept.[66]

It cannot be emphasized too strongly that the claimed benefits of institutional licensure, at this point in time, must be seen and treated for what they are—claims. It would be very unwise to accept them uncritically or, for that matter, to reject them out of hand. The investigations now underway may provide us with better information from which to draw conclusions dependent, of course, on the reliability, validity, and generalizability of their results. More likely, however, the outcomes will not permit a simple "good" or "bad" interpretation.

In assessing the present situation, the National Commission has agreed generally with the national health organizations which have argued for a moratorium on all changes in licensure—including the legislation of institutional licensure—until other cogent developments have been examined. The change from individual to institutional licensure, for example, should not be viewed as a single question. Inevitably, there are ramifications for the entire concept of role congruency and alteration between medicine and nursing and there is good reason to change as few variables as possible, at any one time, or else we may never know those that are positive and those that are destructive.

In the light of the present developments in joint practice and in role expansion for nursing, the National Commission has urged that there be maximum flexibility and the least possible stratification of state licensure laws and procedures. While the studies of institutional licensure now underway should be pursued and the results carefully examined, there should certainly not be premature legislation or reorganization. It was on the basis of this reasoning that the Commission adopted a resolution on December 21, 1972, which stated its opposition to "the extension of institutional licensure to include the regulation of nursing personnel."[67]

More basic, however, than the Commission's concern for flexibility in the face of changing roles is their desire to ensure competence and quality in patient care. Having pointed out the known problems in current approaches to licensure and relicensure, there is still a great deal of question about how well institutional licensure would guarantee competency in practice. As indicated in Table 6-5, the current licensing examinations do tend to bar a significant number of individuals, each of whom possesses the educational background demanded for institutional licensure, from receiving legal designation as a registered nurse. There are, of course, many explanations for the high failure rates demonstrated in Table 6-5—likely, the need for some further clinical experience after completion of preparatory educational programs in order to satisfy demands of the examination elements is a contributing factor. The point to conjure with, however, is that in these two years alone, a total or more than 24,000 individuals were denied nurse registration because of their failure to pass the licensing examination.[68] Any or all of these individuals might have been endorsed under institutional licensure.

Whatever the shortcomings of the current system, we must certainly assure that any change provides at least as much protection and assurance for the patient, if not more. When we review the experiences of both the investigation and implementation phases of the Commission's work, in relation to nursing roles and functions, it cannot be forgotten that our present patterns of institutional utilization have led to such circumstances as that described by Duff and Hollingshead in which patient care is relegated to the least trained health workers while nurses are so involved in systems management that they cannot work directly with the clients.[69] Most of these decisions on manpower utilization and personnel practices were made by the institutions—and their administrators—on the basis of economic and organi-

TABLE 6-5 FAILURE RATES ON STATE LICENSURE EXAMINATIONS FOR REGISTERED NURSES, 1969-1970

Type of Candidate	Percentage of Failures	
	1969	1970
Candidates for first time	20.9	22.8
Candidates who had previously failed an examination	42.3	46.2

Source: *Facts About Nursing, 1970-71 Edition.* New York: American Nurses' Association, 1972.

zational concerns that are demonstrably unrelated to patient care needs. In the scheme of institutional licensure, it is conceivable that we would give these same institutions and administrators even more pervasive powers to affect utilization patterns perversely.

In all of the Commission's efforts to enhance patient care through the redirection of nursing roles and functions, we have necessarily been forced to urge the abandonment of traditional staffing and utilization patterns.[70] To the extent that institutional licensure might well represent an almost reactionary retreat from the new organizational and personnel configurations, it could become the bulwark for making all decisions about patient care on short-run economic and labor perspectives. While no one should reject the study of any new approach, there are fundamental questions and concerns related to institutional licensure that must be faced squarely and answered satisfactorily. To date, this has not been done.

Advanced Competency in Practice

Traditionally, licensure in nursing has been bound up in beginning competency to render safe patient care. As the role of the nurse practitioner has expanded in recent years, there is increased need to determine the standards of performance and competency attached to emerging levels of expertise—such as those of the staff nurse, the clinical nurse, and the master nurse clinician. This is particularly important because of the proliferation of nurse clinician programs in a wide variety of specialty practices, many of which are sharply divergent in length, content, and objectives.

Fundamentally, it would appear there are two general approaches that might be taken. There could be a variety of state nursing licenses reflecting the variety of subspecialties and gradations similar to the certification apparatus employed in elementary and secondary education over many states. A second approach would be to retain a single license, attesting to basic competency, while offering certification, or diplomate, status under professional auspices to denote advanced competency. After weighing these choices, the Commission recommended that:

> In view of the emergence of advanced levels of clinical practice in nursing:
>
> a. A single license be retained for the registered nurse, and
> b. Advanced levels of nursing practice be recognized through some form of organizational or institutional certification.[71]

This conclusion reflected three factors: 1) the desire to retain a clear focus on the objectives of, and procedures for, basic licensure; 2) a recognition that most advanced practice roles in nursing are still emerging and must remain fluid for some time to come; and 3) an intention to encourage the joint development of advanced roles through interaction of nurses and physicians with minimum constraints imposed by bureaucratic givens.

To propose that nursing follow the example of medicine and have advanced certification taken over by something like a specialty practice academy, requires recognition that, at present, there simply is no mechanism by which this can be accomplished. The state boards of nursing are a reality; the alternative approach is still in an embryonic organizational stage. It is for this reason, then, that the Commission has stated:

> One of our greatest concerns, however, lies in the present posture of the nursing specialties . . . in relation . . . with the American Nurses' Association . . . the various groups and the ANA Divisions on Practice [must] work together, plan together, and stand together in the search for new and more meaningful practice patterns.[72]

The Commission then proposed three specific tasks that must be accomplished through interorganizational planning:

> 1. The development of functions and standards for practice as influenced by the findings and recommendations of the National Joint Practice Commission.
> 2. The making of a basic decision on procedures and standards for certifying clinical excellence of nurse practitioners in both episodic and distributive areas.
> 3. The establishment of coherent national patterns to ensure career mobility for the advanced practitioner and maintain assurance of quality health care for the consumer.

Each and all of these activities demand the cooperative planning and joint agreement of one or more specialty groups and the related ANA practice division if we are to avoid absolute confusion and frustration. As the National Commission phrased it:

> It would be disastrous if the promises that lie in the National Joint Practice Commission were to be seared by parochial protestations and organizational opportunism. Consider for a moment the effect on the public and the other health professions if the Nurses Association of the American College of Obstetricians and Gynecologists, the American College of Nurse-Midwives, and the ANA Division of Maternal and Child Health produced conflicting and confounding statements on nurse functions and standards with regard to labor and delivery.[73]

In the period of the implementation, there have been an increasing number of interorganizational discussions taking place concerning the expanded role of the nurse practitioner. Preliminary statements have been published in the areas of maternity care[74] and pediatric nursing.[75] These are likely, however, to be only indicative of what may well come from the efforts of the national and state joint practice committees. It is essential, then, that the nursing organizations strive to anticipate the need both for descriptive standards of advanced practice and certification procedures related thereto. Both the National Nurses' Congress (by whatever name it may become known) and the Academy of Nursing stand as potential bulwarks to ensure that order and harmony prevail.

The National Commission has sought throughout the implementation phase to encourage the development of mechanisms for change; these now exist, including the joint practice bodies. The challenge now facing nursing is to invoke the detailed joint planning that can make the process of certification operational. The profession, the individual practitioner, and the public all deserve a positive response.

STATE HEALTH PRACTICE ACTS

State boards of nursing possess varying degrees of discretionary power dependent upon the enabling legislation under which they are constituted. For some years now, these boards have used the same licensure examination for candidates throughout the country, but have established their own pass/fail scores. Under these circumstances, one might assume, given the sameness of the examination, that there would be a high degree of consistency in nursing practice across the nation. The flaw in this reasoning lies in the fact that the various nursing boards, or other designated agencies, are also administrators of the state nurse practice act which legally defines or limits the practice of nursing throughout the jurisdiction.

While there is common agreement on what might be described as "general hospital nursing" from state to state, there is considerably less consensus on the legality of the emergent role of the advanced clinical nurse practitioner. Generally speaking, nurse practice acts reflect the circumstances and patterns attendant at the time of passage. Traditional acts are generally regarded as legal; unique or innovative acts might well be considered illegal. The more definitive and prescriptive the language of the legislative act, the more possible it is that expanded nursing roles may fall outside the sanctioned areas.

In the past, a number of states have expressed willingness to accept joint statements of practice from nursing and medicine as interpretations of the specific provisions of a health practice act. Thus, if medicine and nursing agree to expand the role of the nurse practitioner in coronary care, a statement of the enlarged functions might be addressed to the state attorney general and treated as an official explication of the statutory provision for that particular aspect of practice. This approach has been invoked in a number of states and has been useful in role expansion for nursing. On the other hand, some states have not utilized these procedures and there is still a question of what might happen if some of these statements were challenged in the courts.

At the very best these joint statements have tended to be so specific and task-oriented that they would be a cumbersome vehicle indeed for broad-scale changes in professional roles. As a result, there has been increasing interest, among both nurses and physicians, in developing new health practice legislation that will permit more latitude for evolutionary development and be less prescriptive in its definition of practice parameters.

Perhaps the most famous of these new practice acts is that of New York State. After heated testimony before legislative committees, the act was passed by both houses and transmitted to the Governor who vetoed it in 1971. In 1972, after some minor revisions in verbiage, the act was passed and signed into law. Two sections of this new nurse practice act deserve particular notice. In one, the practice of nursing is defined as:

> . . . diagnosing and treating human responses to actual or potential health problems through such services as casefinding, health teaching, health counseling, and provision of care supportive to or restorative of life and well-being, and executing medical regimens prescribed by a licensed or otherwise legally authorized physician or dentist. A nursing regimen shall be consistent with and shall not vary any existing medical regimen.[76]

In the other, the practice act provides a definition of the nursing diagnosis which is described as:

> . . . identification of and discrimination between physical and psychosocial signs and symptoms essential to effective execution and management of the nursing regimen. Such diagnostic privilege is distinct from a medical diagnosis.[77]

Thus, there is a general expansion of the functional role of the nurse practitioner along with legal recognition of "nursing diagnosis" although this is still defined as distinct from the medical diagnosis. It was this latter point which evoked much of the controversy over the proposed legislation since many physicians, health administrators, and others have seen "diagnosis" as generically reserved to medicine. The New York statutes provide for a new interprofessional understanding of patient and client assessment based on the emergent capabilities of nurse clinicians.

A very different approach, developed in a vastly more cooperative climate, underlies the revised nurse practice act of Idaho. In this statute, the practice of nursing is defined as follows:

> . . . the performance for compensation of any act in the observation, care, and counsel of the ill, injured, or infirm, or in the maintenance of health or prevention of illness of others, or in the supervision and teaching of other personnel, or the administration of medications and treatments as prescribed by a licensed physician or dentist; requiring specialized judgment and skill based on knowledge and application of the principles of biological, physical and social science. The foregoing shall not be deemed to include acts of medical diagnosis or prescription of therapeutic or corrective measures except as may be authorized by rules and regulations jointly promulgated by the Idaho state board of medicine and the Idaho board of nursing which shall be implemented by the Idaho board of nursing.[78]

The significant aspect of the Idaho statute is that, essentially, nursing practice is whatever the state boards of medicine and nursing agree it is. This, of course, not only provides great freedom for development, but places responsibility for role enlargement on professional interaction between the two largest health practicing professions.

In 1972, the state of Arizona amended its nurse practice act and added two important provisions. The first of these recognized the concept of nursing assessment and evaluation. The second added a new dimension to nursing practice in unordinary contingencies by permitting:

> The performance of such additional acts under emergency or other conditions requiring education and training and which are recognized by the medical and nursing professions as proper to be performed by a professional nurse under such conditions and which are authorized by the board of nursing through its rules and regulations.[79]

An increasing number of states are beginning to reexamine their health practice acts in the light of these statutory changes. Colorado and Pennsylvania, for example, have proposed legislation that is modeled after the New York definition of nursing practice (the Colorado bill also includes a passage similar to the cited Arizona section on "emergency or other" conditions). Other states have moved toward the Idaho form of enactment. All of these developments, however, share a common emphasis on some form of interprofessional planning for role change. With more permissive, less prescriptive health practice acts emerging, the functional alterations proposed by the joint practice committees should be more easily adopted than might have before been the case.

There is some evidence that even the more traditional nurse practice acts are less restrictive than we have imagined them to be. The Secretary's Committee to Study Extended Roles for Nurses initiated a limited inquiry into the probable effects of state practice acts on proposed role changes in nursing. They reported:

> Since each of the states has legal responsibility for control of nursing practice within its borders, several of the items listed as "Functions for Which the Nurse is Now Prepared or Could be Prepared to Assume Further Responsibilities" were excerpted and distributed to state constituents of the American Nurses' Association and State Boards of Nursing in 53 states and territories. Although returns were not complete, the comments of the several respondents indicated that there are no legal barriers related to the functions presented and that these are expected activities although specific authority is lacking. . . . It was indicated that the barriers are more traditional than legal.[80]

In terms of both statutory and common law, there seems to be a firm basis for planned expansion of the nursing role, particularly as it is evolved through joint planning and discussion with medicine. In these circumstances, then, the Commission's emphasis on the joint practice committees may either impel more revisions of health practice acts or point up the lack of need for such legislation. What is most important is that the nursing role expand with adequate protection for the client and the practitioner. Time and the provisions of the various state practice acts will determine whether amendent or revision is really required.

OTHER RECOMMENDATIONS ON NURSING CAREERS

In *An Abstract for Action*, the National Commission proposed nineteen specific recommendations for change in nursing career perspectives. Many of these proposals were subsumed in the NCSNNE's emphasis on the major points of implementation and some were most appropriately directed to other organizations than the Commission and its staff for purposes of action. A number of publications and materials were prepared, however, to aid in gaining public understanding and acceptance of the recommendations.

For example, the Commission proposed that nursing become much more involved in planning for health care delivery and manpower needs. The very development of statewide master planning and joint practice committees encourages the involvement of nurses in comprehensive health and regional medical planning programs. Likewise, the development of conceptual schemes for modified and expanded practice roles in episodic and distributive care has given substance and direction to participants in the various planning groups. While the Commission primarily emphasized the need for an enlarged scope of nursing practice to enhance careers, it is logically related that the recommendations for the divestment of non-nursing functions and operations should be implemented. In order for our health care system to use nursing most effectively and efficiently, it is essential that we do involve nurses in our systems planning and that they, in turn, become active, contributing agents to the reconstruction of our delivery patterns.

One whole area of concern in the Commission's career recommendations dealt with enlarging the programs for disseminating information, and recruiting potential students, into nursing. Working with our advisory committee people from the National Student Nurses' Association and others, we reviewed the minority groups which are presently quite under-represented in nursing, for example—men, blacks, Spanish-speaking and American Indians. In addition, there are the aides, attendants, and licensed practical nurses to whom upward mobility in registered nursing is a natural pathway for career development. There are also the older students, either those making a second occupational choice, or those who have graduated from a baccalaureate program without specific vocational preparation. All of these groups are potentially sound reservoirs for recruitment purposes. The full realization of their capacity, however, is necessarily interrelated with the development of a comprehensive, articulated pattern for nursing education.

A third cluster of recommendations deals with the interrelationships between the various nursing organizations particularly, the American Nurses' Association and the National League for Nursing. For years, these groups have worked cooperatively to meet the diverse needs of American nursing. With the recent growth of the specialty practice groups and the American Association of Colleges of Nursing, there is need for increased concern about duplication and fractionation of effort. The resources, both in finances and in leadership personnel, are still so limited in American nursing that the profession simply cannot afford the extravagance of redundancy or to work at cross-purposes. For this reason, the NCSNNE has urged that the national organizations join in discussion of mutual approaches, and then proceed with serious examination of programs, activities, and possible areas of collaboration.

Most critical of all, however, is the pervasive need, expressed throughout the recommendations on nursing careers, to develop an unambiguous profession based on client care. While society can provide a system in which nurses find challenging roles and functions, individual nurses must respond to that challenge. States can alter licensure or certification; individual nurses must rise to new heights of responsibility in order to make those alterations meaningful. Leaders can bring nursing organizations together; individual nurses must demonstrate trust, respect, and mutual willingness to work out problems. In simplistic terms, "professional is as professional does," and American nursing must now demonstrate its maturity and its purposiveness by enlarging its contribution to our health care system through a career perspective based on meeting client needs. Only through the personal, direct, and overt commitment of the individual nurse to clinical excellence can nursing become all that it might as a profession.

SUMMARY

The National Commission advanced nineteen recommendations in the area of nursing careers. In contrast to proposals in the area of nursing roles and nursing education, many of the specific suggestions on careers had to be long range and quite gradual. At the same time, however, the basic need to establish satisfying and motivating conditions for nurses is so critical that action could not be deferred. The Commission felt that a start had to be made—and very quickly—if we were to alter the prevailing patterns that have been in force. These patterns of reward and utilization have been largely responsible for the malaise of American nursing, the high rates of withdrawal and turnover, and the evident frustration that can be found at every turn.

To the extent that the Commission's hypotheses are correct, and an abundance of evidence in everyday nursing experience confirms them, it is likely that most American nurses find it difficult to meet their lower level needs for security, and beyond those, to satisfy their psychosocial needs for greater contribution, acceptance, recognition, and fulfillment. If we are to escape an endless cycle of personnel shortage, frustration, failure, and conflict, we must make basic, sweeping changes in the reward systems for nursing—both extrinsic and intrinsic. We must provide career patterns that enhance the possibility of self-actualization and, essential to this, provide the opportunity for more nurses to reach higher levels of satisfaction without need to move away from direct patient involvement. For years, we have continued to emphasize the "supply" aspects of nursing without really examining why our shortages persisted. It is essential now, more than ever before, that we get to the root causes of the problem and correct them.

Throughout the implementation phase, the National Commission has sought to inform the health professions, the administrators, and the general public about the shortcomings of the present reward system for nursing. While it is obvious that more must be done to increase economic security, the progress in nursing salaries has induced the Commission to look beyond that level of need and emphasize the next concern—the needs satisfactions that are bound up in professional performance related to client care. In anticipation of what will become the critical issue of the next quarter century, proposals have been generated for new patterns of utilization and recognition that can lead to the intrinsic satisfaction that nurses will be needing. The extent to which these patterns, or viable alternatives, are developed and proffered, may well be the determining factor in whether nursing becomes the professional partner in health care practice that we need, or slips deeper into an occupational mode that is peripheral to our central concerns.

To focus attention on these problems, and to encourage nursing to deal with them, the Commission has supported a variety of interorganizational approaches including the National Nurses' Congress and the Academy of Nursing. While these two groups are less than a year old, they represent increasing awareness of the need for a united "House of Nursing" characterized by excellence in clinical practice. Many real problems and differences remain for the nursing organizations to solve, but the first steps toward resolution have been taken and progress to date is most encouraging.

In the area of licensure, the National Commission has encouraged the idea of a general moratorium on change until a number of ongoing activities have been able to generate data. Issues such as institutional licensure must be studied critically; it would be irresponsible to switch to such a system at a time when initial investigations are still in progress. Similarly, to move toward relicensure with mandatory provisions for continuing education demands both lead time and the provision of adequate opportunities for gaining that education. Relatedly, decision making on certification procedures can undoubtedly benefit from the findings and conclusions generated by the joint practice committees that are just now becoming operational. In all this, the Commission does not suggest that the status quo is idyllic or that there is no need to change. To the contrary, the Commission has been most forthright in pointing out problems of our present system. We simply do not propose to do anything which would not be an improvement or which would, in turn, require corrective action within a short while.

State practice acts have frequently, in the past, been held to blame for prescriptive and restrictive regulations on nursing roles. It is a moot point, perhaps, whether the statute or tradition is the real culprit. The Commission, of course, supports the extended and expanded role of nurse practitioners and the clear legal acknowledgement of that thrust. Each state, however, must examine its own laws and regulations to determine whether new legislation, or amended statutes are necessary. If the answer is "yes," there are a number of model practice acts that can serve as valuable guides for regulating nursing practice with proper concern for the public but without undue constraints on the practitioner.

It is significant, perhaps, that the Commission's recommendations on nursing careers received the highest consensus of all in terms of organized reaction. The NLN Council of Diploma Programs, which indicated nonsupport of some recommendations related to education and roles, expressed no reservation in the area of careers.[81] The NLN task force endorsed fifteen recommendations as stated, three with minor modifications in wording, and endorsed the underlying principle of the remaining recommendation while suggesting that specific action await the final report of the national study of accreditation in the allied health professions.[82] The ANA Commission on Economic and General Welfare voiced its concern that the Commission recommendations failed to emphasize "collective determination" of salary and related matters.[83] Otherwise, most nursing organizations and associations indicated full support of the career recommendations without exception or reservation.

The millennium in nursing careers will not come this year or next; many of the changed patterns advocated in *An Abstract for Action* will likely not be in full form until the 1980s. But every progressive step, taken by nursing, medicine, health management, and the public, to restructure the patterns and rewards for nursing careers can have a tremendous impact on the coming generations of nurse practitioners. To replace the present system with its frustrations and failures is essential. To construct a system in which intrinsic satisfaction and humane practice are exemplified is entirely possible. For the sake of our society, we must try.

FOOTNOTES

1. "20 Filipino Nurses at Baptist Center." *Arkansas Gazette*, January 20, 1973, pp. 1A, 6A.
2. *Technology and Manpower in the Health Service Industry.* Manpower Research Bulletin No. 14. Washington, D.C.: U.S. Department of Labor, 1967, p. 22.
3. Anderson, Odin W. *Toward an Unambiguous Profession? A Review of Nursing.* Chicago: University of Chicago Center for Health Administration, Pamphlet No. A6, 1968, p. 11.
4. Lysaught, Jerome P. "An Epistle to the New Corinthians." *Heart & Lung.* 2:2:180 (March-April) 1973.
5. Maslow, Abraham H. *Motivation and Personality.* New York: Harper & Row, 1954.
6. Herzberg, Frederick, *et al. The Motivation to Work.* Second Edition. New York: John Wiley & Sons, 1959.
7. Source for the data: U.S. Department of Commerce, Bureau of the Census, *Census of Population, 1960 and Census of the Population, 1970*, both published in Washington, D.C.
8. Source: U.S. Department of Commerce, Bureau of the Census, *1970 Census of the Population, Subject Reports, Earnings by Occupation and Education*, PC(2)-8B, Washington, D.C., 1973.
9. ibid.
10. Anderson, Odin W., op. cit., p. 3.

11. ibid., p. 1.
12. Altman, Stuart H. *Present & Future Supply of Registered Nurses.* Washington, D.C.: U.S. Department of Health, Education, and Welfare Publication No. (NIH) 72-134, 1971, p. 60.
13. "No Carrots, No Sticks: Motivation in Nursing." Rochester, New York: The National Commission for the Study of Nursing and Nursing Education, 1972 (pamphlet) p. 11.
14. Anderson, Odin W., op. cit., p. 6.
15. ibid.
16. Yett, Donald E. "Yes, Virginia, There is a Shortage of Nurses–But It's Not Quite as Simple as All That." Paper presented at the Second Conference on the Economics of Health, Baltimore, Maryland, December 5-7, 1968, p. 3.
17. ibid., p. 68.
18. ibid., p. 51.
19. Altman, Stuart H., op. cit., p. 108.
20. ibid.
21. Yett, Donald E., op. cit., p. 68.
22. "No Carrots, No Sticks: Motivation in Nursing." op. cit., p. 5.
23. ibid., pp. 5-7.
24. "Distributive Nursing Practice: Development and Fusion of the Roles." Rochester, N.Y.: The National Commission for the Study of Nursing and Nursing Education, 1971 (pamphlet) pp. 10-11.
25. "Episodic Nursing Practice: Refinement and Expansion of the Roles." Rochester, N.Y.: The National Commission for the Study of Nursing and Nursing Education, 1971 (pamphlet) pp. 14-15.
26. ibid., pp. 10-11.
27. Hughes, Everett M., *et al., Twenty Thousand Nurses Tell Their Story.* Philadelphia: J. B. Lippincott, 1958, *passim.*
28. Maslow, Abraham H., op. cit., pp. 92-106.
29. Davis, Fred (ed.) *The Nursing Profession: Five Sociological Essays.* New York: John Wiley & Sons, 1966, p. vii.
30. Lysaught, Jerome P., "The House Reunited: It Must Not Fall." *American Journal of Public Health.* 62:7:959 (July) 1972.
31. ibid., p. 957.
32. "No Carrots, No Sticks: Motivation in Nursing." op. cit., *passim.*
33. "New Patterns in Nursing Administration: The Vanishing Supervisor." Rochester, N.Y.: The National Commission for the Study of Nursing and Nursing Education, 1972 (pamphlet).
34. "Episodic Nursing Practice: Refinement and Expansion of the Roles." op. cit., pp. 1-4.
35. Treat, Margaret and Marlene Kramer. "The Question Behind the Question." *Journal of Nursing Administration.* 2:1:20-27 (January-February) 1972.
36. Gabrielson, Rosamond C. "New Approaches for Nursing Services." *New York State Nurse.* 41:4:46-51 (April) 1969.
37. Dahlsten, A. M. and F. R. Flood. "No Evening or Night Supervisors." *Nursing Outlook.* 18:1:49-53 (January) 1970.
38. Towner, A. M. "No More Supervisors?" *Nursing Outlook.* 16:2:26 (February) 1968.
39. "No Carrots, No Sticks: Motivation in Nursing." op. cit., pp. 12-14.
40. "New Patterns in Nursing Administration: The Vanishing Supervisor." op. cit., pp. 9-11.
41. Lysaught, Jerome P. "An Epistle to the New Corinthians." op. cit., p. 182.
42. Lysaught, Jerome P. "The National Commission and the Specialty Practice Groups in Nursing." *JOGN Nursing.* 1:3:20 (September-October) 1972.
43. ibid., p. 19.
44. ibid., pp. 19-20.
45. Personal communication from Jerome P. Lysaught, Director, NCSNNE to Presidents and Executives of American nursing organizations listed in the 1972 AJN directory issue, plus additions proposed by NCSNNE advisors, dated September 21, 1972.
46. Zschoche, Donna A. "Introduction to the National Nurses' Congress." *Heart & Lung.* 2:2:177 (March-April) 1973.
47. Lysaught, Jerome P. "An Epistle to the New Corinthians." op. cit., p. 180.
48. Zschoche, Donna A. "Report on the National Nurses' Congress." *Heart & Lung.* 2:2:168-169 (March-April) 1973.
49. ibid., pp. 169-170.
50. Personal communication from Donna A. Zschoche, Executive Director, AACN to Jerome P. Lysaught, Director, NCSNNE dated April 21, 1973.
51. Personal communication from Mary E. Craton, Past-President, AANN to Jerome P. Lysaught, Director, NCSNNE dated April 21, 1973.

52. Personal communication from Ruth S. Miller, Executive Director, EDNA to Jerome P. Lysaught, Director, NCSNNE dated April 13, 1973.
53. Personal communication from Patricia B. Owens, President, NAACOG, to Jerome P. Lysaught, Director, NCSNNE dated April 30, 1973.
54. "National Academy of Nursing Launched; ANA Names 36 Charter Fellows." News release prepared by the ANA for general distribution dated February 6, 1973.
55. The National Commission for the Study of Nursing and Nursing Education. *An Abstract for Action.* Jerome P. Lysaught, Director. New York: McGraw-Hill Book Co., 1970, pp. 141-144.
56. ibid., p. 142.
57. National Advisory Commission on Health Manpower. *Report: Volume I.* Washington, D.C.: U.S. Government Printing Office, 1968, pp. 41-42.
58. *Report on Licensure and Related Health Personnel.* Washington, D.C.: U.S. Department of Health, Education, and Welfare, DHEW Publication No. HSM 72-11, 1971, pp. 75-77.
59. "Open Letter." *RN Magazine*, 35:10:21 (October) 1972.
60. Personal communication from Jerome P. Lysaught, Director, NCSNNE to the Editors of *RN Magazine* dated October 13, 1972.
61. Cooper, Signe. "Should Continuing Education be Mandatory? No!" *American Journal of Nursing.* 73:3:442 (March) 1973.
62. "News in Focus." *American Druggist.* 166-22, November 27, 1972.
63. Zschoche, Donna A. "Report on the National Nurses' Congress." op. cit., p. 169.
64. *Report on Licensure and Related Health Personnel.* op. cit., p. 76.
65. Hershey, Nathan and Walter S. Wheeler. *Health Personnel Regulation in the Public Interest.* Sacramento: California Hospital Association, 1973, p. 5.
66. ibid., *passim.*
67. "Resolution Opposing the Extension of Institutional Licensure to the Regulation of Nursing Personnel." News release of the NCSNNE prepared for general distribution, dated January, 1973.
68. *Facts About Nursing, 1970-71 Edition.* New York: American Nurses' Association, 1972, p. 47.
69. Duff, R. S. and A. B. Hollingshead. *Sickness and Society.* New York: Harper and Row, 1968, p. 374.
70. "New Patterns in Nursing Administration: The Vanishing Supervisor." op. cit.
71. *An Abstract for Action.*, op. cit., pp. 143-144.
72. Lysaught, Jerome P. "The National Commission and the Specialty Practice Groups in Nursing." op. cit.
73. ibid.
74. "The American College of Obstetricians and Gynecologists, and the Nurses Association of the American College of Obstetricians and Gynecologists, and the American College of Nurse-Midwives Joint Statement on Maternity Care," January, 1971.
75. "A Joint Statement of the American Nurses' Association, Division on Maternal and Child Health Nursing Practice and the American Academy of Pediatrics, Guidelines on Short-Term Continuing Education Programs for Pediatric Nurse Associates," January, 1971.
76. State of New York, Senate-Assembly. "An Act to amend the education law, in relation to the practice of nursing." S.8274, A.9422, dated February 9, 1972. Section 6902.
77. ibid., Section 6901.
78. State of Idaho, House Bill No. 46. "An Act relating to the practice of nursing . . ." Signed by Governor Cecil Andrus, February 11, 1971. Section 54-1413.
79. State of Arizona, Senate Bill No. 1098. "An Act relating to professions and occupations, defining the practice of professional nursing . . ." Approved May 4, 1972. Section 32-1601.
80. "Extending the Scope of Nursing Practice." A Report of the Secretary's Committee to Study Extended Roles for Nurses. Washington, D.C.: U.S. Department of Health, Education, and Welfare. November, 1971, p. 26.
81. Personal communication from Frances K. Peterson, Director, Department of Diploma Programs, NLN, to Jerome P. Lysaught, Director, NCSNNE, dated May 15, 1972.
82. "Report of the Task Force to Study the Implications of the Recommendations Presented in *An Abstract for Action.*" *Nursing Outlook.* 21:2:116-118 (February) 1973.
83. "Statement of the Commission on Economic and General Welfare on the Findings and Recommendations of the National Commission for the Study of Nursing and Nursing Education." Enclosure to a memorandum from Alice L. Ahmuty, Director, to Executive Directors, State Nurses' Associations, dated October 7, 1971.

SEVEN | SUMMARY AND PROLOGUE

To conclude any lengthy work generates its own admixture of feelings. Whatever the satisfactions of accomplishments, there are the disappointments of shortcomings and there are the nagging regrets over the many things still left incomplete and the few things not begun. Perhaps the greatest exhilaration upon completing the implementation phase of the National Commission's work lies in the recognition that this is not, and cannot be the termination of activities related to the accomplishment of aims advanced in *An Abstract for Action.* We have reached the end of one stage; we have already begun another. Too many processes have been set in motion; too many projects are generated for any consideration of limitation or conclusion. At the same time, transition and continuation must be planned, assigned, and assumed or progress will be slowed and efforts diffused.

As a preliminary step toward the next phase of implementation, it may be useful to review succinctly and candidly what has been essayed, how much was accomplished, wherein lay the shortcomings and disappointments, and what might reasonably constitute the next set of work priorities to be undertaken. No one, of course, can speak with precision about all the strands woven into such a broad-scale effort to effect social change. It is possible, however, to discern emerging patterns from which reasonable projections may be inferred. By assessment of these outcomes, succeeding national, state, and local bodies may be better able to guide and select their continuing efforts at implementation.

This comparative analysis of progress and impasse, achievement and shortcoming, will be limited to the priority goals described in Chapter 1 of this volume. These include all the major concerns and primary points of issue. In addition, a detailed summary of status and progress on each individual recommendation is provided in Appendix B and an account of each state's activities is contained in Appendix C. From these combined compendiums, it is possible to develop a feeling for the general state of progress, the differential accomplishments attained toward specific goals, and the regional or national patterns of "contagion."

To accentuate the problems and shortcomings—for these constitute the concerns of continued implementation—each of the focal areas of the Commission's work will be discussed in a point-counterpoint fashion rather than by a general grouping of "successes" and "failures."

INFORMATIONAL AND EDUCATIONAL PROCESSES

Emphasized the first year of implementation, and continued throughout the entire period, was the effort to inform and influence nursing, other health professions, educators, administrators, and consumer representatives about the root problems uncovered in the NCSNNE investigation and the need to take corrective action as outlined in *An Abstract for Action.* To accomplish this end, and to gain endorsement and support for change, the Commission and its staff initiated a lengthy series of report meetings, statewide informational conferences, individual organizational contacts, and written materials.

Accomplishments of Implementation

In anticipation of the initiation of an organized effort at implementation, the NCSNNE staff had, in early 1970, begun direct involvement and elicited participation of a number of groups and organizations in the examination of findings and draft recommendations. The results of that period indicated that there was a good deal of consensus on the conclusions of the investigation and the proposed actions for change. While many people had assumed basic incompatibility of viewpoints among the interested "publics," the survey outcomes suggested that these had been overestimated and that agreement far outweighed conflict of viewpoints. As indicated in the sample of opinions displayed in Figure 7-1, there was a certain symmetry and harmony of reactions across traditional "party lines."

The opinions sampled and reported in Figure 7-1 are related to the area of education, and are displayed here because that particular set of findings produced the *greatest amount of disagreement.* Learning this, the staff was strongly encouraged, in the early implementation phase, to begin building on the broad foundation of consensus and educate for the relatively smaller areas of uncertainty and disagreement.

Over the course of the implementation period, this effort resulted in estab-

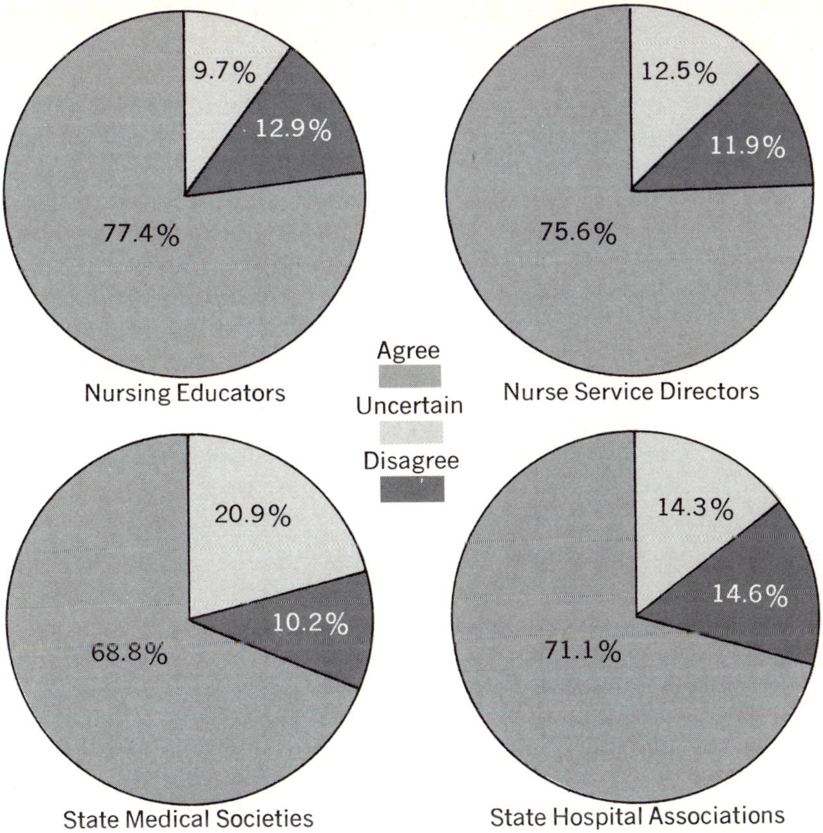

Figure 7-1. Comparison of Reactions Among Various Sample Groups to Findings Reported by NCSNNE Staff

Source: The National Commission for the Study of Nursing and Nursing Education, *An Abstract for Action: Appendices*. Jerome P. Lysaught, Director. New York: McGraw-Hill Book Co., 1971. "Appendix C. Tabulation of Reactions to Third Draft Findings, Study Area B," pp. 61-64.

lishing strong organizational backing for change processes. Given an opportunity to discuss, question, and criticize the data and recommendations presented in *An Abstract for Action*, a large number of groups found that they could support most of the recommendations and lend their aid to the central thrust of the changes proposed. In the first few months of the implementation period, an unprecedented number and variety of national and regional organizations went on record as stating their approval and support for the basic concepts of the National Commission report. Table 7-1 provides a partial listing of those organizations which announced their general support of the report from the time the advance summary was published in the spring of 1970 to the end of the first year of implementation in October, 1971.

Over this same period of time, a number of state, district and local groups expressed their support, and, subsequently, so did an increasing number of national organizations. The critical point from the standpoint of the National Commission, however, was that this display of consensus allowed us to avoid much of the confrontation politics that some people had anticipated. It facilitated work with the state organizations in nursing, medicine, and health management, and it encouraged a spirit of collaboration at all levels. No one thought for a moment that a series of supportive statements or outright endorsements implied absolute agreement with each and every recommendation. Rather, these actions cleared the air, established that there was a considerable amount of common ground, and allowed everyone involved to begin collaboration on areas of agreement and initiate discussion on areas of difference.

One immediate outcome of the supportive statements was cooperative planning in the development of statewide informational meetings for the purpose of sharing information on *An Abstract for Action* and eliciting local and personal involvement in its implementation. While nurses most frequently took the lead in proposing such meetings and follow-up, there is abundant and eloquent testimony to the support provided by physicians, health management people, societies and associations outside nursing, regional medical plans, comprehensive health planning groups, and a goodly number of interested consumers.

TABLE 7-1 NATIONAL AND REGIONAL ORGANIZATIONS INDICATING SUPPORT OR ENDORSEMENT OF *AN ABSTRACT FOR ACTION*, APRIL, 1970–OCTOBER, 1971

Organization	Date of Action
Executive Committee, Board of Directors, National League for Nursing	April, 1970
House of Delegates, American Nurses' Association	May, 1970
Council of the Conference of Catholic Schools of Nursing	January, 1971
Board of Trustees, American Medical Association	February, 1971
New England Board of Higher Education	April, 1971
Council on Nursing Education, Southern Regional Education Board	April, 1971
General Council, American Hospital Association	May, 1971
Board of Directors, American Public Health Association	July, 1971
American Association of Deans of College and University Schools of Nursing	October, 1971
American Association of Industrial Nurses	October, 1971

These initial informational contacts were quite frequently followed up by establishment of ad hoc planning groups and district and local meetings. They were supplemented by a planned series of NCSNNE pamphlets, articles, and monographs relating to identified areas of concern and disagreement. Later, as demand spread for speakers and change agents, a volunteer group of advisers, regional associates, and involved individuals was enlisted to expand the coverage. Audio-visual materials were developed and made available, without cost, so that the background of the Commission, its findings and recommendations, and its plans for implementation could be conveyed to even the smallest local groups.

Many of the nursing associations and publications took up responsibility for informing their members, readerships, and the public about Commission activities. Over the same time span, the NCSNNE staff prepared and distributed a stream of press releases, special mailings, and selected publications to computerized address lists of thousands of individuals classified into various interest groups. More than 136,000 reprints and pamphlets alone were distributed by the Commission staff over the course of the implementation.

In terms of specific outcomes, there was evidence of widespread participation by nurses, other health professionals, and consumer representatives in the discussion and implementation of *An Abstract for Action.* Statewide information meetings were held in forty-four states and many of these had regional and district follow-up. Fifteen national organizations took formal action, over the implementation period, in support of the NCSNNE proposals for change as did numbers of regional and statewide groups. These many organizations represented nursing, medicine, health management, higher education, and, in many cases, included consumers and lay people. From all this, one can conclude that thousands of individuals were informed about, and many subsequently involved in, the work of implementation.

Shortcomings and Difficulties

To review the volume of activity in terms of informational and educational processes is to sense the enormity of the work that lies unaccomplished. Health care is an ultimate concern of every American. Yet, try as the Commission and staff might, every informational meeting, every discussion, every presentation found a paucity of lay people and consumer representatives. It is little consolation to know that this is a problem which affects all the health groups, and is found commonly on each health issue taken up across the country. The fact is that the National Commission has enjoyed circumscribed success in developing lay understanding or consumer support for its recommendations.

In large measure, this may simply be a statement of the public's priorities. Health, and concern for health, may only be in sharp focus when we are personally threatened by illness or injury, or when we are acutely reminded of the costs of treatment. In other times and circumstances, the average citizen finds many other concerns more engrossing.

More frequently than consumers, there was involvement on the part of physicians, administrators, and health planners. Unfortunately, far too often, such participation was of short duration and limited depth. This could often be understood in terms of the job demands and time pressures under which these persons worked. In part, however, it reflects a limited understanding of what the "fuss" is all about in nursing. Some administrators and even more physicians still feel that all the "girls" want is someone to occasionally show up at a meeting, tell them they are doing a fine job, and reassure them that they are valued. This perception simply misses the entire concern over the plight of the health care system, the roles and functions of nurses within it, and the genuine desire to effect fundamental change.

While nurses in great numbers participated in the implementation activities, sober reflection impels us to realize that the majority of American nurses today still remain uninvolved. Most of the nurses we worked with directly are ones who have affiliations with one or more professional groups. However, somewhere between one-third and one-half of all active nurses do not belong to any professional organization and we have no way of gauging how many of these "independents" have read about, heard about, or care about *An Abstract for Action.* Our concern here is not with numbers alone. If there were some random distribution of involved nurses across all lines and levels, the problem would not be so acute. The probability, however, is that involvement is skewed, with leadership in education and service "over" represented, and staff practitioners correspondingly "under" represented. Naturally the desire is to get greater dispersion of information and understanding, and this requires that there be participation down to the grass roots. Success in this endeavor has been only partial.

Another area of limited accomplishment lay in the matter of informing and involving political and administrative decision makers at both state and federal levels. Many of the occupants of these positions—with some notable exceptions—have little understanding of the problems and potential of nursing. Although most of these people with whom the NCSNNE staff came into contact are positively disposed toward nurses and nursing, their perspective is quite traditional and, in the light of rapidly changing practice, bordering on the antiquated.

Continuing Needs

The work of the Commission in the area of information and education clearly demonstrates that three years of intensive and extensive effort is insufficient to effect all of the attitudinal and thought changes we wished. While more, perhaps, could have been done, and what was done might have been done more wisely and well, nursing must continue to deal with the fact that there are deep-seated misconceptions, or lacks of conception, about the profession which will require continuous programs of information and education. For too long a time, the public has shared a restricted image of nursing. As the director of the NCSNNE staff describes it:

> . . . American nursing has long been subjected to a set of cultural constraints that ordained organizational failure. American nurses, even when they were men, were seen as "females" in a society which perceived man to be the naturally superior and commanding figure. American nurses were seen as "attendants" in a system which placed the physician and the surgeon atop the pillar of acclaim. American nurses were seen as non-intellectuals in a society in which excessive attention was given to the academic trappings of the culture. We have placed nursing in a subordinate position and then accused it of lack of independence; we have "trained" nurses for motor-skill activities and then berated them for lack of judgment. . . .[1]

As suggested in Figure 7-1, many of those persons most closely involved with nursing share, to a large extent, similar concerns and convictions. There is, however, a pervasive perception throughout our society, with regard to nursing, that must be changed—and can be changed—over time. The public must be made aware of what has happened in nursing practice and education, what is happening, and, most importantly, what will be happening as even more fundamental developments take place in role enlargement and joint practice.

In doing this work of informing and educating, organized nursing must work together, but not alone. The involvement of other health professions, educators and planners, and an ever-increasing number of lay persons will not only add quantitatively to the effort, but can help to convey more acutely the concerns and the wants of health care consumers. Information on nursing can then be directly related to the felt needs of the client and communication can be more effectively established.

No single item should be higher in nursing's list of priorities than a developmental program of information, education, and persuasion aimed at influencing the public, health policy makers, and other health professionals about the contributions and potential of this largest of the health practitioner groups. The efforts of the National Commission over the recent past have sensitized many groups and individuals to the changes now taking place. Organized nursing must raise and expand the consciousness level.

NURSING ROLES AND FUNCTIONS

For the period of implementation, the National Commission established four primary goals in the area of nursing roles and functions. These were:

1. Establishment of a National Joint Practice Commission.
2. Establishment of counterpart state joint practice committees.
3. Stimulation of interest in distributive nursing practice to broaden health care coverage.
4. Stimulation of interest in new utilization patterns for nurses within both distributive and episodic practice to improve client care.

Whereas the first two of these goals were designed to develop the apparatus and agencies for change, the others were intended to point out the directions and patterns for future utilization of professional nurses. During the second year of the implementation phase, the priority emphasis of the NCSNNE was placed on the erection of the national and state joint practice committees; provided throughout the implementation phase was the presentation of information and experimentation on episodic and distributive practice.

Accomplishments of Implementation

Toward the end of the first year of implementation, in August of 1971, members of the AMA Committee on Nursing and the ANA Congress for Nursing Practice, together with their staff personnel, met with NCSNNE representatives to discuss arrangements and guidelines for the establishment of a national joint practice commission. That first meeting resulted in a memorandum of agreement subsequently approved by the boards of the parent organizations. The understanding specified that there would be equal numbers of nurses and physicians, most of whom would be practitioners involved in direct patient care, and that there would be a joint effort to improve health care through alterations in the roles and functions of *both* professions.

Members were named over the late fall of 1971, and on January 20-21, 1972, the National Joint Practice Commission held its inaugural meeting in St. Louis, Missouri. Over the next few months, the NJPC has met at periodic intervals, developed its operating procedures, established bylaws and organizational objectives, and moved on to substantive programs. With interim funding from the parent organizations, the NJPC has successfully moved to secure long-term support, and has begun to establish a headquarters and staff of its own. It has conducted its first national conference of state joint practice committees at which forty-seven states were represented, the majority by nurse-physician pairs. Most recently it has appointed three task forces to assess roles and functions in: care of the aging, rural health care, and interdisciplinary education for joint practice.

The rapid development of the NJPC has been paralleled by the growth of statewide joint practice committees. By April, 1973, there were no less than twenty-seven states with operational groups, three more were designated but not yet functioning, and fourteen additional states had liaison, or preliminary, committees. Only three states had, to the best knowledge of the NCSNNE staff, failed to initiate some steps toward establishment of a medical-nursing group to examine joint concerns. Many of these groups have already begun to play a significant part in health practice acts, demonstration projects, new practitioner patterns for rural health care, and a variety of other activities. They constitute a vital and vigorous new force in health planning.

In the case of proposing and developing the concepts of episodic and distributive care, the National Commission's recommendations appeared in conjunction with, and congruent to, Esther Lucile Brown's[2] two-volume report on emergent nursing roles and Secretary Richardson's[3] document on extending the role of nurses to enhance health care delivery. Through a series of speeches, pamphlets, and articles, the NCSNNE staff attempted to emphasize that nursing, in common with most of the American health care system, is largely committed to a medical service, hospital-based model of treatment. Unfortunately, this approach takes too little account of *health care* in its emphasis on *patient cure.* The maintenance of health and the prevention of disease are just as important to the nation as the treatment of an acutely ill person lying in a hospital, yet over 85 percent of our active nurse practitioners are involved in episodic care while less than 15 percent are involved in distributive practice.

So pervasive has been our concentration on cure that we have often labelled hospital nursing as "general practice" when, in reality, it is surely as specialized a set of roles and functions as school nursing, occupational nursing, or community nursing. As one observer notes,

> . . . hard as it is to admit, it is fact that the delivery system we built around our activity has not kept pace with increase in technology, expanding population and changing social attitudes. . . . The system is full of inequity in terms of both quality and availability of its product-service.[4]

At the heart of improving both quality and availability of health care lies a reformulation of nursing's contribution to that practice which "is generally continuous in nature, seldom acute, and increasingly will take place in community or emergent institutional settings."[5] By documenting the expanded roles of nurse clinicians in distributive care, the Commission and its staff have provided input that can now be utilized by national and state joint practice committees in developing new configurations of care that include health maintenance as well as cure activities on an equal scale of importance.

In the area of changed utilization patterns, the Commission documented that expanded role demands in both episodic and distributive care, as well as the development of clinical career opportunities which provide for continuing direct client contact, can not only produce higher qualities of care, but greater practitioner satisfaction; there was also some indication of lowered per capita costs through reduced care periods, improved adherence to treatment regimens, and lowered readmission rates to treatment centers.[6] In a number of hospitals and in community care facilities, there was evidence of positive professional response to the divestment of non-nursing functions and the expansion of clinical activities.[7] Again, these are materials and data that can be utilized by the joint practice groups, and by individual facilities, addressing the refinement of health care delivery.

Shortcomings and Difficulties

It is captious to complain of the amount of progress of the National Joint Practice Commission. One could always wish that even further advances might be recorded, but so much has been accomplished in building a new structure and program that to expect more would be presumptuous.

In terms of the statewide joint practice committees, it is more reasonable to say that success could have been greater. Three states have no reported progress. In four more states, medicine and nursing meet together under the aegis of a "physician-nurse-allied health personnel" committee that has little concern and less power over the congruent roles of nurses and physicians. In another fourteen states, medicine and nursing meet together in liaison committees rather than joint practice bodies—these terms are not synonymous. As the state groups and the NCSNNE have defined them, joint practice committees are those that adequately reflect the objectives and program of the NJPC including the provision for a majority of practitioners from the participating professions. Liaison committees frequently reflect the leadership of the state medical society and nurses' association. Thus, the nurse members are more likely to be educators, deans, directors of nursing service—but not practitioners and clinicians.

Much more should be done in organizing joint practice committees in the remaining states, either by developing them *ab initio* or, where practicable, reorganizing existing liaison committees to reflect the concentration on roles, functions, and joint practice. There is still a noticeable tendency in some states toward mutual avoidance among physicians and nurses, and there is certainly a strong indication that meeting together is not going to solve anything unless there is joint commitment to planning for change. The millennium is not reached by designation of a nurse-physician committee. There must be willingness to share decision making and there must be willingness on both sides to risk change. The differential success, to date, of state joint practice committees indicates that some have operated largely as discussion groups while others have set out to make fundamental improvements in the health care system.

Perhaps no other proposal of the National Commission evoked so much controversy as that which recommended nursing roles be developed in both episodic and distributive practice. To the NLN Task Force assigned to study the Commission's recommendations, "The specific meaning of the terms episodic and distributive was ambiguous to the committee and created confusion when implications and implementation were considered."[8] To Christy, Poulin, and Hover, the development of two career patterns for nursing practice represents "one of the more drastic and divisive items in the report as well as one of the more historically tenuous."[9] In letters to the editor and in questions from the floor at state and district informational meetings, it was evident that specialty concentrations in practice were disturbing to many nurses.

It was the opinion of the National Commission and the staff that much of this reaction was of the muscle reflex type. Nursing had for so long regarded hospital nursing as "general" nursing that it found itself unable to see the specialized elements involved in such practice. Had the concept of episodic and distributive care been less important, it might have been tempting to eschew the debates that necessarily followed, but the Commission felt strongly that nursing must evolve a primary commitment to practice that would meet the full range of societal needs, including those for health maintenance and disease prevention, as well as those for treatment and cure. In the months of implementation, then, a great number of articles, pamphlets, and discussions were devoted to episodic and distributive care. Gradually the issue softened, and the terms began to appear in the literature as useful conceptual formulations.[10] It is nevertheless true that continued explanation and demonstration is very necessary for these terms and their underlying importance to achieve common currency and acceptance.

From the outset, the National Commission recognized that the recommendation for fundamental reevaluation of practice patterns would cause anxiety. Halfway through the implementation phase, the director emphasized the developmental aspects of the change process:

> We have a great commitment to the validity and usefulness of this concept [episodic and distributive practice]. At the same time, we know that such a fundamental reorganization, and the changing of a pattern of thinking that goes back over three-quarters of a century, is neither lightly nor easily accepted. Moreover, the Commission's own thinking is open-ended in that no one knows precisely what might constitute the . . . specialties.[11]

It is to be anticipated that the ANA Congress for Nursing Practice, the several specialty practice groups, and the state and national joint practice committees will empirically define the parameters of episodic and distributive care more usefully than any theoretic discussion might hope to accomplish. In terms of the implementation effort, it is fair to say that the terms "episodic" and "distributive" have lost much of their threatening aspects. This, however, is only the first step. Only a handful of educational institutions and health care facilities have become involved in studying and experimenting with change models for these concepts. In the terms employed by the group dynamics people, we have warmed the situation sufficiently so that the status quo is unfrozen and permits movement. We have not, however, overcome inertia sufficiently to see more than very slight progress.

In terms of the proposals for changed utilization patterns for nurses in both episodic and distributive care—patterns that would encourage more direct involvement in patient care over the course of a professional career—there was little in the way of opposition or rejection. An increasing number of service institutions and advanced clinical practitioner programs have tended to support the concept of increased involvement of nurses in direct client care with a corresponding divestment of non-nursing functions. This is, however, a long-term process and one in which more remains to be done, by far, than has been accomplished to date. Through the publication of site visits to demonstration projects, and the presentation of data on quality and cost effectiveness of new nursing roles, the NCSNNE was able to fan interest. It still remains for this to be translated into overt action and organizational repatterning.

Continuing Needs

Success of the National Joint Practice Commission is most likely the key to implementation of the entire set of recommendations relating to nursing roles and functions. If the NJPC can begin, through its task forces and programs, to effect change in congruent roles between medicine and nursing, then all other things will likely come about as well. This is not because of some "domino theory" game plan. It is simply that success on the national level would strengthen and support success at the statewide level which would, in turn, encourage further activity by the NJPC. There is a strong reciprocal relationship that must be fostered and extended.

In addition to the relationships between national and state joint practice committees, organized medicine and nursing must continue—and increase—their commitments and assistance to the state joint practice committees. Many of these bodies have operated on the barest kind of financing; some have borne expenses personally to help in setting up and organizing the groups. State medical societies and nurses' associations must recognize the importance of joint planning and activity in health care and provide support for the state committees. Expenses are modest, but they are essential.

Nursing must continue to examine its posture and response to the broad spectrum of health care needs across the nation. Episodic and distributive practice, as terms, are far less important than their references in the real world. There is a large proportion of our population whose health care needs are better classified under the headings of "health maintenance" and "disease prevention" than under our current model of cure and treatment. Nurses could become the primary care practitioners for many of these people through interdependent planning with medicine, other health professionals, and the public. A solution must be found and nursing, with its large resources in clinically capable personnel, is in a key position to respond. At the same time, nursing must maintain and enlarge its contributions to our traditional episodic care areas. Taken together, these are invigorating challenges to excellence. The response of nursing must be positive.

There is great need, too, for continuing reexamination of our utilization patterns in nursing practice. Continuation of a career should not mean inevitable removal from direct client care. Our withdrawal and turnover rates are tragic testimony to the outcomes of our present system. Demonstrations and experimental models have shown that there are better ways to provide excellent care and professional satisfaction while reducing per capita costs. These must be examined more broadly and implemented as quickly as results are verified.

Perhaps, in essence, the National Commission is saying that one element of professionalism is the commitment to continuing change in the face of emerging needs, altered technology, and expanded knowledge. Nursing is not, and cannot be, exempt from such demands.

In the last year of the implementation phase, the NCSNNE staff met with the combined advisory groups that assisted the Commission and staff in planning and evaluating activities and programs. After review of what had been done, and what was projected for the final months of work, the advisors were asked, through a conference and forced choice technique,[12] to project the continuing aims of implementation over the period ahead. The results of the individual decisions were then grouped to provide a rank-ordered set of priorities according to the combined weightings suggested by the participants. The results in the area of nursing roles and functions are indicated in Table 7-2.

These proposals for continuing implementation efforts obviously are addressed to nursing in particular, and to society and the other health professions generally. They provide a set of guidelines for the next stage of implementation, based on the considered judgment of persons from many disciplines and viewpoints who have followed closely the developing approaches to activating the National Commission's work. As such, they deserve careful consideration by the various nursing organizations as they contemplate the immediate and long-range future.

TABLE 7-2 RECOMMENDATIONS FOR CONTINUING IMPLEMENTATION ACTIVITIES RELATED TO NURSING ROLES AND FUNCTIONS

Number	Relative Weight	Recommendation
1	(28)	Development of support for research designed to study the impact of nursing practice on patient care
2	(26)	Presentation of ongoing, systematic, and well-documented data on nursing practice, including the expanded role of the nurse, to health administrators, legislators, planners, and physicians
3	(16)	Continual review of all the individual recommendations in *An Abstract for Action* with periodic updating of those which have been accomplished, those which need continued effort, and those which should constitute the next set of priorities
4	(14)	Development of nursing leadership at the local level to bring practitioners and clinicians into decision-making processes
5	(13)	Creation of institutional and management support structures to enable health care practitioners to concentrate on practice
6	(11)	Emphasis on research on joint or multidisciplinary roles and functions for health care practitioners to develop a centralized source of information on the results of such research and experimentation

NURSING EDUCATION AND PATTERNING

To focus the efforts of the staff in working for change in nursing education and its patterns, the National Commission established, at the outset of the implementation phase, four priorities; all were related to an overall plan to establish statewide master planning committees for nursing education throughout the country to guide and effect the changes contemplated. The four chief aims were:

1. Positioning of nursing education within the collegiate system of higher education.
2. Articulation of programs and curricula between junior and senior colleges involved in nursing education.
3. Development of curricular concentrations in episodic and distributive practice within all collegiate nursing programs.
4. Enhancement of advanced and continuing education programs for nursing, particularly those aimed at expanding practice excellence.

As indicated, the establishment of statewide master planning committees was considered to be an important fulcrum to the realization of each of the four primary goals. This was true not only because the states legally are the designated creators of educational policy, but also because they represent viable planning units for assessing needs and resources, determining goals and timetables, and organizing transitional approaches to the accomplishment of long-range objectives. National committees and groups may propose policy, but the formulation of that policy into specific ways and means involves local participation, involvement, and execution.

Accomplishments of Implementation

There was continuing effort over the three years of implementation to assist states in forming and organizing statewide master planning committees. One of the first publications of the NCSNNE was a guide to developing such groups,[13] and, with the designation of the target states, the Commission staff became immersed in the details of planning committee organization. By the third year of the implementation phase, this became the primary area of activity to ensure continuation of work and planning beyond the termination of the Commission itself.

As a result of the contribution of nurses and other individuals, at the state level primarily, and with the assistance of NCSNNE staff, our regional associates, and advisors, it was possible to determine that by April 1, 1973, no less than twenty-six states had operational statewide master planning committees. Some activity was underway in twenty-one other states, and there were only four in which, to the best of our knowledge, there was no progress to report. Many of these groups had received some formal recognition or designation; most were working with the cooperation and acceptance of state health boards, state planning and health officials, and the various health professions and associations within the state.

All are involved in assessing the present state of nursing education, its needs and problems, and the developmental tasks that must be undertaken to provide a comprehensive pattern for its institutions and levels.

To supply grist for these statewide planning groups, the NCSNNE has attempted to furnish data, operational alternatives, and information on educational innovations that can, in turn, permit better decision making and long-term planning.

In terms of moving the educational patterns for nursing into the collegiate system, for example, the National Commission recommended basically what every national study of nursing has proposed since 1923. This time, however, the NCSNNE staff has worked with institutions and hospital schools to develop planned alternatives and phased implementation. Over the three-year period from 1970 to 1973, some 155 hospital schools of nursing were closed—a decline of approximately 22 percent. For the most part, however, these institutions have continued some role in nursing education. In one case, a hospital school transformed itself into a college pursuant to suggestions in *An Abstract for Action.* In several instances, former hospital schools joined in interinstitutional arrangements with colleges to strengthen collegiate programs through improved facilities and opportunities for clinical instruction. In almost all cases, the hospital continued to have student nurses learning inside its walls. Within the time period of implementation, collegiate programs for the first time became the "majority partner" in American nursing education with more than 55 percent of the programs and the enrolled students located in colleges.

As the hospital schools decline and transform, the Commission anticipated that the next most problematic issue would be that of educational articulation between two- and four-year colleges. Historically, nursing education in the junior college was perceived as "technical" and "terminal" whereas the baccalaureate nursing program was seen to be "professional" and "open-ended." Leaving aside the entire question as to whether there ever was, in fact, any basis for this distinction, the present patterns of institutional growth and development indicate that more and more students will complete their preparatory nursing education in a community or junior college and that increasing numbers will then be seeking admission to upper division courses in senior colleges to extend their personal and professional horizons. To plan for this and to provide access to soundly articulated programs for advancement is essentially a societal requirement with evident ethical overtones. Nursing education must react—positively.

Over the course of the implementation, the NCSNNE staff has been able to document a growing awareness and willingness of nursing education to respond to the challenge. A small, but increasing number of "two plus two" programs are emerging in senior colleges. These are specifically designed for facilitating the transfer of graduates from associate degree nursing programs by providing similar courses and clinical experience in the first two years of a baccalaureate program. Thus both transfer students and "generic" students from the home institution can begin the third year of the upper division on reasonably related levels. Other institutions are providing specialized upper division courses for ADN graduates and are planning their entire educational sequence in terms of junior, senior, and graduate instruction of those who have already passed licensure examinations.[14] Perhaps the key concept in all this is greater flexibility. What was once a rather monolithic approach to baccalaureate nurse education has become much freer, much more individualistic, and much more responsive to demands for articulated progression.

This very essence of flexibility has begun to affect the Commission's proposals for educational electives and concentrations in episodic and distributive care. The long historic association of hospitals and nursing education tended to focus all curricular emphasis on the medical service model of the hospital wards. The use of distributive practice and facilities as an alternative approach to clinical instruction was more unrecognized than opposed. After some brief flurry over what is and what is not "general" nursing, an increasing number of educational institutions at both the junior and senior levels are providing electives and concentrations in episodic and distributive nursing practice.[15] This not only relates to defined and recognized societal needs, but promises to provide more alternatives and more individualized opportunities for the nursing student in determining career paths and settings. It opens the way to a recognition that all nursing is not the same and cannot be taught in the same ways. Expanding knowledge, enlarging roles, and developing client needs all militate against "one best way" to prepare a nurse. Rather, the challenge is to ensure that quality is built into all preparatory and advanced programs and that quality of care provided by the graduate becomes the most important measure of success.

Continuing and advanced education have made remarkable progress over the three years of implementation. This, of course, is due to the nurse leaders involved with the National Commission and its staff playing more the role of advocate and cheerleader than change agent. The evolution of the informal organization on continuing education into a full-blown commission of the American Nurses' Association paralleled the time span of the National Commission; our frequent interchanges and cooperative activities reinforced our shared commitment to improved continuing and in-service education. The growth of advanced practitioner programs in graduate nursing education was a development soundly applauded by our Commission which sought primarily to provide improved and increased support for such developments.

Largely through the activity of the NLN Council of Baccalaureate and Higher Degree Programs, the ANA Commission on Education and the interstate compacts in the south, the northeast, the midwest, and the west, the tempo of change in nursing education is noticeably more accelerated. With continued experimentation and development at the institutional level, new patterns of articulation and advancement will become even more rational and comprehensive. The thrust is clearly discernible; and movement is already well underway.

Shortcomings and Difficulties

Obviously, the task of forming and establishing statewide master planning committees is incomplete. Moreover, many of the groups "in process" of organization are still seeking direction, goals and objectives, and some operational mechanisms that will give substance to the form they are creating. There is still a great spatial distance between hope and reality.

Most of the excitement in the implementation of the National Commission's recommendations for nursing education has been generated by the reactions to the proposals for moving all institutions into the collegiate mainstream. The reactions were rather predictable from those organizations that represented the hospital schools of nursing. The NLN Council of Diploma Programs voted "nonsupport" of the recommendations while the AHA Assembly of Hospital Schools of Nursing sought an "official statement repudiating those groups and individuals who are alluding to the phasing out of diploma programs of nursing education."[16] When neither of these approaches seemed to reverse the steady diminution of the ranks of hospital schools, antagonism turned to hopeful allegation. After one report on the closures and projected closures of diploma programs, the newsletter of the AHA Assembly asserted:

> If any conclusions are to be drawn from the discussion, they are that there are still sharp differences of opinion between Type VIII (hospital school) members and the commission, and that the majority of the assembly believes that hospital schools will continue to grow in strength, vigor, and excellence.[17]

At the biennial meeting of the NLN in 1973, the Council of Diploma Programs sounded a similar hopeful note:

> The Executive Committee of the Council of Diploma Programs . . . believes that the future potential of hospital-based schools is limitless. . . .[18]

If, at either meeting, notice was taken of the decreasing number of hospital programs, this was not generally communicated. While the Commission is pleased over the progress that has been made, it is still concerned to see that the remaining 540 diploma institutions begin transitional planning. It is the students who attend and graduate from these programs who are faced with the problems of mobility and opportunity. It is the students who suffer from the lack of comparability of institutions and their programs. And it is a sobering fact that thousands of individuals have graduated from this bifurcated system of nursing education over the course of the implementation period. All those who prepared in hospital schools might have graduated from collegiate programs with clearer paths for advanced educational opportunities. All of them might have graduated from significantly different educational environments that could have broadened and deepened their personal horizons. It is little satisfaction that 22 percent of the institutions have transformed; it is critical that we get on with the work of full resolution of this gnawing separatism.

If there was anger and emotionalism over the proposals to disestablish the hospital schools, there certainly was excitement and nervousness over the Commission's recommendation that two- and four-year programs be articulated and jointly planned. For years, the ADN and BSN associations have met separately to discuss their individual concerns. Many nurse educators took it almost as a matter of revealed truth that associate degree programs had nothing in common with baccalaureate curricula. Labels like "technical" and "professional" were treated as though they were taxonomic terms that truly distinguished observable behavior in the real world. Most importantly, however, the recommendations threatened the psychological distance and mystique that had long enshrouded the generic, baccalaureate programs. The prospects of interinstitutional planning, of "outside meddling" with baccalaureate programs, and, perhaps, the exposure of weakness in all programs caused a great deal of concern and frustration.

Many baccalaureate programs are still uninvolved in the plans for articulation. Many have shown themselves to be more than reluctant to accept transfer students from associate degree programs or to encourage challenge examinations or advanced placement procedures. This laggardly reaction to required change has already resulted in legislative or administrative intervention in some state educational systems, and could lead to more. It is essential that, at the very minimum the institutions for nursing education examine the experience of those upper and lower division programs that are involved in study and demonstration of change.

As in the case of articulation, the Commission's concerns in terms of curricular flexibility and alternative concentrations are bound up in the relatively small number of institutions that have begun to grapple with the emergent problems of the age. It can only be hoped that the combination of joint practice committees, consumer demands, and ongoing reexaminations of the nursing curriculum can combine to encourage greater individuality in collegiate nursing education and the proffering of elective concentrations to the students. It is not so much a matter of opposition as it is one of slow progress and great inertia.

In contrast, one can hardly be critical of developments in continuing education in nursing. The progress and vision established over the past six years has been a remarkable testimony to a small number of dedicated, energetic, committed people. Progress in graduate education has likewise been steady and positive, the most problematic factor being the question over continuing financial support for such programs.* The Commission has expressed concerns over the length and complexity of many graduate programs for nurses, but these are matters that are being addressed and resolved.

*Note: for a discussion of the entire impact of recent federal proposals for the financial support of nursing, see pp. 251-253.

Continuing Needs

The statewide master planning committees, organized nursing, educators, involved lay persons and others must press on with the analysis of educational needs and resources for nursing. Needs can be found rather easily. The challenge is to develop sound answers within the scope of available resources while seeking to strengthen the entire system.

We must cooperatively press on toward the goal of centering all nursing education within the collegiate pattern. The trend is clearly set and the wheels are in motion.

> The question to be resolved is whether reason and reasonableness will govern the change, or whether the rhetoric of anger and frustration will continue to exact its toll for every step of progress.[19]

Statewide master planning committees must encourage the development of a collegiate pattern, but they must also help to ensure that the resultant arrangement includes planned articulation between two- and four-year programs, as well as enlarged flexibility in individual electives and concentrations. Nursing education, itself, must do the specific planning and determination, but it needs the encouragement, support, and perhaps the prodding of others to get on with the essential tasks at hand.

Likewise, the master planning committees must look beyond preparatory education, that has for so long held center stage, to examine the needs and resources for continuing and advanced nursing education. These areas are vital to the development of excellence in nursing practice, and they have long been neglected by those who saw preparatory education as the only solution to cries of nursing shortage. Wise regional and statewide development of advanced programs in nursing education is required to maintain and expand practitioner roles and functions. They are too critical to be viewed on any less than an equal plane of importance.

At the request of the NCSNNE staff, the combined advisory committees to the Commission and staff reviewed progress and problems in the implementation of recommendations related to nursing education and its institutional patterns. After considerable discussion, the advisors were asked to rank individually their suggestions for continuing activities, and the grouped results were then collected. Priority items for consideration by organized nursing and others are presented in Table 7-3.

These long-term priorities are proposed for examination and action by the various nursing organizations at both national and state levels. They offer a program, not only for further implementation of *An Abstract for Action*, but a continuing program of involvement and participation in decision making that materially affects nursing over all the years to come. To confront change rather than merely experience it is, in the last analysis, the only way that nursing can adequately keep its educational programs and patterns relevant to the nation's needs.

TABLE 7-3 RECOMMENDATIONS FOR CONTINUING IMPLEMENTATION ACTIVITIES RELATED TO NURSING EDUCATION

Number	Relative Weight	Recommendation
1	(38)	Plan transition of the implementation efforts to effective national, state, and local groups in order to obtain even greater "grass roots" involvement in effecting change
2	(30)	Strongly encourage existing nursing organizations to assist in developing relevant educational programs that will unify the profession, through the development of realistic standards of practice, related competencies of nurse practitioners in episodic and distributive care, and guidelines for utilization so that nursing education will have a basis to proceed on curricular planning
3	(24)	Encourage organized nursing to become involved with all health care issues being discussed in order to contribute to the understanding of nursing's role in care provision and in order to see that changing demands for practice are quickly reflected within the nursing curriculum
4	(20)	Seek active involvement in the politics and planning of higher education by working with state higher education and coordinating agencies in the development of master planning for nursing education
5	(17)	Develop areawide interinstitutional consortia for the coordination of continuing education programs, with a specific focus on interdisciplinary education aimed at involving all the health professions in joint learning experiences
6	(16)	Plan a continuing program of communications and consultation with nurses and with nursing students to ensure continuing movement toward accomplishment of the Commission's recommendations in the area of nursing education

NURSING CAREER PERSPECTIVES

Inasmuch as the area of nursing careers, by the very nature of the Commission's recommendations, required the longest time perspectives, it was obvious that only the beginnings could be realized over the three-year period of NCSNNE implementation. Economic and social patterns are often more difficult to alter than the functional relationship of two practitioners, or even the transfer of educational responsibility from one institution to another. Simply because many of our patterns are familiar and comfortable, we fail to see the fundamental flaws they contain. Yet corrective action or change requires, first of all, that problems be identified and recognized.

Throughout the implementation period, the Commission has attempted to inform and educate nurses, other health professionals, health management and other policy makers as to the basic paradoxes and absurdities that affect career perspectives in nursing. In particular, four primary aims were selected for emphasis:

1. Dissemination of information on motivation in nursing and the effects of depressed economic and skewed psychosocial rewards on nursing careers.
2. Encouragement of nursing organizations to cooperate in interpreting the profession to the public and to other health groups and to effect greater internal consensus and unity.
3. Advocacy of increased individual commitment to an active role in professional development through participation in nursing organizations.
4. Encouragement of greater organizational involvement in issues like licensure, relicensure, and certification.

By working on these four principal objectives, some progress could be realized in the general domain of all nineteen specific recommendations of the Commission related to nursing careers. Moreover, the combination of better knowledge about nursing's needs together with a stronger, more unified organization, could ensure both a direction and an impetus for prolonged change. Succeeding years could bring the resolution of matters that presently can only be outlined and illumined.

Accomplishments of Implementation

Over the course of the implementation phase, the Commission's effort to inform and educate the public and relevant agencies about the problems in nursing careers received a series of supportive assists. The ANA Commission on Economic and General Welfare had already sensitized many nurses and health administrators to underlying problems of security. This was heightened by an upsurge in collective bargaining activities across the country, and these, in turn, secured sizeable advances in compensation for nurses. The appearance, at this point, of two economic analyses of nursing's career perspectives—one by Altman[20] and one by Yett[21]—clearly indicated that most of these advances were really only a belated catching up with other female occupations and that there must be some plan for action rather than reaction. The impact of the feminist movement now added its weight by raising the consciousness level throughout society that females generally are militated against in the present economic system and that nursing, as one of the female occupations, suffered in comparison with any male groups in the health professions.

Taken all together, these factors underscored what the National Commission reported out of its investigative phase relative to financial reward and security. Nursing has long been depressed in comparison with other women's occupations, has been greatly depressed in comparison with other female professions, and has simply not even been in a comparative structure with male professions. Progress over the past decade is quite encouraging, but there is still much that needs to be done to reflect adequately the demands of society on nursing in the compensation levels afforded the profession.

The Commission's concern, however, was to anticipate the succeeding levels of motivation that must be satisfied once minimal security needs have been attained. In this regard, the Commission emphasized that the traditional "career patterns" in nursing have invariably led the practitioner away from the patient or client and that this would be a destructive force even in a well-compensated profession. Case examples, demonstration projects, and economic data were advanced to show that withdrawal, turnover, frustration, and apathy could all be reduced and the quality of care advanced through reorganized professional and structural patterns that would permit advancement through patient care rather than away from direct client involvement. This aspect of the Commission's concern for motivational problems of the profession received support from the contemporary reports of Brown[22] and Secretary Richardson's task force on extended roles in nursing.[23] Both these analyses recognized that poor utilization and misutilization of nurses in the past have prevented us from receiving all the benefits we might have in terms of health care. To encourage nursing to extend its reach beyond its grasp is both to ensure greater professional satisfaction and better public satisfaction with resultant increments of care.

Through the medium of statewide meetings, contacts with the health professions and organizations, and an extensive series of articles and pamphlets, the NCSNNE staff has worked to provide basic information on these matters. No measuring rod can be applied to the results, but thousands of decision makers have received data and cases that document the Commission's position.

More tangible evidence is afforded in the case of the effort to build a "house of nursing" that could provide greater unity and consensus. Through simultaneous actions of the American Association of Critical-Care Nurses and the American Nurses' Association, two meetings were held in 1972-73 which laid the groundwork for a continuing series of conferences with participants from virtually all the national organizations of nursing. The ANA, NLN, specialty practice groups, and federal nurses' agencies have begun to regularize their relationships and to press for joint action on issues and concerns. At the so-called National Nurses' Congress held at San Clemente in January of 1973, the participating groups reached a number of consensual decisions and set a date for their next convening session in June of the same year. Out of greater experience and cooperation can come the basis for a united attack on common problems. In time, there may develop a house of nursing envisioned by the Commission—its form and structure to be determined by the associations now beginning, as never before, to work together.

One specific outcome of the Commission effort toward this objective lay in the accelerated involvement of the nurse specialty practice groups in the implementation of the National Commission's work. Most of these associations had been positively oriented toward *An Abstract for Action*; some took early action to support its program of change. As more of the specialty groups looked toward continuing implementation efforts, however, there was a definite quickening of organizational activity designed to ensure that the termination of the National Commission's work would not mean the end of nursing's commitment to effecting implementation. Of the eleven specialty practice groups present at the San Clemente meeting, no less than eight have taken positive action to support the implementation of the Commission's recommendations. The three remaining groups have indicated that their boards will consider action at the next scheduled meeting or national convention. The associations which have taken action to date are listed in Table 7-4.

This expression of common purpose is one more indication of the growing awareness of consensus in American nursing. In their shared concerns for continuing implementation, the nurse specialty practice groups, as well as the other professional organizations, have generated whole new areas for joint action and cooperative movement.

TABLE 7-4 SPECIALTY PRACTICE GROUPS INDICATING SUPPORT OR ENDORSEMENT OF *AN ABSTRACT FOR ACTION*, 1971-1973

Organization	Date of Action
American Association of Industrial Nurses	October, 1971
Department of School Nurses—National Education Association	September, 1972
Association of Operating Room Nurses	October, 1972
American Association of Critical-Care Nurses	April, 1973
Emergency Department Nurses' Association	April, 1973
The Nurses' Association of the American College of Obstetricians and Gynecologists	April, 1973
American Association of Neurosurgical Nurses	April, 1973
American Urological Association—Allied Membership Division	May, 1973

At every opportunity, the National Commission has encouraged nurses and student nurses to assume professional responsibility for joining their national and local organizations and to participate fully in their activities. It is encouraging to note that one of the outcomes of the national meeting of nurse associations in 1973 was a consensual determination to increase recruiting activities to enlist nurses in at least one of the professional bodies. This kind of effort, cooperatively mounted, could materially strengthen nursing's ability to communicate with the public and become a full partner in determining health care policies and plans.

Finally, the Commission has taken an active role in the debates on relicensure, institutional licensure, certification and related issues. Frequently, it has been required to play the role of advocate for *planned* change. Such a posture is not designed to preserve the status quo—hardly a likely move on the part of a general change agency. There is concern, however, over too quick a legislative or administrative response to proposals in these areas. Institutional licensure, for example, is currently being studied in a few areas; already, however, there are advocates for nationwide implementation of the concept in advance of findings and results. The same is true in mandated continuing education for relicensure. Some proposals are in process to require statewide compliance with regulations—but without the educational system that would permit individual conformity.

Shortcomings and Difficulties

Perhaps the greatest difficulty in implementing recommendations in the area of career perspectives is the agonizingly slow pace of change in some critical concerns and the contrasting willingness of persons and organizations to fly off swiftly in response to proposals in others. While nursing has made some hearty financial advances, for example, there is great reluctance among health administrators to face the fact that nursing is still poorly compensated in comparison with most other occupations having similar preparation and job responsibilities. These same administrators, however, may herald institutional licensure as a salvation for hospitals and care facilities. The coupling of these two considerations leads one to wonder seriously what effect institutional licensure might have on the beginning gains toward a career compensation pattern for the nursing profession.

There is a paradoxical, if not downright absurd, quality to the fact that most institutions utilizing nurse practitioners have not formulated a career pattern that permits the individual to stay in direct care activities, but in one state—and soon likely to be in more—we have mandated continuing education for relicensure using as one argument the need for maintenance of individual practice skills. It is not that the Commission is opposed to some form of documented practice level in association with relicensure; rather, there should be some greater evidence that practice skills will be utilized as well as examined. So long as head nurses and supervisors spend less time in direct patient care than nursing students, aides, and orderlies, there is a fundamental flaw in our career usage of nurses that cannot be solved by continuing education or any other regulatory device. Our system needs fundamental restructuring before any peripheral adjustment can have worthwhile impact.

In the matter of nursing organization membership and individual support, there is conflicting evidence. Some of the growth in nursing associations is real; some of it involves a membership switch from older organizations to the newer specialty practice groups. Altogether, there are hundreds of thousands of nurses who belong to no organization and have abdicated their right to participate not only in nursing decisions, but in the larger arena of public policy and health care delivery determination. So long as these many people remain uninvolved, the profession will always be at a disadvantage in acting as a full and responsible partner with the other health organizations.

There must be continuing willingness among the health organizations, and in their relations with state health and planning bodies, to defer action of a determinative nature on many of the present proposals related to licensure, relicensure, and certification. The studies are underway in some cases; the joint practice committees and other relevant bodies are just beginning in others. The effort to concretize legislation is not only inappropriate but dangerous because we don't know what the outcomes might be. To study institutional licensure is appropriate and right; to legislate it at this time is ridiculous. The same could be said of many of the other proposals to enact untried systems and mandates into law.

Continuing Needs

Out of the combined wisdom of the master planning and joint practice committees, as well as the results of institutional experimentation and demonstration, we must evolve a career pattern in nursing that allows for the satisfaction of economic and psychosocial needs through the provision of quality patient care to the full extension of the nurses' individual capacities. Nurses must be permitted to "stay" in patient care and find there the compensation patterns and recognition and esteem that should be accorded the proper aim of the profession—the care of people. Our traditional patterns and organizations have not worked! They must be replaced—and quickly. There are models already available from which selections or variations might be developed, but there is need to get on with the long unfinished agenda of career perspectives in nursing.

There is need for nurses to address the long-term erection of a house of nursing that can encompass the viewpoints and concerns of the entire profession. This cannot be a monolithic organization, but neither can nursing afford a fractionated approach to matters substantive to its very existence. A house, large enough to permit diversity, strong enough to permit the various stories and rooms required for living together—this is what must be built. The expanding common concern and cooperative course taken by nursing's professional organizations points the way to some future method of consolidation, the precise nature of which is still undetermined. The need is too paramount, however, for some form of constructive building not to take place.

In assessing the gains and the shortcomings of the NCSNNE implementation phase, the combined advisory groups attempted to predict the next succeeding efforts that should be mounted in the area of nursing careers. Their six priority items are shown in Table 7-5 along with the weights attached to their rank-ordering.

In the long run, it is at least as much to the public's interest as it is to nursing to see that there is an attractive and rewarding career perspective in nursing practice. Only by fundamental rearrangement can we overcome the problems of alienation, frustration, and induced apathy that have so long been evident throughout the profession. Career patterns must be clarified and revitalized. Then, and only then, can the promise of nursing be fulfilled.

In the future look at careers, one of the critical areas must be that of licensed practical nursing. In the investigative stage of *An Abstract for Action*, primary focus was on the roles, education, and career of the registered nurse. It was the

TABLE 7-5 RECOMMENDATIONS FOR CONTINUING IMPLEMENTATION ACTIVITIES RELATED TO NURSING CAREERS AND PERSPECTIVES

Number	Relative Weight	Recommendation
1	(30)	Encourage nurses and their organizations to become more involved in the development of health policies at the national and state levels
2	(17)	Promote the nursing career ladder concept in both educational institutions and practice settings
3	(14)	Expand the career horizons of nurses through the development of state joint practice committees and through periodic readjustment of health practice acts reflecting their recommendations for expanded roles
4	(14)	Urge a moratorium on all legislation concerning licensure and relicensure pending the outcomes of current studies on the impact of such legislation and the results of controlled trials
5	(12)	Encourage more frequent communications among the various nursing organizations in order to promote unity and consensus
6	(10)	Encourage nursing to define the roles of the nurse practitioner at staff and advanced levels so as to relate these to educational preparation and experience for the purpose of promoting career perspectives and planning

Commission's considered opinion that the problems uncovered there would be generic and would differ in degree rather than kind from those of the licensed practical nurse. Particular attention was paid to the educational mobility of the LPN through available programs that could provide access to the RN license.[24] These activities were not fully satisfactory to the LPN organizations which felt that there ought to be more overt inclusion of them and their members in the planning of change and the establishment of new patterns for nursing practice and education. The Commission and the staff conducted a series of discussions with LPN spokesmen and, in 1972, held an invitational conference to examine the implications of *An Abstract for Action* for licensed practical nursing, and to discuss what might be done to satisfy the felt needs of these groups. In Appendix E of this volume, there is contained a report on the outcomes of that conference including material related to a study proposal prepared by the NCSNNE staff as a possible future activity of the combined LPN organizations. At this time, no specific follow-up is planned, but it remains something for further thought and action.

NURSING AND THE FEDERAL GOVERNMENT

No discussion of the implementation stage, with its successes and shortcomings, would be complete without reference to the present relationship between American nursing and the federal government. The ambivalence of the current situation demands resolution, but the proper role of the National Commission delimits clearly the extent to which it can, or should, participate in the process of debate. It is essential, however, to provide objective information on two things: the enlarged demands on nursing proposed by the federal government; and the simultaneous proposal to reduce the support provided nursing through federal funding. It is in the logical conflict of these two positions that the National Commission finds its greatest concerns.

Extension of the Nursing Role

In 1971, Eliot Richardson, then Secretary of Health, Education, and Welfare, established the Secretary's Committee to Study Extended Roles for Nurses.[25] Serving as chairman of the distinguished, multidisciplinary group of health leaders, was Dr. Roger O. Egeberg, then Special Assistant to the Secretary for Health Policy. In the body of the report, there are a number of specific proposals for altered roles and functions in nursing for primary, acute, and long-term practice.

Perhaps the tone of the entire report may be succinctly summarized in the last paragraph of the preface to the specific comments and recommendations. The committee wrote:

> We believe that the future of nursing must encompass a substantially larger place within the community of the health professions. Moreover, we

> believe that extending the scope of nursing practice is essential if this Nation is to achieve the goal of equal access to health services for all its citizens. Our hope is that this report will hasten progress toward so worthy and necessary a goal.[26]

In transmitting the report of the committee to the Secretary, Dr. Egeberg and Dr. Leroy A. Pesch, Co-Chairman and Special Consultant for Health Manpower in the Office of the Secretary, commented on the development and goals of the report:

> We send you herewith a paper, not official in the sense of binding any groups to verbatim statements but a collaboratively prepared paper which states the thought, conclusions, and recommendations of professionals in nursing, medicine, hospital administration and the allied health organizations. The persons you selected brought to these meetings many years of experience, thought and previous deliberations in this area. There is a need among the professions to know what these people think and recommend. This is therefore, a statement of an ethic intended to be approached, a suggestion of a modus operandi.
>
> Nurses in extended roles are crucial to President Nixon's goal if making health care available to all our citizens is to be reached. It is the Committee's hope that its deliberations will prove helpful to the health professions, Congress, and the Administration.[27]

In his statement accepting the report, Secretary Richardson wrote:

> One of the guiding principles of the Administration's health strategy is that we must build on the strengths inherent in the American health enterprise while we work to overcome its weaknesses . . .
>
> Without doubt, the nursing profession can and must occupy a larger and more effective place in the delivery of health services for the American people . . . While the number of nurses will have to increase substantially to catch up and keep pace with the expanding demand for nursing services, it will be necessary at the same time to enable professional nurses to extend the scope and range of their contribution to health care, to assume duties that involve increased responsibility for the care of patients, and to collaborate more effectively with physicians and other health professionals . . .[28]

This positive attitude toward the extension of the nurse's role in providing care seemed both a natural progression of previous federal policies and a recognition of experimental developments already underway in community care facilities and in hospitals.

Reduction of Federal Support

Federal support for nursing, particularly nursing education and research, has shown steady expansion over the past quarter century. In 1950, nursing education received approximately one quarter of a million dollars. By 1970, over $80 million was provided to nursing through the Health Manpower Act for loans, scholarships, traineeships, construction grants, and other purposes. The Nurse Training Act of 1971 continued to increase funding for nursing with appropriations of $144 million in fiscal 1972 and $112 million in fiscal 1973. In much of this period of time, there were considerable differences among budgetary requests, Congressional authorizations, and final appropriations so that the generally upward trend was marked, as well, by uncertainty, prolonged debate, and some rancor. In this regard, nursing was no different from other health professions and organizations which received federal funding.

It should be noted, too, that the increased appropriations for nursing were not unduly large by most standards. In 1970, for example, when nursing received a sharp boost in federal funding through the Health Manpower Act, its total support was approximately one-eighth of the then current level of federal aid supplied medical education. At that time, nursing enrolled four times as many students as medicine—in ten times as many institutions. Nursing received less than the Peace Corps, and one-fifth of what was allotted for the removal of surplus commodities.

It is against this background that the administration's budgetary figures for fiscal 1974 must be viewed. The request transmitted by Secretary Weinberger is for approximately $53 million. Student assistance funds would be continued in reduced amounts, but most funds for institutional support would be eliminated, and research funding dropped completely. In commenting on the general approach to budgetary construction, the Secretary stated:

> Apart from the consideration of overall budget constraints, it is essential to clarify the federal role in social programs . . . We have not just made a series of reductions in the budget to meet a spending ceiling determined by a responsible fiscal policy.[29]

In applying this policy to nursing education specifically, the Secretary went on to remark:

> Nursing education, of course, has been funded through state and local support, private sources, and portions of patient care revenues. We believe the substitution of federal financing for these more traditional means of support is undesirable.[30]

Predictably, the administration's proposals and rationale have generated strong reaction from nursing. Both the ANA and the NLN have pointed out that, in their opinion, the proposed reductions in federal support would be destructive, particularly in relation to the expanded role for nursing. Much of the impact of the budgetary cuts would fall on the graduate and advanced programs for nursing education in which clinical specialists are currently being prepared, and these programs, many of them quite new, have not had time to develop institutional support similar to that enjoyed by many preparatory programs.

Toward a Resolution

While it is outside the prerogatives of the National Commission to enter the debate over the broad issue of revenue sharing and federal-state relations, there is reason to believe that the findings which led to the initial recommendations of *An Abstract for Action* still obtain and that there is a national interest in, and need for, the kinds of federal support outlined in the Nurse Training Act of 1971. In its summary report in 1970, the Commission stated:

> Nursing, in common with other clinical professions, is among the more expensive fields of education. The need for laboratory sciences, along with supervised student experience, almost insures that instructional costs will far exceed tuition charges. This is an acute problem for nursing because most of its educational institutions lack endowment or outside financial support. To alleviate these constant difficulties, the Commission recommends that:
>
> > *Federal, regional, state, and local governments adopt measures for the increased support of nursing research and education. Priority should be given to construction grants, institutional grants, advanced traineeships, and research grants and contracts. Further, we recommend that private funds and foundations support nursing research and educational innovation where such activities are not publicly aided.*
>
> Considering the importance of national health and the significance of nursing for the system of care, an increased public investment in nursing education would appear to be fully justified in light of the probable return.
>
> Nursing may well be the key to whether our entire system for health care remains viable and responsive to the requirements it faces. It is essential, therefore, that the nation which makes these demands prove itself willing to support the efforts required to meet them.[31]

In 1970, the National Commission recommended that no less than $110 million, and desirably $125 million be appropriated by the federal government to support nursing education and research. At the time, organized nursing thought these figures too small. The Commission, however, based them on objective consideration of needs and resources and arrived at the specific figures on the basis of modest projections from the Health Manpower Act, the National Advisory Council on Nurse Training, and actual expenditures from appropriated funds reported by the Division of Nursing. As a result, the Commission felt that the proposed amounts were reasonable and based on factual analysis. At the same time, the Commission stated that the amounts would need to be enlarged in the future.

In 1973, the Commission continues to believe that federal support is required for nursing to meet the national demands for health care, and that the need for expanded roles in nursing practice is a natural evolution in the enhancement of patient care. The projections made in 1970 were consistent with the Nurse Training Act of 1971 and with the anticipated expenditures that legislation conveyed. In that light, the Commission would repeat:

> With the levels of support suggested here, we would have the capability of getting on with the conduct of research and educational development that are required to bring nursing up-to-date and into partnership in the delivery of quality health care. We believe that nursing, given that opportunity, can generate more increased support for itself in future years.[32]

Through review and reexamination of our health care needs and the potential contribution of a strengthened profession of nursing to help meet them, it would seem that a long-term, realistic program of public support could be developed. The Commission's projections on federal funding represent an objective appraisal for use as a measuring rod against which other analyses and projections might be placed. It is our earnest hope that, now and in the future, support levels will be matched to demand requirements and that American nursing will receive the aid it most surely needs to meet the commitments we ask of it.

A STATEMENT OF FAITH, HOPE, AND LOVE

In the concluding portion of *An Abstract for Action*, the National Commission, after reviewing the previous national inquiries into the problems of American nursing, stated:

> This time, neither the public nor nursing can afford to fail. We must provide the means by which nursing can succeed. Furthermore, nursing must take the opportunity afforded by these recommendations, capitalize on them, and emerge as a full profession, dedicated and capable. Any less achievement will represent less than optimum health care for all Americans, in all likelihood, for generations to come. Reveille sounds not for nursing alone, but for all those who want American society to enjoy the promise of the best health care, sensitively and humanely dispensed.[33]

Over the past three years, this Commission has worked with nurses, other health professionals, and with large numbers of committed lay persons in the pursuit of objectives outlined by the National Commission. The fact that so much progress has been made is a tribute to their efforts and to their concern over the needs of health care in these United States.

Any effort to effect change is bound to encounter resistance from those organizations and individuals who are entrenched in their own behavioral patterns. Any report that sets out, simultaneously, to alter professional roles, educational patterns, and career perspectives is bound to encounter resistance. Perhaps the clearest insight into why some of the previous nursing studies have not realized their goals is afforded by Hardin who says:

> It is one of the peculiarities of the warfare between reform and the status quo that it is thoughtlessly governed by a double standard. Whenever a

> reform measure is proposed it is often defeated when its opponents triumphantly discover a flaw in it . . . worshippers of the status quo sometimes imply that no reform is possible without unanimous agreement, an implication contrary to historical fact.[34]

Diedrich has refined this "double standard" into a formulated method of problem evasion. "We must not move too rapidly." This avoids getting started. "There is no simple answer." This is intended to eliminate *any* answer. "The problem cannot be separated from others." No problem can be solved until *all* problems are solved. And so forth.[35]

But change does occur in society, so there are ways of overcoming inertia and evasion. Sargent and Williamson emphasize that all social change is mediated by individuals, particularly those who are deviants within the culture. As they describe the agent of social change, he or she is:

> . . . the deviant individual [who] may or may not be maladjusted, discontented with society, or driven by manic energy, neurotic anxiety, or obsessive-compulsive tendencies to change the world around him. But one thing stands out: he is certainly nonconformist and unorthodox . . .[36]

While a prettier picture of a social change agent might be painted, it is undoubtedly true that the implementation processes of the National Commission have been forwarded by those individuals and groups that have a lively sense of dissatisfaction with the status quo and have striven to give a world of reality to alternatives that promise a better system of care and a more rewarding career perspective. In the Commission itself, in its staff, in its advisory groups, regional associates, and local supporters, there was a strong desire to move, to act, to accomplish. If the motto of the investigatory phase was "Why?" then the battle cry of the implementation was "Why not?"

The transition of agitation into actual social change can only be accomplished, however, when the time is right and conditions favor the direction proposed. Organized nursing in the early seventies in these United States, as well as many of the individuals within and without the professional associations, was ready for change. The demonstrated capability of some nurses in experimental settings to give vastly expanded care became a rallying point for practitioners who were tired of misutilization and under-utilization. Curricular innovation in educational programs challenged the old tenets and patterns. A new sense of social worth and personal contribution to health care generated a heightened concern over career perspectives and the development of an unambiguous profession that would become a full partner in the health care system. Out of this came a greater felt need in nursing for consensus and a united front.

This fact was critical to any plan for change. Each time in the past that a major effort was mounted to solve the underlying problems of nursing, there had been so much factionalism, parochialism, and negativism that the work was diffused and blunted. Now, however, nursing moved with unprecedented agreement to work together on the general thrust of the National Commission's recommendations and let the future determine the points of disagreement or concern. In concert with this approach, relevant "others" including medicine, hospital administration, and consumers lent their support at critical times and places.

A Statement of Faith

From the outset of the formal implementation phase, it was obvious that some progress could be made on many of the recommendations, but that few could be "completed" in the time period before us. The Commission determined a set of priorities and focused its efforts on accomplishing those objectives that would most likely generate their own succeeding follow-up. In this arrangement, we had to place our faith in nursing to carry out the work of implementation beyond the beginnings. We believed strongly that the sense of accomplishment and self-worth gained through the early effort of organizing joint practice and master planning committees, for example, would be so rewarding as to generate their own need for continuation.

The Commission's primary goal in implementation was to achieve so much progress, through the efforts of our change agents, as to overcome the inertia and adversity of the status quo in significant measures in each of the three areas marked out for restructuring. Beyond that point, it is up to nursing, its leaders, and its organizations to maintain momentum and to accelerate the processes of social action.

We believe that American nursing is resolved to continue and expand upon the work so far completed. And in the process of building and changing, it may well be that better ideas and solutions are generated—ones not anticipated at this point in time. It has been said that nurses are sometimes their own worst enemies. If this is true, then its corollary must also be true. If the more than 1,400,000 nurses of this nation, banded together as their own "best friends," could not bring to our society a new era in health care, then nothing could. Our Commission has faith that nursing will unite in action to complete its journey toward a rendezvous with destiny.

A Statement of Hope

Our primary purpose in studying nursing, and then implementing the Commission's recommendations, was to enhance health care delivery through increasing nursing's contribution to our health system. This concept has been the standard for comparison by which each proposal and each activity was measured. It remains, today, the central concern and hope of the National Commission.

As we enter the last quarter of the twentieth century, it is obvious that American health care needs cannot be met without better utilization of our human resources, particularly that large body of professionally prepared, whom we harnessed for so long with poor patterns of utilization.

Proper use of nursing, to all of its powerful potential, however, means first of all a commitment on the part of that profession to unlimited excellence in clinical practice—practice which is widened to encompass the whole range of patient needs across that continuum which we have described as episodic and distributive. It is our great hope that nursing will take up this challenge.

Second, there must be standardization of levels and functions in the various care specialties so that consumers and other health professionals may reasonably identify the capabilities of the "new" nurse practitioner, and so that the nurse, in turn, can reasonably fulfill the expectations held of her. Nursing must assume this responsibility.

Third, there must be far greater cooperation, communication, and consensual decision making among the many groups and bodies that now speak for nursing. Out of this must come agreed systems, not only for standards and functions, but processes and patterns for the education and certification of advanced clinicians so that order and reasonableness will prevail in the development of expanded patient care. Nursing, again, must accept the task.

Finally, there must be recognition that no profession stands alone and that no final determination of practice and function can ever be made. Rather, nursing, in becoming a full profession, commits itself to research designed to change its corpus of knowledge and its particulars of practice. It increases its responsibility for joint planning with other health professions toward the end of enhanced patient care, and assumes the onus of continuous self-assessment and experimentation. In short, challenge and change are the ingredients that will continue to face each health profession in the years ahead and nursing must live up to the hopes and expectations accorded it.

It is the confident hope of this Commission that nursing, given the support to which it is entitled, will meet these demanding requirements, and those now unarticulated by society, in the years ahead. For all our sakes, and for our future generations, it is essential.

A Statement of Love

To have worked six years with American nursing is to become fully aware of the remarkable potential and vitality of this profession. It is also to become aware of the paradoxes, the problems and the frustrations that beset this largest of all the health practitioner groups.

As a society, we have much to answer for in our treatment of nursing. We have under-compensated, mis-utilized, and bullied the profession for years. Hardly any proposal for improvement has not been attacked; almost none have been implemented. Nursing has found us inordinately unresponsive to suggestions to expand practice, improve education, or enhance career attractiveness. We have viewed them as a "female occupation" with all the connotations that identity has developed in a male dominated society. We have perceived them as "handmaids" to the ascribed important figures in health care—the physician and the surgeon. We have derogated the intellectual content of nursing and have played up the "mother surrogate" image with all of its saccharine flavor.

The wonder in all this is that American nursing has survived as well as it has. To those nurses who have endured, this society owes a great debt. To those nurses who have managed against all odds to strengthen professional commitment and purpose, this society owes even more. In the last quarter of the twentieth century, we now begin to realize that our societal needs for health care are largely dependent upon the quantity and quality of help that nurses can provide. With an increased population enjoying greater life expectancy, we suddenly recognize that nurses must play a major part in keeping us well and caring for us when we are ill or injured. Belatedly, we see that the more than 700,000 active nurses are our only pool of professionally trained practitioners large enough and competent enough to make a fundamental difference in health care.

It is to the eternal credit of the nursing profession that it has continued to struggle against great odds to contribute more than we recognized or appreciated over the past 100 years. If we are only wise enough to give them the tools they truly need, and the support which they have long merited, we may yet attain the lofty aims we have espoused concerning the right of all Americans to proper health care.

The recommendations of the National Commission are not the product of bleeding hearts or soft sentimentalists. They are a critical, hard-headed analysis of where we are, where we ought to be going, and how to get there. What we have learned more than anything else, is that American nursing contains remarkable human resources that lie untapped, that it possesses remarkable strength that stands unused, and that it holds genuine talent that we have not sought. Properly supported and aimed, American nursing can and will help us solve our dilemmas in health care; unsupported and left alone, nursing will cease to be a determinative factor in making health care a national reality.

Over six years of study and work, of accomplishment and disappointment, this Commission has been taught by American nurses how much can be done in the face of adversity. If empathy has turned to affection and then to love, who could fail to understand? It is this special feeling for nursing that impels us to possess the faith and hope we have for its increased contribution to American health care. In the face of all the problems and all the difficulties of continuing implementation, the Commission would speak to nursing in the words of Padraic Pearse:

> Ye shall call for a miracle . . .
> And for this I will answer, O people, answer here and hereafter,
> O people that I have loved shall we not answer together?[37]

The final determination of our health care system awaits nursing's answer.

FOOTNOTES

1. Lysaught, Jerome P. "An Epistle to the New Corinthians." *Heart & Lung.* 2:2:182 (March-April) 1973.
2. Brown, Esther L. *Nursing Reconsidered: A Study of Change. Part I. The Professional Role in Institutional Nursing.* Philadelphia: J. B. Lippincott Co., 1970, and *Nursing Reconsidered: A Study of Change. Part II. The Professional Role in Community Nursing.* Philadelphia: J. B. Lippincott Co., 1971.
3. "Extending the Scope of Nursing Practice." A Report of the Secretary's Committee to Study Extended Roles for Nurses. Washington, D.C.: U.S. Department of Health, Education, and Welfare. November, 1971.
4. Dorsey, Harry N. "The Mental Hospital," in *The Changing Composition of the Hospital System.* A Report of the 1969 National Forum on Hospital and Health Affairs. Durham, N.C.: Duke University Graduate Program in Hospital Administration, 1969.
5. The National Commission for the Study of Nursing and Nursing Education. *An Abstract for Action.* Jerome P. Lysaught, Director. New York: McGraw-Hill Book Co., 1970, p. 92.
6. "Episodic Nursing Practice: Refinement and Expansion of the Roles." Rochester, N.Y.: The National Commission for the Study of Nursing and Nursing Education, 1972 (pamphlet) and "Distributive Nursing Practice: Development and Fusion of the Roles." Rochester, N.Y.: The National Commission for the Study of Nursing and Nursing Education, 1971 (pamphlet).
7. "New Patterns in Nursing Administration: The Vanishing Supervisor." Rochester, N.Y.: The National Commission for the Study of Nursing and Nursing Education, 1972 (pamphlet).
8. "Report of the Task Force to Study the Implications of the Recommendations Presented in *An Abstract for Action.*" 21:2:112 (February) 1973.
9. Christy, Teresa E., Muriel A. Poulin, and Julie Hover. "An Appraisal of *An Abstract for Action.*" *American Journal of Nursing.* 71:8:1579 (August) 1971.
10. Thurston, Hester I. "Education for Episodic and Distributive Care." *Nursing Outlook.* 20:8:519-523 (August) 1972.
11. Lysaught, Jerome P. "The House Reunited: It Must Not Fall." *American Journal of Public Health.* 62:7:960 (July) 1972.
12. Delbecq, Andre L. and Andrew H. Van de Ven. "A Group Process Model for Problem Identification and Program Planning." Madison, Wisc.: The University of Wisconsin Graduate School of Business. (mimeo, undated).
13. "A Guide for Establishing Statewide Master Planning Committees." Rochester, N.Y.: The National Commission for the Study of Nursing and Nursing Education, 1970 (pamphlet).
14. "Individualization, Articulation, Concentration: Emergent Forces in Nursing Education." Rochester, N.Y.: The National Commission for the Study of Nursing and Nursing Education, 1971 (pamphlet).
15. ibid.
16. "The Diploma Nurse, the Hospital School, and the National Commission." Rochester, N.Y.: The National Commission for the Study of Nursing and Nursing Education, 1972 (pamphlet), p. i.
17. "A Special Report on the Fifth Annual Meeting of the Assembly of Hospital Schools of Nursing." *AHA Newsletter for the Hospital School of Nursing.* 6:1:16 (January) 1973.
18. "Resolution of the Council of Diploma Programs." Adopted by the Council for Presentation to the NLN Board, May 9, 1973, at the Biennial Convention of the NLN in Minneapolis, Minnesota (mimeo, undated), p. 1.
19. "The Diploma Nurse, the Hospital School, and the National Commission." op. cit., p. 15.
20. Altman, Stuart H. *Present and Future Supply of Registered Nurses.* Washington, D.C.: U.S. Department of Health, Education, and Welfare Publication No. (NIH) 72-134, 1971.
21. Yett, Donald E. "Yes, Virginia, There Is a Shortage of Nurses—But It's Not Quite as Simple as All That." Paper presented at the Second Conference on the Economics of Health, Baltimore, Maryland, December 5-7, 1968.
22. Brown, Esther L., op. cit.
23. "Extending the Scope of Nursing Practice." op. cit.
24. The National Commission for the Study of Nursing and Nursing Education. *An Abstract for Action.* Appendices. Jerome P. Lysaught, Director. New York: McGraw-Hill Book Co., 1971. See Appendix P. "Career Enhancement Programs for the Licensed Practical/Vocational Nurse," pp. 395-399.
25. "Extending the Scope of Nursing Practice." op. cit.
26. ibid., p. vii.

27. ibid., pp. i-ii.
28. ibid., frontispiece unnumbered.
29. "Administration Gives ABC's on Funding Policies." *American Journal of Nursing.* 72:5:764 (May) 1973.
30. ibid., p. 765.
31. "National Commission for the Study of Nursing and Nursing Education: Summary Report and Recommendations." *American Journal of Nursing.* 70:2:287-294 (February) 1970.
32. *An Abstract for Action*, op. cit., p. 126.
33. ibid., p. 164.
34. Hardin, Garrett. "The Tragedy of the Commons." *Science.* 162:3859:1243-1248 (December 13) 1968.
35. Diedrich, Paul. "How to Run Away From an Educational Problem." *Progressive Education.* 19:8:167-168 (March) 1942.
36. Sargent, S. Stanfeld and Robert C. Williamson. *Social Psychology, An Introduction to the Study of Human Relations.* Second edition. New York: The Ronald Press, 1958, p. 515.
37. Pearse, Padraic. "The Fool," in Kathleen Hoagland (ed.) *1000 Years of Irish Poetry.* New York: Grosset & Dunlap, 1962, p. 649.

Appendix A PUBLICATIONS RELATED TO *AN ABSTRACT FOR ACTION*

BOOKS AND ARTICLES

An Abstract for Action: Appendices to the Report of the National Commission for the Study of Nursing and Nursing Education. Jerome P. Lysaught, Director. New York: McGraw-Hill Book Company, 1971.

An Abstract for Action: Report of the National Commission for the Study of Nursing and Nursing Education. Jerome P. Lysaught, Director. New York: McGraw-Hill Book Company, 1970.

Aydelotte, Myrtle K.: "Nursing Education and Practice: Putting It All Together." *The Journal of Nursing Education.* 11:4:21-27. November, 1972.

Bullough, Bonnie: "You Can't Get There from Here: Articulation in Nursing Education." *The Journal of Nursing Education.* 11:4:4-10. November, 1972.

Dechow, Georgeen H.: "Future Directions for the AD Nurse." *Nursing Outlook.* 21:2:108-109. February, 1973.

de Tornyay, Rheba: "Today's Nurses are Reaching for a Larger Part in Medical Care." *California's Health.* 28:7:6-10. January, 1971.

Johnsen, Gordon N. and Carol M. Eady: "How Much Does Diploma Nursing Education Really Cost?" Part 1: As the Administrator Sees It; Part 2: As the

Nursing School Director Sees It. *Nursing Outlook* 20:10:658-664. October, 1972. In addition, see Letters to the Editor from Harold R. Rowe and from Jerome P. Lysaught, *Nursing Outlook,* December, 1972.

Lysaught, Jerome P.: "From Abstract into Action: Progress Report from the National Commission for the Study of Nursing and Nursing Education." *Nursing Outlook.* 20:3:173-179. March, 1972.

——: "Assistance for the Physician: Nurse Clinician or Physician Assistant." *Journal of Nursing Administration.* 1:6:10-11. November-December, 1971.

——: "Assistance for the Physician Nurse Clinician or Physician Assistant." *Utah Nurse*. 22:4:13, Winter, 1971-72.

——: "Assistants–How Many Kinds Do We Need in the OR?" *The Surgical Team.* 1:1:18-23. August-September, 1972.

——: "Bell, Book and Candle: The National Commission and the School Nurse." *Today's Education.* 62:1:23-24. January, 1973.

——: "Continuing Education: Necessity and Opportunity." *Journal of Continuing Education in Nursing.* 1:3:5-10. September, 1970.

——: "Distributive Health Care Needs and the Occupational Nurse." *Occupational Health Nursing.* 20:11:7-11. November, 1972.

——: "Eleven Months to Ennistymon!" *The Journal of Nursing Education.* 11:4:46-48. November, 1972.

——: "An Epistle to the New Corinthians." *Heart and Lung.* 2:2:180-184. March-April, 1973.

——: "The House Reunited: It Must Not Fall." *The American Journal of Public Health.* 62:7:957-961. July, 1972.

——: "The National Commission and the Specialty Practice Groups in Nursing." *Journal of Obstetric, Gynecologic, and Neonatal Nursing.* 1:3:13-21. September-October, 1972.

——: "The National Study of Nursing and Nursing Education and Its Relationship to the Concept of the Physician's Assistant." *Federation Bulletin.* 59:3:107-123. March, 1972. Presented during the annual meeting, Federation of State Medical Boards, Chicago, February 12, 1971.

——: "No Carrots, No Sticks: Motivation in Nursing." *Journal of Nursing Administration.* 2:5:43-50. September-October, 1972.

——: "Role Articulation: Primary Target for the Future." *Association of Operating Room Nurses Journal.* 15:4:109-124. April, 1972.

——: "The Vanishing Supervisor: Bad News from NCSNNE?" *Supervisor Nurse.* 3:8:19-24. August, 1972. In addition, see Letters to the Editor, *Supervisor Nurse,* October, 1972.

"National Commission for the Study of Nursing and Nursing Education: Summary Report and Recommendations." *American Journal of Nursing.* 70:2:279-294. February, 1970.

Russell, Charles H.: "Issues in Continuing Education for Nursing." *Ends and Means: The National Conference in Continuing Education in Nursing–1970.* McHenry, Ruth W. (ed.) pp. 8-20. Proceedings of the Second National Conference on Continuing Education in Nursing, Sagamore, New York, October, 1970.

——: "The Nursing Service Administrator and The Report of The National Commission for the Study of Nursing and Nursing Education." *Journal of Nursing Administration.* 1:1:12-16. January-February, 1971.

_____ : "Recommendations of Commission on the Study of Nursing and Nursing Education on Career Development." Novello, D. (ed.) *Report on First State-Wide Institute on Career Development Within the Occupational Field of Nursing.* June 10-12, 1970. Sponsored by Committee on Education of the Pennsylvania Nurses Association. pp. 24-29.

Schaefer, Marguerite J.: "Toward a Full Profession of Nursing: The Challenge of the Educator's Role." *The Journal of Nursing Education.* 11:4:39-45. November, 1972.

Smith, Kathryn: "Episodic and Distributive Nursing in an Emergent Curricular Plan." *The Journal of Nursing Education*. 11:4:11-20. November, 1972.

: "A Special Report on the Fifth Annual Meeting of the Assembly of Hospital Schools of Nursing." *AHA Newsletter for the Hospital Schools of Nursing.* 6:1. January, 1973.

Thurston, Hester I.: "Education for Episodic and Distributive Care." *Nursing Outlook.* 20:8:519-523. August, 1972.

Werley, Harriet: "Research in Nursing as Input to Educational Programs." *The Journal of Nursing Education.* 11:4:29-37. November, 1972.

_____ : "This I Believe . . . About Clinical Nursing Research." *Nursing Outlook.* 20:11:718-722. November, 1972.

REVIEWS AND CRITIQUES

"Abstract for Action: Nursing Commission Reports." *Nursing Research Report.* 6:1:5. March, 1971.

Baker, Mary: "Lysaught?!! Students View the National Commission for the Study of Nursing and Nursing Education." *Imprint.* 18:4:18. November-December, 1971.

_____ : "Lysaught?!! Part 3: Students View the National Commission for the Study of Nursing and Nursing Education." *Imprint.* 19:2:17. March, 1972.

Brown, Esther Lucile: "Decisions and Directions: Determinations No Longer To Be Deferred." (Editorial) *The Journal of Nursing Education.* 11:4:2-3. November, 1972.

Christy, Teresa E., Muriel A. Poulin, and Julie Hover: "An Appraisal of *An Abstract for Action*." *American Journal of Nursing.* 71:8:1574-1581. August, 1971. See also, Lysaught, Jerome P. "Let the Recommendations of the National Commission be Judged on Their Merits, Not on the Basis of Whether Nursing Originated Them or Not." *American Journal of Nursing* 71:10:1914ff. October, 1971. In addition, see Letters to the Editor, *American Journal of Nursing,* October and November, 1971.

de Tornyay, Rheba: " 'A Flexner Report' for Professional Nursing." *California Medicine.* 113:3:81-85. September, 1970.

Grigg, Sherry: "Lysaught?!! Part 2: Students View the National Commission for the Study of Nursing and Nursing Education." *Imprint.* 19:1:16. January, 1972.

_____: "Lysaught?!! Part 4: Students View the National Commission for the Study of Nursing and Nursing Education." *Imprint.* 19:3:16. May, 1972.

Kelisch, Beatrice J.: *An Abstract for Action. Library Journal.* October 15, 1970. (a review).

Kelly, Dorothy N. (ed.): "The Vanishing Supervisor." (Editorial) *Supervisor Nurse.* 3:8:6. August, 1972.

Lewis, Edith P. (ed.): "Editorial: In Perspective." *Nursing Outlook.* 20:3:163. March, 1972.

_____: "Lysaught Report Revisited." *Nursing Outlook.* 21:2:93. February, 1973.

Murry, Ruth Neil: *An Abstract for Action. Nursing Outlook.* 19:6:380. June, 1971. (a review).

"Report of the Task Force To Study the Implications of the Recommendations Presented in *An Abstract for Action*." *Nursing Outlook.* 21:2:111-118. February, 1973.

Schumann, Mary Jean (ed.): "Imprint Editorial." *Imprint.* 19:5:8. December, 1972.

Singleton, Estelle: "Guest Editorial." *Colorado Nurse.* 71:12:1-2. December, 1971. In addition, see Letters to the Editor from Jerome P. Lysaught, *Colorado Nurse*, 2:5:11. May, 1972.

Smith, Kathryn M.: *An Abstract for Action. American Journal of Nursing.* 71:4:814-818. April, 1971. (a review).

Sorenson, Gladys: *An Abstract for Action. Nursing Research.* 20:2:173-174. March-April, 1971. (a review).

"Statement on Report of National Commission for the Study of Nursing and Nursing Education." *Hospitals.* 45:10:131. May 16, 1971. See also, *AHA Newsletter for the Hospital School of Nursing.* 4:4. April, 1971.

"Summary Report and Recommendations: National Commission for the Study of Nursing and Nursing Education." *Nursing Outlook.* 18:2:46-47. February, 1970.

"Type VIII Members Meet, Assembly of Hospital Schools of Nursing hears Dr. Lysaught, Charter members of last-man's club?" *Hospitals.* 47:1:94-95, 114. January 1, 1973.

MONOGRAPHS

All of the following were published in Rochester, New York by and for the National Commission for the Study of Nursing and Nursing Education.

Lysaught, Jerome P.: "Abbreviated Summary Report, *An Abstract for Action*." _____ 1970.

*_____: "Bell, Book and Candle: The National Commission and The School Nurse." 1972.

*_____: "Continuing Education in Nursing: Necessity and Opportunity." 1971.

_____: "Costs of Nursing Education and A Case for its Greater Support." 1970.

*Asterisked items are reprinted from authored articles, see "Books and Articles" section preceding.

_____: "The Diploma Nurse, The Hospital School, and The National Commission." 1972.

_____: "Distributive Nursing Practice: Development and Fusion of the Roles." 1971.

_____: "Episodic Nursing Practice: Refinement and Expansion of the Roles." 1971.

Lysaught, Jerome P.: "A Guide for Establishing Statewide Master Planning Committees." 1970.

_____: "A Guide for Establishing Statewide Joint Practice Commissions." 1970.

_____: "Individualization, Articulation, Concentration: Emergent Forces in Nursing Education." 1971.

_____: "The National Joint Practice Commission: New Bottles, New Wine." 1972.

*_____: "New Patterns in Nursing Administration: The Vanishing Supervisor." 1972.

*_____: "No Carrots, No Sticks: Motivation in Nursing." 1972.

*_____: "Nurse Clinician and Physician's Assistant: The Relationship Between Two Emerging Practitioner Concepts." 1971.

_____: "Professional Partnerhood in Health Care: The Need for Research into Nursing Practice." 1971.

Lysaught, Jerome P. and Sydney Anne Sutherland: "From Diploma School to College: Two Case Studies on Changing Patterns Within Institutions for Nursing Education." 1970.

Appendix B

RECOMMENDATIONS OF THE NATIONAL COMMISSION AND PROGRESS TOWARD THEIR ACHIEVEMENT

In *An Abstract for Action,* the National Commission presented fifty-eight specific recommendations related to nursing roles and functions, education, and career perspectives. Out of these many proposals, the Commission and staff selected a smaller number for intensive implementation efforts, and these activities are reported in detail throughout Chapters 4, 5, and 6 of this volume. To provide a summary review of the entire range of implementation actions, this appendix contains a thumbnail sketch of status and progress on each recommendation as well as a brief statement on further suggested activities.

Because these summaries are based on staff observation and interaction with our advisory committees and regional associates, there is built-in emphasis on the work of the NCSNNE and its extensions. What must be recognized, however, is that each step of progress on each recommendation was made possible only through the tremendous energy and cooperation of individuals at state and local levels. Most of these were nurses, some from state associations or leagues, and some from speciality practice or student groups. Many of the persons who became involved in state and local implementation, however, were physicians, health administrators, educators, and concerned lay persons. Their contribution simply cannot be singled out or measured. The accomplishments recorded, however, are surely theirs.

The summary reports are grouped in three sections according to the development of the original investigation:

Section I. Recommendations Related to Nursing Roles and Functions
Section II. Recommendations Related to Nursing Education
Section III. Recommendations Related to Nursing Careers

Section I
NCSNNE Recommendations
Related to Nursing Roles and Functions

1. The federal Division of Nursing, the National Center for Health Services Research and Development, other governmental agencies, and private foundations appropriate grant funds and/or research contracts to investigate the impact of nursing practice on the quality, effectiveness, and economy of health care.

Implementing Agencies
Federal and state agencies and private foundations.

Status and Progress
Over the first three years of the implementation, federal appropriations for nursing research totaled more than $11.5 million. The amounts were fairly stable from year to year, and the total appropriated is compatible with the Commission's recommendation that a desirable level of support over the period should be approximately $12 million. As a result, the NCSNNE staff met only on occasion with officials from the Division of Nursing and the National Center for Health Services Research—generally to exchange information and to discuss areas of priority in nursing research. No systematic follow-up or developmental project was initiated by the NCSNNE.

In the light of the budgetary requests for fiscal 1974, which make no provision for nursing research funds, the National Commission has appointed an ad hoc committee of members to consider how best to emphasize the importance of support for nursing and, particularly, for nursing research. Recognizing that the various health organizations, including but not limited to those of nurses, must primarily be involved in the debates over future support systems, the National Commission nevertheless is concerned that its independent and objective analyses be considered. Further action is still under consideration.

In order to involve more foundations in the support of nursing research, the Commission staff prepared an informational pamphlet, "Professional Partnerhood in Health Care: The Need for Research into Nursing Practice." This was supplied to all major private foundations with an interest in the health fields, and, through the cooperation of state and regional nursing groups, was distributed to additional foundations and governmental agencies at the more local levels.

Suggested Further Action

The nursing profession, through concerted action by all its associations and organizations, should establish *regular* formalized discussion with federal and state agencies concerned with funding, grant support, and research. Cooperative planning should also be given to the possibility of enlarged private and voluntary support of nursing research through joint organizational support of the American Nurses' Foundation, the Fund for Graduate Nursing Education, and the Academy of Nursing.

It is further suggested that the American Nurses' Foundation be designated as the profession's primary spokesman in circulating information on the effects of research into nursing, its benefits to clients derived, and its impacts on costs of patient care. The ANF, with the support of the several nurse associations, should endeavor to keep public agencies and private foundations well-informed and aware of the outcomes of nursing research. All of the nursing organizations, in turn, should encourage their members to take new initiatives in developing research consciousness related to clinical practice so that quality proposals can be generated and supported.

2. Federal funds be supplied through the ERIC program, or through the Division of Nursing, as well as private and state funds, to the American Nurses' Foundation so that it might become a national clearinghouse for the collection and dissemination of information about research and innovations in nursing.

Implementing Agencies

American Nurses' Foundation and other nursing organizations.

Status and Progress

Pursuant to this recommendation, a number of discussions and meetings were held with Dr. Martha Pitel, Director of the American Nurses' Foundation. The ANF subsequently developed and submitted a proposal to a private foundation for the funding of a National Nursing Information Center that would function as a clearinghouse on research and innovation in nursing. The NCSNNE staff has indicated its willingness to participate in any requested follow-up activities or to assist ANF in any other way.

In other action related to this recommendation, the American Nurses' Association independently has prepared and submitted a proposal to the USPHS Division of Nursing for the development of a "National Inventory of Nursing Research."

This, of course, would supply the beginning corpus of materials for a centralized clearinghouse.

Suggested Further Action

The National Nurses' Congress* should take formal action to designate the ANF as the central clearinghouse agency for information on nursing research. This would materially strengthen the ANF's position for subsequent contacts with public agencies and private foundations to secure support funding.

In anticipation of the clearinghouse designation, ANF should begin an informational campaign among private foundations to interest them in the possibilities of nursing research for improving the health care delivery system of the nation. Digests of theses and dissertations completed by nursing graduates would be basic material for such an effort.

3. The Division of Nursing, the National Center for Health Services Research and Development, and state and private funds allocate increased monies for applied research and demonstration grants that would examine new methods, procedures, settings, and personnel relationships for improved nursing practice. We further recommend that the following guidelines be used in expending funds:

a. Innovation and demonstration projects in patient care should be based on preceding research;

b. Innovations should be conceived and focused to improve methods of meeting patient needs, rather than designed primarily to answer professional problems;

c. All grants and contracts for applied research and demonstrations should include an allocation for the evaluation of results;

d. All innovations and demonstrations should be weighed against alternative courses of action that might produce similar results. Both quality of care and comparative costs should be considered.

Implementing Agencies

Federal and state agencies and private foundations.

Status and Progress

The Commission has not initiated any systematic follow-up to this recommendation other than to assist individuals, institutions, and organizations that contacted us concerning study proposals they were developing related to *An Abstract for Action.* In each of those cases, professional consultation, critiques, and advice on funding

*A group which met in San Clemente, California in January, 1973, representing seventeen nursing organizations and associations, for the purpose of discussing nursing's focus and methodology in meeting the challenges faced.

possibilities have been supplied. As a direct result, a number of studies and demonstration projects have been funded and are currently in progress.

One of the features of the ANF proposal for a National Nursing Consultation Service would be the provision of a continuing consultation service to nurse practitioners interested in pursuing clinical nursing research. This would be an important added dimension to the ANF support of increased research into nursing practice.

Suggested Further Action

Federal and state agencies and private foundations should endorse collaborative efforts with the ANF in order to develop an effective and efficient national program of nursing research.

ANF should explore the sponsorship of regular regional conferences across the country focusing on the application of research findings to nursing practice. Other organized nursing groups, including the specialty practice bodies, should incorporate programs on applied research into their meeting and convention agendas.

Nursing organizations should encourage innovative interdisciplinary projects at both student and practitioner levels so that medicine, nursing and other health groups might become more involved in joint research on improved health care delivery.

All nursing organizations and associations should make a stronger effort to publish research studies, findings, and subsequent applications to practice in their professional journals and magazines.

> 4. A national joint practice commission be established between medicine and nursing to discuss and make recommendations concerning the congruent roles of the physician and the nurse in providing quality health care, with particular attention to the rise of the nurse master clinician; the introduction of the physician's assistant; the increased activity of other professions in areas long assumed to be the concern solely of the physician and/or the nurse.

Implementing Agencies

American Nurses' Association and American Medical Association.

Status and Progress

The National Joint Practice Commission (NJPC) is established and functioning with the approval and support of the parent bodies. The NCSNNE has published a descriptive account of the development and organization of the body in a pamphlet entitled, "The National Joint Practice Commission: New Bottles, New Wine." This publication includes a summary of the objectives, program, and structure of the NJPC.

In addition to its own organizational processes, the NJPC has already conducted the first National Conference of State Joint Practice Committees, held in November of 1972. At that meeting, representatives attended from forty-seven states. Currently, the NJPC is setting up three task forces to recommend ways to improve: rural health care, care of the aging, and interdisciplinary education for joint practice.

Funding has been assured for the continued operation of the NJPC and a permanent staff director has been named. Throughout the interim period, the NCSNNE will continue, with the assistance of staff from AMA and ANA, to serve the needs of the NJPC as it increases the tempo of its activities.

Suggested Further Action

The NJPC should continue its efforts to organize state joint practice committees across the country and to develop new task forces in additional areas of health concern as time and finances permit.

The NJPC must consider how best to bring their findings and recommendations to the appropriate professional bodies for implementation and, in doing so, it must determine how best to involve additional groups beyond the AMA and ANA in the work of the task forces and the NJPC itself.

5. Counterpart joint practice commissions be established in each state between medicine and nursing to consider the congruent roles of physicians and nurses, and to recommend to state legislatures and to the national joint practice commission such changes or alterations in basic health practice acts, licensure, and other regulations as they deem necessary to ensure the provision of quality health care.

Implementing Agencies

The National Joint Practice Commission, AMA and ANA staff, NCSNNE staff, state medical and nursing associations, along with the statewide groups involved in implementation of *An Abstract for Action.*

Status and Progress

In order to provide some initial assistance to individuals and groups, the NCSNNE published and distributed the pamphlet entitled, "A Guide for Establishing Statewide Joint Practice Commissions," for use within the states. As of April 1, 1973, the following progress had been made:

Operational State Joint Practice Committee	27
SJPC in Process of Organizing	3
Liaison Committee Between Medicine and Nursing	14

Some Other Committee or Organized Contact	4
No Organized Group or Committee	3
(total includes the District of Columbia)	

Continuing communications are now taking place between the national and the state joint practice committees and further organizational efforts are being planned to establish committees in those states which have not as yet taken action. Follow-up surveys have been conducted among participants of the 1972 National Conference of State Joint Practice Committees and the results circulated so that information on organization and programming could be shared. NCSNNE staff are continuing to meet and work with developing state groups.

Suggested Further Action
The NJPC, in cooperation with state committees, should develop informational literature and guides for distribution among the states. These materials should identify problems in organizing, ways to overcome them, and suggestions for goals and short term programs.

As quickly as NJPC develops its own full-time staff, it should provide consultative help and institute a planned organizational campaign to assist the remaining states to organize and develop active committees.

Particular emphasis should be placed on attracting more nurse and physician *practitioners* into active involvement, and efforts should be made at the state level to encourage local facilities and institutions to establish joint practice groups at the very grass roots.

6. As early as progress in these joint discussions indicates, the national and state joint practice commissions should invite health management executives, other professions and allied health personnel, as well as the rising number of groups involved in health maintenance, disease prevention, and patient care to join in planning for optimum working relationships and concerted role performance that will assure the best delivery of quality health care.

Implementing Agencies
NJPC and state joint practice committees.

Status and Progress
At the national level, the NJPC has already begun involving other disciplines (including law, dentistry, health management and education) and consumer representatives in the composition of the initial task forces. It is anticipated that this will be continued and broadened as future committees are formed.

At the state level, several of the joint practice committees have already invited other health practitioners, administrators, and public representatives to participate in their planning activities. Osteopaths, dentists, clinical pharmacists, licensed practical nurses and social workers are among the relevant professions represented on some of the state committees.

Suggested Further Action
Both the NJPC and the state joint practice committees must maintain their awareness of the need for broad involvement and participation by all those concerned with role changes and care delivery. It is particularly important, too, that consumers be brought into the process of determining better functions and systems for providing care.

7. Two essentially related but differing career patterns be developed for nursing practice:

a. One career pattern, episodic, would emphasize the nursing practice that is essentially curative and restorative, generally acute or chronic in nature, and most frequently provided in the setting of the hospital or in-patient facility;

b. The second career pattern, distributive, would emphasize the nursing practice that is essentially designed for health maintenance and disease prevention. This is generally continuous in nature, seldom acute, and increasingly will take place in community or emergent institutional settings.

Implementing Agencies
Professional nursing organizations, particularly specialty practice groups; health care facilities; educational institutions; continuing education programs.

Status and Progress
Considerable emphasis has been placed on the development of informational materials that serve to explain the terms "episodic" and "distributive" and the importance the Commission attaches to their acceptance and exploitation. Two pamphlets have received wide circulation:

1. "Episodic Nursing Practice: Refinement and Expansion of the Roles."
2. "Distributive Nursing Practice: Development and Fusion of the Roles."

In addition, a number of journal articles were prepared for the nursing press explaining these concepts and applying them to the particular concerns of nurse practitioners. Specially aimed monographs were developed for school nurses, obstetrical and gynecological nurses, occupational nurses, and public health nurses.

Documentation was obtained on demonstration projects in both nursing education and practice to show that episodic and distributive care is a viable concept and one directly related to problems in current health care delivery. An increasing number of educational institutions and care facilities are showing interest in experimentation related to these areas, and more and more frequently the terms and the concepts are beginning to appear in nursing literature.

Suggested Further Action

More educational institutions and care facilities must become involved in the study and testing of episodic and distributive care patterns. Specialty practice groups, particularly, have to encourage the enlarged functional role involved in these patterns, and both two- and four-year colleges must examine the provision of concentrations and electives in a parallel track system.

> 8. Both nursing career patterns should be so organized that recognition, reward, and increased responsibility for practice are based on increasing depth of knowledge and demonstrated competence to perform in complex clinical situations.
>
> 9. Within each functional specialty, episodic or distributive, a career plan should be developed by which beginning nurse graduates would start at an entry level (staff nurse) then move to increased levels of competence (clinical nurse). In this position, the nurse might function as a nursing team leader in clinical practice. With proper experience and advanced study, an individual could be recognized as a master clinician capable of organizing and providing complex care using initiative and individual judgment.

Implementing Agencies

Professional nursing organizations, health care facilities, educational institutions, health administrators, and the public.

Status and Progress

The NCSNNE staff has prepared a number of articles and monographs detailing the need for some better system of career growth in nursing practice. In particular, two pamphlets describe the shortcomings of our present approaches and suggest new departures that should be employed:

1. "Nurse Clinician and Physician's Assistant: The Relationship Between Two Emerging Practitioner Concepts"
2. "No Carrots, No Sticks: Motivation in Nursing"

In addition, the materials prepared to explain episodic and distributive nursing practice include case examples of career progression based on growing excellence in care and patient management. The pamphlet entitled, "New Patterns in Nursing Administration: The Vanishing Supervisor," contrasts the traditional and the emergent patterns for nursing careers and cites specific examples of new approaches to keeping nurses in clinical contact with clients.

Suggested Further Action
Organized nursing, particularly through the practice associations, should make a major commitment to the development of career patterns that keep the nurse in contact with the patient or client.

Hospitals and other health care facilities should study and test the new patterns for nursing careers and determine whether early findings on economy, reduced turnover, and improved care quality are substantiated. If they are, then major changes in staffing and utilization patterns for professional nursing should be made.

> 10. All clerical, technical, and routine supportive functions which are not therapeutic be performed by non-nursing personnel. These would include the provision of supplies, maintenance of records, supervision of housekeeping services, and related activities.
>
> 11. Continuous study be given to the provision of ward clerks, unit managers, self-contained departments, automated services, and other organizational departures that can release nurses from non-nursing functions while maintaining nursing control over the delivery of nursing care.
>
> 12. Each change in handling and procedure be accompanied with educational programs and followed by evaluative procedures to ensure that organizational changes are accompanied by actual increases in nursing time for health delivery and by qualitative improvements in care.

Implementing Agencies
Clinical directors of nursing service; health care facilities and health administrators.

Status and Progress
No systematic effort was developed for implementation of these recommendations because they were seen as corollaries to the effort exerted to enlarge the practice role of nurses. Nevertheless, the emphasis on keeping nurses in clinical contact with clients requires that more attention be placed on the provision of supporting services and personnel. In the reported case studies on expanded nursing roles in both episodic and distributive practice, some comment was included on supporting roles, but these must be studied in far greater depth.

Suggested Further Action
Experiments and demonstrations of expanded clinical nurse roles must include the consideration of supportive personnel and services that will permit nurses to divest

non-nursing functions. Evaluation and follow-up should be conducted to ensure that savings in nursing time are translated into increased patient contact and enhanced patient care.

Professional organizations and specialty practice groups in nursing should conduct investigations and follow-up analyses on proposals to provide better support for nursing in non-care functions. Nursing must reemphasize its commitment to providing client care directly rather than through "agents" and must determine what configurations of support personnel and aid are required to give nurses the most freedom to provide professional care.

> 13. Institutional policy-making and administrative bodies in health care facilities (both episodic and distributive) should be so organized that the clinical director of nursing service has a voice in planning and decisions that affect the provision of health care, and that medicine, nursing, and health administration join together for mutual discussion of their common concerns in optimizing care delivery.

Implementing Agencies

Clinical directors of nursing service; health care facilities and health administrators.

Status and Progress

The NCSNNE staff prepared, in both the pamphlets on episodic practice and new patterns in administration, case examples which detail the enlarged role of nursing administration in clinical decision making—including instances in which nursing, medicine and health administration developed triads for cooperative planning of patient care.

In furtherance of this proposal, the NCSNNE staff gave testimony before an AMA committee studying the systematic inclusion of nurses on joint boards for accreditation and related actions. Both the Commission and staff have vigorously presented these concepts at statewide planning meetings and interdisciplinary conferences held to discuss *An Abstract for Action.*

Suggested Further Action

Directors of nursing service, health administrators and medical directors must begin to reexamine the roles and functions they share in the provision of patient care. They should examine the emerging patterns of those institutions and facilities which have increased the responsibility and authority of nursing to determine whether the reported improvement in patient care is realized—and if so, how best to restructure their own organizational patterns to obtain similar benefits.

14. Nursing leadership work actively to bring education and service together in joint planning and decision making, and that where practicable

a. Nurse practitioners and clinical directors of nursing service receive significant appointments to (or relevant association with) institutions for nursing education, and

b. Nursing faculty in institutions for nursing education be given responsibility for providing or organizing significant elements of nursing care.

Implementing Agencies

Professional nursing organizations, educational institutions and health care facilities.

Status and Progress

In all of the monographs, pamphlets and articles prepared by the NCSNNE staff throughout the implementation phase, there has been repeated emphasis on the need to bring nursing education and service back into close relationship. Examples of joint appointment and shared responsibility have been cited and case studies reported. State master planning committees have been encouraged to look into better means for integrating nursing education and service so as to end the bifurcation that now exists in so many cases.

Suggested Further Action

Both educational institutions and health care facilities must exercise initiative to see that there is a close professional link between these two services. Joint appointments, dual responsibility, and organizational structuring can be invoked to ensure that no false dichotomies are established or preserved. Professional nursing organizations must take the lead in encouraging and supporting more closely integrated relationships between education and service.

15. Nurses seek to use technology in their activities for two primary purposes:

a. To eliminate as much routine as possible, allowing them to achieve maximum personal contact with their charges;

b. To enlarge the monitoring and feedback systems that can supply information on individual conditions and reactions, thus facilitating further nursing intervention.

16. Clinical nurses, in both episodic and distributive settings, assume responsibility for:

a. Seeing that every nursing action evidences an interest and concern for the individual;

b. Facilitating the efforts of other health care personnel in providing for the needs of an individual.

17. Nursing educators and practitioners place continuing emphasis on the role of the nurse:

a. As a central figure in the provision of psychosocial as well as physical care for the patient and his family;

b. As a representative of the individual care recipient and his interests in inter- or multidisciplinary approaches to the delivery of health care.

Implementing Agencies

Professional nursing organizations and individual nurses.

Status and Progress

Throughout the investigation phase of the National Commission's work, there was evidence that the American health care system was perceived as being impersonal and unconcerned for the individuals who came for help. This is, of course, a very broad generalization, but one that must concern us all. For this reason, the emphasis throughout the implementation was to stress greater involvement by professional nurses in actual delivery of care coupled by more nurse-patient contact and communication. Both the art and science of nursing are important in caring for people, and this point has been repeated consistently in NCSNNE publications and presentations.

Suggested Further Actions

Professional nursing, through its organizations, educational institutions, and health care facilities, must continually emphasize the need for human and personal concern in every aspect of health care delivery. In both episodic and distributive care settings, there are tremendous opportunities for nurses to aid clients and their families to understand and comply with care and treatment regimens. Nursing must view patient contact and advocacy as a vital aspect of all professional activities.

Section II
NCSNNE Recommendations Related to Nursing Education

1. Each state have, or create, a master planning committee that will take nursing education under its purview, such committees to include representatives of nursing, education, other health professions, and the public, to recommend specific guidelines, means for implemen-

tation, and deadlines to ensure that nursing education is positioned in the mainstream of American educational patterns with its preparatory programs located in collegiate institutions.

Implementing Agencies
State nurses' associations and constituent leagues with assistance from ANA, NLN, and NCSNNE staff. In many states, hospital associations, medical societies, health planning groups, educators, and citizens have assisted.

Status and Progress
The NCSNNE staff prepared a pamphlet, "A Guide for Establishing Statewide Master Planning Committees," to assist groups seeking to organize local SMPCs. This was supplemented by information and material developed out of the experience gained in working with the nine target states designated by the National Commission. As of April 1, 1973, the following progress in organization was indicated:

States with Operational SMPCs	26
States in the Process of Organizing	21
Unorganized	4

(total includes the District of Columbia)

Seven of the model states have developed informational brochures on their development of master planning committees, and all nine of them have contributed to a lengthy survey developed by the NCSNNE staff. The information provided will be organized into a "how to" manual for those states still organizing their planning committees.

Suggested Further Action
Many of the SMPCs need more multidisciplinary input in order to broaden their representation and their approach to problem solving.

The ANA and NLN should consider the development of regularized progress reports so that experiences could be shared and progress hastened among the states still attempting to organize.

Relationships between the SMPCs and state departments of health and higher education should be strengthened and some regularized form of progress reporting should be instituted so that implementation of recommendations could be facilitated.

2. Those hospital schools that are strong and vital, endowed with a qualified faculty, suitable educational facilities, and motivated for

excellence be encouraged to seek and obtain regional accreditation and degree granting power.

Implementing Agencies
Individual institutions assisted by NCSNNE staff.

Status and Progress
Over the course of the implementation, the NCSNNE staff has worked with the project group at Labouré Junior College in Boston on the transition of a hospital school of nursing into a collegiate institution. The early portion of that experience, along with the successful transition of St. Mary's College, in Minneapolis, was reported in the pamphlet entitled, "From Diploma School to College: Two Case Studies on Changing Patterns for Nursing Education."

In the past three years, NCSNNE staff and regional associates have consulted with institutions in California, Illinois, Massachusetts, Minnesota, and New York that have set up study or project groups to consider such a course of action. To our knowledge, however, only the two cited institutions have culminated the process.

Suggested Further Action
There are a number of hospital schools of nursing that might well consider this recommendation as one possible alternative in the face of changing educational patterns. Some of these might consider a consortium arrangment that would reduce per capita costs and significantly increase the available resources. It remains that only unusually motivated and innovative schools are likely to follow this course of action.

3. All other hospital schools of nursing move systematically and with dispatch (under the guidance of the state master planning committee), to effect interinstitutional arrangements with collegiate institutions so that:

a. Graduates of the nursing preparatory program will receive an academic degree from the educational institution upon completion of their course of instruction;

b. Joint planning takes place between the academic institution and the hospital on the articulation of instruction so that optimum use is made of clinical teaching facilities.

Implementing Agencies
Statewide master planning committees, individual institutions, regional and area consortia of schools.

Status and Progress

Over the course of the implementation phase, somewhat more than 22 percent of the hospital schools of nursing announced their closing or intent to close. Most of these have gone into some joint arrangements with collegiate nursing programs to provide clinical facilities and experiences for the students. Whereas in the past most of these arrangements have been between individual institutions, more frequently we find local or regional consortia being explored so that two or more hospital schools may phase their programs out and replace them with an enlarged and strengthened collegiate school.

Two pamphlets prepared by NCSNNE staff discuss specific transitional concerns: "The Diploma Nurse, the Hospital School, and the National Commission," and "Individualization, Articulation, Concentration: Emergent Forces in Nursing Education." These supplement and expand on the basic recommendations of the Commission and provide case examples and updated information on the process of change.

Staff members from NCSNNE, regional associates, and advisors have worked with a large number of individual institutions and regional groups to consider alternatives and arrangements to the status quo. In addition, the NCSNNE staff maintained contact with the hospital school organizations of both the NLN and the AHA so as to provide some dialogue on the acceleration of change.

Suggested Further Action

Educational institutions and their people must become increasingly involved in examining the processes for establishing a comprehensive, collegiate system of nursing education. The statewide master planning committees can facilitate this through objective and independent counsel.

All nursing organizations, including those composed of the hospital schools of nursing, must assess both the direction and velocity of change, and consider well the impact on the student so long as a bifurcated system is maintained.

State boards of nursing, accrediting agencies, and organized nursing must accept responsibility for moving with purposive speed toward the establishment of a collegiate pattern for professional nursing education.

4. Junior and senior collegiate institutions cooperatively develop programs and curricula that will preserve the integrity of these institutions and their aims while facilitating the social and professional mobility of the nursing student.

Implementing Agencies

Statewide master planning committees, individual institutions, educational associations, and area groupings of schools.

Status and Progress

In the pamphlet entitled "Individualization, Articulation, Concentration: Emergent Forces in Nursing Education," the NCSNNE staff expanded upon the rationale for this recommendation and supplied case examples of new, emergent relationships between the two- and four-year institutions.

Staff from the Commission have worked with both the Southern Regional Education Board and the Orange County curriculum projects in preliminary fashion to develop a concerted study of educational articulation between the junior and senior colleges; in addition, the NCSNNE has worked quite closely with a number of collegiate institutions beginning experimental or developmental projects.

Furthermore, the staff has met from time to time with such groups as the ANA Commission on Education, the NLN Council of Baccalaureate and Higher Degree Programs, and the American Association of Colleges of Nursing to emphasize the necessity of developing planned articulation and transfer between the two levels of collegiate education for nursing.

Suggested Further Action

Statewide master planning committees and state boards of higher education should place strong emphasis on the need to articulate two- and four-year programs in nursing.

The national nursing organizations must develop overt activities to foster improved relationships and articulation between the two- and four-year institutions. The NLN Councils of Baccalaureate and Higher Degree Programs and Associate Degree Programs must begin joint deliberations and planning for change. Similarly, the American Association of Colleges of Nursing must make a commitment to articulated programs between the two levels.

The National Student Nurses' Association should exert every effort to encourage and support activities in this area.

5. The state master planning committees be charged with drawing up a plan for each state to determine the number and minimum size of institutions to receive institutional and individual student aid.

6. Small programs be terminated or consolidated into larger programs in order to reduce the per unit costs of education and in order to make better allocation of qualified faculty.

7. Nursing education institutions be encouraged and given federal and state awards and support grants proportional to the number of students enrolled, such moneys to be used to defray the expenses of operation and expansion, and to provide salary support for qualified faculty.

Implementing Agencies

State master planning committees, federal and state funding agencies, accrediting agencies, organizations of nurse educators, and individual educational institutions.

Status and Progress

In its pamphlet entitled, "Costs of Nursing Education and a Case for Its Greater Support," the NCSNNE staff developed documented evidence that per capita costs in nursing education differ significantly with larger programs providing education at far lower per capita costs. The fact that there are more than 1,350 preparatory programs in nursing, many of them very small in terms of students and graduating class size, militates against cost effectiveness and efficient use of resources.

We must make every effort—consistent with sound planning and reasonable transition—to enlarge some programs and eliminate others so that better allocation of resources and personnel can be provided. Many of the schools that have closed over the span of the implementation effort have been among the smaller in enrollment. The state master planning committees, however, must take more active roles in assessing needs and resources and attempting to match them.

Over the first two years of implementation, encouraging progress was made in terms of federal support of the concept of capitation and institutional support. This has been eliminated in the administration's request for fiscal 1974 and would accordingly represent a real blow to the support of nursing education. Nursing organizations are seeking now to restore these funds, but their loss would be felt heavily.

Over the course of the implementation, NCSNNE staff have worked with a number of institutions planning various consortia arrangements by which smaller programs could coalesce and develop the savings and resources enjoyed by larger institutions. Several consortia are on the drawing board and could be realized by 1975.

Suggested Further Action

Planning groups and institutions must take a hard, objective look at per capita costs and new interinstitutional arrangements for nursing education. Needs must be balanced by resources and some reduction in small programs is almost mandatory.

Nursing organizations must develop educational efforts aimed at fighting the assumption that we need more and more nursing programs to eliminate the nursing shortage. Even if we need more nurse graduates, we should provide them through enlarging and strengthening our present institutions unless there is a true, compelling reason for initiating a new program.

8. Federal and state grants for building and construction of facilities be sharply increased to up-date and enlarge laboratory and classroom areas. There should, however, be an effort made at each institution having multiple preparatory programs to encourage and plan joint, cooperative use of buildings, laboratories, etc.

22. Federal, regional, state, and local governments adopt measures for the increased support of nursing research and education. Priority should be given to construction grants, institutional grants, advanced traineeships, and research grants and contracts. Further, we recommend that private funds and foundations support nursing research and educational innovations where such activities are not publicly aided. We believe that a useful guide for the beginnings of such a financial aid program would be in the amounts and distribution of funds authorized by Congress for fiscal 1970, with proportional increases from other public and private agencies.

Designated Agencies

Federal and state legislatures, administrative agencies, professional nursing organizations, citizens.

Status and Progress

With the passage of the Health Manpower Act of 1968 and the Nurse Training Act of 1971, there was a progressive federal policy toward the support of nursing and nursing education, generally, and a beginning effort toward support of institutional construction through grants and interest subsidies. The latter were never more than $20 million per annum, but they had the promise of some long-term public commitment. The expectation they accorded was swept away with the administration's request for fiscal 1974 which eliminated funds for construction and reduced those for loan guarantees and interest subsidies to $1 million.

While no one can tell at this point the ultimate level of appropriations and expenditures, this reversal of policy has severe consequences for the institutions of nursing education.

Suggested Further Action

Organized nursing, in conjunction with other health professions and associations, is seeking to restore the reduced funds through federal appropriations. At the same time, alternative approaches to state agencies receiving revenue sharing funds, and other sources of support must be examined and developed. Nursing must, through its organizations and associations, become more involved in the policy-making process. Increased knowledge and information on activism and involvement must be shared by nurses and their organizations.

Regardless of the outcomes of fiscal 1974, it is essential that nursing develop less dependency on federal funds through cultivation of other kinds of support from various public and private sources.

> 9. Both state and regional committees explore the possibilities of sharing and increasing scarce faculty resources. A state, for example, might employ faculty through its university system to serve at several institutions for nursing education, while both state and regional associations could develop programs for the professional advancement of current and future faculty personnel.

Implementing Agencies
Statewide master planning committees, interstate compacts for higher education, regional associations, and individual institutions.

Status and Progress
The NCSNNE staff has examined the Inter-Collegiate Center in Spokane and worked with preliminary project proposals in Tennessee, Pittsburgh, and Syracuse. Each of these efforts includes a pooling of faculty and the optimum allocation of resources. Materials relating to these projects have been made available to the statewide master planning committees, and these groups will now have an opportunity to assess the possibilities for state or regional sharing of scarce faculty and instructional resources.

Suggested Further Action
In the planning of the curriculum studies for the Southern Regional Education Board and the Orange County consortium, there is built-in opportunity to study and test new educational arrangements and relationships. It would be possible, particularly in the SREB area, to test some methods for sharing faculty and institutional resources as proposed in this recommendation. Likewise, some statewide master planning committees could propose state models for trial and evaluation.

> 10. A national committee be initiated by joint action of the American Nurses' Association and the National League for Nursing to study and make recommendations for future accrediting of nursing programs considering this commission's recommendations for changed institutional patterns and the several current proposals for altering accreditation procedures in other health fields.

Implementing Agencies

The American Nurses' Association, the National League for Nursing, state boards of nursing, educational organizations and associations in nursing.

Status and Progress

Despite impassioned denials, there are problems in the accreditation of nursing programs. Many of the guidelines and rulings (such as the specification that the nursing major should be concentrated in the upper division of the baccalaureate program) were developed at a time when articulation between two- and four-year programs was hardly considered—if not condemned. Moreover, it is essential that practitioners have stronger input into educational decision making and this is best accomplished by joint planning of accreditation rules and procedures.

The ANA and the NLN already possess a coordinating council that could initiate action in this area, or propose an ad hoc group that could devote its entire attention to concerns in accreditation. The reports of the national study on accreditation in allied health schools (SASHEP) is one resource that could be utilized, but accreditation procedures and guides from the other health professions should be examined as well.

Suggested Further Action

Accreditation must be viewed as a positive incentive to institutional improvement and innovation rather than a punitive or narrowly prescriptive procedure. Particularly, accreditation procedures should advance educational articulation and curricular concentrations rather than canonize the status quo. The ANA and NLN, joined by other specialists, should review the basic intent and the real effects of current accreditation and provide for continuing reexamination on a periodic basis.

11. No less than three regional or interinstitutional committees be funded for the study and development of the nursing curriculum to develop educational objectives, universals, alternatives, and sequences for instruction. These committees should seek to specify appropriate levels of general and specialized learning for the different types of educational institutions.

12. Federal, state, and private funds be invested in a small number of grants for the specific purpose of demonstrating, testing, and evaluating the proposed curricula emanating from the study committees.

17. The federal Division of Nursing, the National Center for Health Services Research and Development, other governmental agencies, and private foundations provide research funds and contracts for basic and applied research into the nursing curriculum, articulation of educational systems, instructional practices, facilities design, etc., so

that the most functional, effective, and economic approaches are taken in the education and development of future nurses.

Implementing Agencies

Regional compacts or associations of institutions, public and private funding agencies, statewide master planning committees, and boards of higher education.

Status and Progress

Two projects related to these recommendations are currently underway. The Southern Regional Education Board and the Orange County Articulated Program in Nursing are both exploring curricular arrangements for articulating and sequencing collegiate programs in nursing.

A third project has been begun, but is currently inactive. The Coordinating Council for Higher Education of the State of California received a legislative mandate to identify levels of nursing practice and then to relate those levels to the academic preparation required. This would result in a curricular plan for both sequencing and relating general and specialized learnings. While the work was in progress, the legislative request was withdrawn; the project could, however, be renewed at any time.

Suggested Further Action

Reports from the two major projects should be widely disseminated and studied upon their conclusion. Moreover, present efforts at articulation as reported in "Individualization, Articulation, Concentration: Emergent Forces in Nursing Education" (NCSNNE pamphlet) should be examined and tested in an increasing number of junior and senior collegiate programs.

13. The state master planning committee for nursing education be particularly concerned that the number of graduate programs in nursing be consistent with human and economic resources, and that the inauguration or expansion of weak programs not be permitted.

16. Federal, state, and private funds be extended to support a limited number of institutions to establish or expand doctoral programs in nursing science. These programs should focus on developing research capabilities for the study of nursing practice and nursing education, and should undertake the specification and development of nursing theory and knowledge.

Implementing Agencies

Statewide master planning committees, interstate educational compacts, individual institutions.

Status and Progress

The NCSNNE staff has discussed this recommendation and attendant concerns with statewide master planning committees in all of the target states and is developing material for the remaining SMPCs. Relatedly, the Nahm study of graduate education for the Southern Regional Education Board has information and documentation that would be helpful in considering the problems of advanced programs.

Suggested Further Action

The New England, Southern and Western interstate compacts on nursing education should initiate leadership in strengthening graduate programs and in preventing the proliferation of small, intrinsically weak programs. The ANA and NLN should lend their support and strength to this effort, while state master planning committees outside the compact regions should seek to enforce the concern for quality in their areas.

14. The Congress continue and expand such programs as the Health Manpower Act to:

a. Provide educational loans to nurses pursuing graduate degrees with provision for part or whole forgiveness based on subsequent years of teaching;

b. Provide postmaster and postdoctoral fellowships and traineeships for nursing faculty and master clinicians to permit added professional development and continuing reorientation to changing practice and developing health care delivery systems;

c. Provide earmarked funds for faculty members of schools of nursing to enable them to obtain additional formal academic preparation equal to that required for regular appointment to faculty posts in collegiate institutions. These funds should have similar forgiveness features based on years of continuing service.

Implementing Agencies

Federal government and state agencies receiving revenue sharing funds.

Status and Progress

Earlier progress in the funding of these particular needs for advanced education in nursing through the Health Manpower and Nurse Training Acts has been slowed in the administration proposal for fiscal 1974. While loans for students would be continued at 1972 levels, scholarships and traineeships would be greatly reduced and research grants for graduate students would be eliminated.

In the face of the need for faculty, clinical administrators, and nurse clinicians, all of whom need advanced preparation, it is imperative that funds be restored or supplied through revenue sharing or other new sources. Provision of aid to hospital school faculty is particularly critical in the present repatterning of preparatory education.

Suggested Further Action
Nursing organizations must present a united and vigorous educational campaign to establish understanding of needs and priorities that are so directly related to the health care delivery system. Both federal and state agencies and lawmakers should be provided with clear and concise information on the effects of sharp reductions in support of graduate and advanced programs in nursing so that they can make valid decisions–now and in the future.

15. Federal, state, and private funds be made available to nursing institutions:

a. In the form of small research grants or contracts to assess and evaluate the effectiveness of new media and technology for nursing education and to disseminate the results;

b. In the form of grants and stipends to support short-term workshops to acquaint faculty members with new media and instructional materials;

c. In the form of institutional grants or matching funds to permit the purchase and installation of media systems and the required technicians to maintain and operate them;

d. In the form of demonstration grants to develop a limited number of centers so that faculty members may visit and have "actual" experience with these new media and materials.

Implementing Agencies
Federal, state, and private funding agencies.

Status and Progress
In the investigation phase, the NCSNNE staff developed information on the costs of nursing education which indicated, because of the clinical content and low faculty-student ratios, that per capita expense is much greater than the average liberal arts or science program. It seems, then, that investigations should be made into any possible cost savings through instructional media, technology, or other forms of educational innovation.

In cooperation with the Rochester Clearinghouse on Self-Instructional Materials for Health Care Facilities, an annotated bibliography on materials and research related to instructional technology is now under development for dissemination to statewide master planning committees and educational institutions. The NCSNNE staff is also assisting the American Institute for Research on an investigation of the effectiveness of instructional technology in applications to nursing education.

Suggested Further Action
More small grants should be made available to foster developmental and demonstration projects that could hold the promise of improving instruction and reducing per capita expense. Individual institutions and instructors should explore the possibility of developmental efforts in collaboration with publishers or commercial organizations so that materials might be disseminated and developmental costs recouped.

> 18. The institutions for nursing education develop new approaches to the matter of admissions, including:
>
> a. Development of both written and performance examinations to assess the quality of prior nursing experience and practice for the purposes of credit and advanced placement;
>
> b. Development of achievement, placement, and diagnostic examinations in academic subjects to provide credit and proper placement of individuals within instructional programs.
>
> 19. To decrease student withdrawals and academic failures, nursing preparatory institutions:
>
> a. Study their application procedures, academic advising, and student completion data for the purpose of developing better selection and counseling;
>
> b. Investigate the development of more individualized programs of instruction that require accomplishment of curricular objectives, but permit variance in student rate of learning and in the number of courses taken at any one time.

Implementing Agencies
Individual educational institutions, state boards of higher education, interstate educational compacts.

Status and Progress
An increasing emphasis is being placed on the development of new admissions and diagnostic procedures that can individualize the programs of nursing education in the light of new societal needs and expectations. In the NCSNNE pamphlet, "Individualization, Articulation, Concentration: Emergent Forces in Nursing Education," there are vignettes of institutional efforts to maximize advanced placement, give proper individual recognition, and establish variable programs that take into account the varied interests and time factors involved in student learning. The New York State external degree program in nursing, for example, incorporates a number of these features.

A staff review of selecting procedures and screening tests for nursing student admission failed to reveal any valid and reliable instruments that could provide clear guides to success in career choice or academic admission.

Suggested Further Action
Educational institutions and organizations must explore greater individuality in admissions, placement, and advancement through the nursing programs. The Southern Regional Education Board and Orange County curriculum projects, as well as the results of the New York State external degree program, should be examined for guides to future developments in these areas.

20. The state master planning committee for nursing education identify one or more institutions to be responsible for regional coverage of continuing education programs for nurses within that area, and further that:

a. Federal and state funds be utilized to plan and implement continuing education programs for nursing on either a statewide or broader basis (as suggested by the current interstate compacts for higher education); and

b. In the face of changing health roles and functions, and the interdependence of the health professions, vigorous efforts be taken to have continuing education programs jointly planned and conducted by interdisciplinary teams.

21. Health care facilities, including hospitals, nursing homes, and other institutions, either individually or collectively through joint councils, provide professional training staffs to supervise and conduct in-service training and provide released time, facilities, and organizational support for the presentation of in-service nursing education as well as that for other occupations.

Implementing Agencies
Statewide master planning committees, educational institutions, health care facilities.

Status and Progress
Over the course of the implementation phase, perhaps no area of nursing has moved so rapidly and dramatically as continuing education and in-service training. From being "stepchildren" of the profession, they are now in the forefront of consideration due to the mandating of continuing education for relicensure in one state and the prospect of that being extended throughout the country.

Nationally and regionally, continuing education has been receiving both attention and direction. The informally organized "conference group" on continuing education is now a commission of the ANA. In the midwest and upper midwest, new interstate compacts have appeared for the specific purpose of developing and improving continuing education offerings and programs.

In furtherance of this effort, the NCSNNE staff prepared and distributed the pamphlet, "Continuing Education in Nursing: Necessity and Opportunity," which highlighted the developing needs for programs in this area.

Suggested Further Action

Statewide master planning committees and local educational institutions, should work with the emerging regional groups in continuing education to build strong programs that have planned curricular thrust and sufficient support to ensure long-term coordination.

In-service education should be planned in conjunction with continuing education so that effective and efficient programming can be accomplished. More in-service education should be planned on an interinstitutional basis so as to reduce per capita costs and permit better course development.

Section III
NCSNNE Recommendations Related to Nursing Careers

1. Nurses be appointed to, and hold full membership in, groups involved in health manpower planning at all governmental and regional levels.

2. Manpower planning in nursing be premised on the concept that nursing is primarily a clinical practice directed to the care of people. An adequate supply of practitioners, plus the effective and efficient utilization of this resource, requires more than general planning projections.

a. Planning should take into account the developing types and levels of nursing, including the pattern of staff, clinical, and master clinician nurse, and the functional distribution of nurses into episodic and distributive fields;

b. Planning should include the categories of non-nursing personnel (clerks, housekeepers, receptionists, registrars) required to free nurses from tasks not related to the direct care of people;

c. Planning should also take into account those categories of health workers required to provide routine personal and therapeutic services—those currently known as practical nurses, aids, auxiliaries, attendants.

Implementing Agencies

Planning and manpower agencies, nursing organizations, individual nurses.

Status and Progress

The vigorous development of interdisciplinary planning and joint practice committees in more than half the states, and the preliminary activities now underway in almost all the others, is intended to spark activity not only in nursing, but in participation by nurses in all other kinds of health and social planning.

The numerous pamphlets and articles prepared by the NCSNNE staff have highlighted the many persistent misconceptions that prevail about nursing. The misinterpretation of a nursing shortage, the poor patterns for career development related to nursing practice, the overemphasis on episodic as opposed to distributive practice are all cogent reasons why nurses must respond to each and every opportunity to join planning agencies. When they have participated actively in these committees, they have been valued and contributing members.

Suggested Further Action

Each nursing organization should make individual and association involvement in planning and policy making a key objective for the years ahead. The inclusion of nursing input is essential if decisions are to reflect the best contributions of the profession. The NSNA should endeavor to widen its already active program to involve student nurses in interdisciplinary and public planning so that future generations of nurses will be committed to and skilled in these activities.

3. Health management administrators and clinical directors of nursing service build on current improvements in starting salaries to create a strong reward system for remaining in clinical practice by developing schedules of substantially increasing salary levels for experienced nurses functioning in advanced capacities.

4. Personnel policies in all health care facilities should be so designed that they:

a. Differentiate levels of responsibility in accord with the concepts of staff nurse, clinical nurse, and master clinician with appropriate intermediate grades. These levels should be designed according to the content of the position and the clinical proficiency required for competent performance;

b. Provide for promotion granted on the basis of acquisition of the knowledge and demonstrated competence to perform in a given position.

Implementing Agencies

Nursing organizations, directors of nursing service, health administrators, and health associations.

Status and Progress
Significant improvements in nursing salaries have been realized over the past ten to fifteen years. Nursing salaries remain depressed in comparison with other female professionals and, most assuredly, in comparison with male professionals.

Nevertheless, as indicated in "No Carrots, No Sticks: Motivation in Nursing" (NCSNNE pamphlet), we must begin now to develop those career perspectives that will provide for motivational satisfaction at the higher levels of psychosocial need. If we are ever to realize the full potential of American nursing, it will be when we formulate a career perspective that permits true upward mobility attached to direct patient care.

In the many monographs and articles of the staff, and in the nursing literature as a whole, there are increasing numbers of demonstrations and experiments on new staffing, utilization, and career patterns. Administrators and directors must begin to innovate and change.

Suggested Further Action
Nursing organizations, other health associations, and policy makers in the public and private domains must study more seriously than ever before the present reward systems in nursing and relate them to our economic and psychosocial knowledge of human behavior.

> 5. Health management administrators and clinical directors of nursing service establish conditions to promote optimum opportunity for excellence in nursing practice by providing such elements as sufficient staff to develop and execute a personal care plan for each individual, the opportunity to discharge appropriate nursing functions in client teaching, counseling, and rehabilitation, and the surveillance and evaluation of the nursing plan for care.

Implementing Agencies
Nursing organizations and health care facilities.

Status and Progress
In the NCSNNE pamphlets on episodic and distributive care, a number of case examples of new staffing patterns and broadened responsibility for nursing practice were cited. The resultant economic and social savings were remarkable.

The rise, throughout the implementation period, of the nurse clinician and the continuing efforts of the National Joint Practice Commission to study the extended role of the nurse would indicate that administrative and organizational change must be initiated now if we are to make proper use of the opportunities afforded by these nurse practitioners.

The companion development of the patient oriented record and the interest of the Joint Commission on Hospital Accreditation in the auditing of nursing service also supports the development of better models and organizational arrangements.

Further Suggested Activities
Nursing organizations and health associations must begin to work jointly to anticipate the rapidly expanding role of the nurse in both episodic and distributive care areas. In most instances, our present utilization patterns would be limiting and prescriptive. In those demonstration projects reported in NCSNNE publications, however, there are new departures that would unleash the personnel potential of nursing. We must accomplish that end through organizational innovation.

6. Local health care facilities adopt policies that provide for orientation and continuing education programs (including in-service and formal course work), more flexible employment policies respecting part-time work, maternity leaves, assistance for education to qualify for advancement, and leaves for education to encourage both the retention and reactivation of qualified practitioners.

Implementing Agencies
Nursing organizations, local nurse associations, health associations and health care facilities.

Status and Progress
Considerable activity has taken place in the development of improved in-service education for nursing. The hospital and nursing journals suggest, too, that some increased flexibility in regulations, hours, and staffing has occurred but that this has not been generalized to a majority of the institutions and facilities that employ nurses.

Further Suggested Activities
The ANA-NLN-AHA liaison committee should explore whether some joint committee or other approach might be helpful in determining the effects of some of the experimental and demonstration programs reported in the literature and whether these could not be more widely adapted.

7. The professional health organizations, including those in nursing, take responsibility individually and collectively for interpreting the characteristics of contemporary nursing to the public and direct their appropriate offices to undertake the task.

Implementing Agencies

All nursing organizations plus statewide planning and joint practice committees.

Status and Progress

Much of the first year of the implementation program involved Commission and staff effort to inform and educate. This has been continued during the entire implementation phase through the pamphlet series, articles and monographs, and speeches.

More recently, a tape-slide presentation on *An Abstract for Action* has been made available to nursing organizations and implementation committees. Coupled with the development of a speakers' bureau, this is designed to give support to local programming and information activities.

An increasing number of articles in the nursing press have begun to give visibility and support to many of the Commission proposals relating to nursing roles, education, and careers.

Further Suggested Activities

Nursing must continue to provide educational and informational material on its professional mission, roles, accomplishments and concerns. To some extent, the Commission and its staff have performed missionary work with many outside organizations and with the public. The organized bodies in American nursing, however, must see this work as one concomitant with professional development.

8. State nurses' associations and state leagues for nursing undertake more effective dissemination of information to high school guidance counselors on the changing status of nursing, the opportunities for expanded clinical practice, the improving salary levels, and other career aspects of the profession.

Implementing Agencies

State and local nursing associations, leagues and student nurses' groups.

Status and Progress

No systematic effort was mounted in relation to this recommendation because it must, by its nature, be carried out at state or even the most local levels. Materials were reviewed, however, and one brochure from the Ohio State Nurses' Association was particularly helpful in providing the kind of information that a vocational or guidance counselor might need.

Further Suggested Activities

State and local groups should develop materials and programs (possibly including the NCSNNE tape-slide presentation) to inform counselors and prospective students about nursing, its career offerings, and its educational patterns.

All of the nursing organizations share these concerns, but it seems a particularly relevant project for NSNA.

9. Public and private agencies and health facilities:

a. Seek to identify talented individuals in lower job classifications who, despite probable shortcomings in formal education, display outstanding motivation, competence, and intelligence;

b. Encourage and assist these individuals to obtain the necessary preparation to enter nursing education programs; and

c. Provide scholarships and grants-in-aid to such individuals in amounts proportional to their demonstrated achievement.

10. Institutions for nursing education develop career enhancement programs for licensed practical (vocational) nurses to furnish these individuals with added opportunities for professional growth through sequences leading to academic degrees and registered nurse licensure.

Implementing Agencies

Educational institutions and health care facilities.

Status and Progress

In Appendix P to *An Abstract for Action,* there is a report on the development of educational programs for registered nursing that recruited from the LPN and aide ranks. More recently, the report of the Hunter College Municipal Nursing Program showed a most successful upward mobility program from LPN to RN levels.

The development of advanced placement challenge examinations and the development of the External Degree program in New York State are indicators of what can be done to provide flexibility and mobility within the current framework of nursing education.

Further Suggested Activities

Expansion of the challenge testing program and increased institutional involvement in articulation and mobility are key ingredients. As indicated in the Hunter College program, the probability of success is good if innovation is first initiated. Tradition is perhaps the greatest problem to be overcome.

11. Institutions for nursing education provide:

a. Expanded counseling services for mature individuals seeking initial entry into nursing preparatory programs; and

b. More preparatory programs for recent liberal arts and science graduates seeking a professional career in nursing.

12. Recruitment of men into nursing be fostered through efforts to modify the sex-linked occupational image of the profession by the national and state organizations, and the adoption of specific policies and goals to increase the percentage of males entering nursing preparatory programs by those institutions that offer them.

Implementing Agencies
Nursing organizations, educational institutions and student nurse groups.

Status and Progress
Throughout the implementation phase, the NCSNNE staff has emphasized the need for recruitment into nursing from the traditional underrepresented minorities including men, blacks, American Indians, and others. Among the significant "others" are older women now looking for an occupation, college graduates without occupational training, and individuals making a second career choice. All of these may come from social and economic groups that also are underrepresented in nursing.

There has been little systematic evidence gathered on most of these groups; there currently exists only one Master's program in nursing designed for the arts and science baccalaureate graduate (New York Medical College). Over the past three years, however, there has been greater institutional interest in all these "new" students and the National Student Nurses' Association has evidenced a broad interest in recruiting from all stations and levels of society.

Further Suggested Activities
Educational institutions and student groups should adopt, as a general long-term goal, that nursing recruit in such ways that the profession broadly reflects societal composition. Thus, men should be recruited as should blacks and others. No short-term, high-impact program is likely to work, however, and the commitment must be maintained over time. The more diversified the input into the profession, the more reference groups it will possess and the more likely it will reflect total societal needs.

13. All remaining states without mandatory licensure laws for registered nurses immediately adopt appropriate regulation to this effect.

14. All state licensure laws for nursing be revised to require periodic review of the individual's qualifications for practice as a condition for license renewal.

15. The language of licensing laws in nursing and medicine be couched in flexible terms to permit role evolution in accord with the emerging features of health service.

Implementing Agencies
Nursing organizations, state boards of nursing, and other relevant state agencies.

Status and Progress
Over the course of the implementation period, the NCSNNE staff has participated in discussion of both licensure laws and health practice acts, and has, on request, been of some assistance to state nurses' associations and state boards of nursing in the case of particular legislation.

The Commission has adopted a resolution opposing the extension of institutional licensure to nursing personnel at this time and has generally agreed with the adoption of a moratorium on changes in licensure pending the outcome of recommendations from the National Joint Practice Commission and various other studies now in progress.

Further Suggested Activities
The Commission would urge continuation of the licensure moratorium until NJPC task forces begin their reports and recommendations. All changes should be to provide greater flexibility and role expansion while maintaining guarantees of safety for the consumer.

Mandatory continuing education for relicensure should also be held in abeyance until the report of the ANA ad hoc committee is thoroughly reviewed and discussed.

16. In view of the emergence of advanced levels of clinical practice in nursing,

a. A single license be retained for the registered nurse; and

b. Advanced levels of nursing practice be recognized through:

1. Designation by approved bodies for such purposes, presumably the Academy of Nursing;
2. State licensing standards for health service units;
3. Qualifications for personnel specified in accreditation standards; and
4. Institutional personnel policies for appointments, promotion, and compensation.

Implementing Agencies
The ANA Congress for Nursing Practice, specialty practice groups in nursing, and other nursing organizations.

Status and Progress
The meeting in January, 1973 of seventeen major nursing organizations provided strong impetus to interorganizational planning and agreement on standards,

certification, and specialized practice. The National Commission feels that these groups, supplemented by the contributions of the National Joint Practice Commission and the Academy of Nursing, contain the essential elements to proper decision making.

Further Suggested Activities

As quickly as possible, and utilizing input from the NJPC task forces, standards and certification requirements should be developed through joint organizational efforts between ANA and the specialty practice groups. This is already in the discussion stages, and it must be facilitated.

17. The national nursing organizations press forward in their current study of functions, structures, methods of representation, and interrelationships in order to determine:

a. Areas of overlap or duplication that could be eliminated;

b. Areas of need that are currently unmet; and

c. Areas or functions that could be transferred from one organization to another in light of changing systems and practices.

18. Nursing organizations, in effecting any of the changes that might come out of their current self-study, maintain their focus on responsiveness to health care consumers through the principle (perhaps unique to this profession) of providing for lay representation on their policy-making and deliberative boards.

Implementing Agencies

The national organizations in nursing.

Status and Progress

The holding of the so-called National Nurses' Congress and the plan to continue these planning meetings and discussions is the necessary first step toward better cooperation and coordination of efforts among the many nursing organizations. It is essential to the establishment of a united "house of nursing."

At the same time, the National Commission has urged that nursing involve public representatives in its deliberations so that professional concerns are always viewed in light of public good and societal need. Nursing is unique in its record of concern for consumer welfare, and this could become a very strong point in the future of this profession's development.

Further Suggested Activities

Out of the planning meetings of the nurses' associations, the National Commission would hope to see increased, and closer, organizational cooperation. Much of the information effort directed during the implementation phase toward nursing was intended to underline the importance of this effort. The individual nursing organizations must now demonstrate their commitment to professional growth through mutual assistance.

19. Individual nurses make a professional commitment to their organizations by joining and supporting one or more of them, at the same time ensuring that the organizations become more surely representative and more truly the designated spokesmen for nurses.

Implementing Agencies
Individual nurses and nursing students.

Status and Progress
The NCSNNE staff has consistently urged, in speeches and publications, the need for individual commitment and involvement in the organizations for nursing. Perhaps only one out of every three practicing nurses now belongs to any of the nursing groups, but this is still somewhat more than would have appeared on membership lists six years ago. The rise of the specialty practice groups has been instrumental in many ways in involving previously uncommitted practitioners, and all organizations in nursing have agreed to foster recruitment of members.

Further Suggested Activities
Nursing organizations, educational institutions, care facilities, and student groups must emphasize that professionalism begins with commitment and participation in the work of the profession. This demands personal involvement and membership in the associations and organizations of nursing. Through mutual campaigns and cooperative planning among the nursing organizations, considerable headway can be made.

Appendix C
SUMMARY OF IMPLEMENTATION PROGRESS WITHIN THE STATES

Over the course of the investigation period, members of the Commission staff visited the District of Columbia and all but one of the fifty states. This frequent involvement with the grassroots problems of nursing, plus the recognition that we possess fifty-one laboratories for experimentation in education and practice, convinced the commissioners that national implementation must necessarily involve strong participation by the several states.

The problems of determining specific nursing needs and resources, concern for developing comprehensive and articulated educational patterns, need for planning continuing learning experiences, and the necessity for congruent role functioning between the health practicing professions are all national in scope; answers, however, must be attuned to regional variations, economic and social requirements, and a host of other specific conditions.

For this reason, the Commission recommended the establishment of statewide master planning and joint practice committees in each of the states to determine priorities, set goals and aims, and implement the needed changes called for in *An Abstract for Action*, within their boundaries. There is, of course, no state that is exempt from the problems of health care, so all of the states could benefit from the workings of these committees. Realistically, however, there are degrees of readiness and limitations of money and personnel. To initiate involvement in implementation, the Commission selected nine states, in April of 1971, to serve as demonstration centers, or "target states." It was our hope that we could learn, from their combined experience, helpful information that would facilitate and expedite the ensuing efforts of other states to emulate their progress.

The nine target states are: California, Georgia, Illinois, Kansas, Maine, North Carolina, Pennsylvania, Texas, and Wyoming. Among them, there is contained a broad range of economic, geographic, and social patterns that mirror the problems across the nation. With the help of a supplemental grant from the W. K. Kellogg Foundation, the Commission staff sought to assist each of these states in organizing state committees, setting up goals, and beginning to effect the recommendations of *An Abstract for Action.*

Our broader hope was that progress in these states would serve as a stimulus and a model for their neighbors to begin organizing and planning. This has begun to materialize, particularly in the third year of the national implementation effort. By April of 1973, more than half of all the states had statewide committees for educational planning and for joint practice. Most of the remaining states had made progress toward formal establishment of such groups, and only a half-dozen states, or less, were without any discernible activity.

In organizing this undertaking, it is impossible to give sufficient credit to nurses throughout the country. As individuals and as organizations, nurses have taken up the challenge to organize for action and to become involved in the hard work of effecting change. In every instance, however, where there is real accomplishment to report, it is also true that physicians, health administrators, other health professionals, educators, planners, consumers, and many others have played a significant part in the process. The understanding and cooperation thus generated may be at least as important as specific actions taken by the statewide committees, for they build a foundation for continuing attack on problems throughout our health care system.

In the following pages, an abbreviated summary of state activities is provided.* The reports of the states are grouped alphabetically in two parts:

Section I. Target States
Section II. Non-Target States and the District of Columbia

At the end of Section II, there is a tabular presentation of the status of statewide organization for planning as of April 1, 1973.

*The information reported here was obtained from a series of five surveys conducted by the NCSNNE staff between September 1, 1971 and April 1, 1973. State Nurses' Associations and state implementation committees provided the updating of these surveys.

Section I Target States

CALIFORNIA

SMPC: In Process *SJPC: Operational*

In 1971, an ad hoc group began meeting to assess the nursing needs and resources in California. This group included: representatives of the California Nurses' Association (CNA), the California League for Nursing, the Directors of Nursing Service of the Hospital Council of Southern California; individual nurse leaders in the state, including directors of educational programs; members of the NCSNNE's advisory groups; and two NCSNNE regional associates.

One of the first activities of the ad hoc committee was to arrange five meetings throughout the state, attended by multidisciplinary representatives, for the purpose of informing the state of the NCSNNE report and recommendations and, particularly, to spearhead the development of a SMPC for nursing and nursing education in California.

Meanwhile, the ad hoc committee learned of a legislative mandate to the state's Coordinating Council of Higher Education, to implement educational planning for previously defined levels of nursing practice. In essence, the Coordinating Council was charged with doing a follow-up study to one conducted by the Bureau of Nursing (within the Department of Public Health). The study, like the previous one, was to identify levels of nursing practice and then relate the skills designated to those levels, to the academic nursing community. Hopefully, this joining of practice skills to appropriate educational levels would provide for needed articulation between nursing practice and education in the state.

At that time, the Chief Higher Education Specialist of the Coordinating Council was planning to appoint an advisory committee. Learning of this, the ad hoc committee approached him with the NCSNNE recommendations concerning establishment of a SMPC. They mutually agreed that the advisory committee would be established along the NCSNNE guidelines—in other words, the advisory committee would be multidisciplinary, and thus acceptable both as a SMPC and as an advisory committee to the Coordinating Council.

It was this multidisciplinary advisory committee that then began the preliminary steps in conducting the mandated study of levels and scope of nursing practice, relating them to nursing education. However, in early 1972, the legislative committee withdrew its charge from the Coordinating Council and the work of their advisory committee came to a premature halt.

Following the establishment of the advisory committee and the successful completion of the five state implementation meetings, the ad hoc committee wrote a proposal recommending a Governor's Conference on Nursing which would provide an impetus for the development of a statewide plan for nursing education, based on the final report of the Coordinating Council's advisory committee.

The ad hoc group then disbanded because, at that point, the advisory committee was established, the state informational meetings had been held, and the Governor's Conference was being considered. Unfortunately, it was at this juncture that the advisory committee was required to discontinue its work. Thus, the Governor's Conference never materialized since it was to have been contingent upon the finished report of the advisory committee.

In June, 1972, the NCSNNE staff met in San Francisco with a new ad hoc group of approximately fifteen persons representing the various health professions (including vocational nurses) and organizations in the state. This group discussed issues and problems involved in establishing a master planning committee in California. By mutual agreement, this voluntary group offered to serve in a liaison and advisory capacity to the NCSNNE for further planning of implementation efforts in the state. They also approved the idea of encouraging and supporting the reactivation of the Coordinating Council's advisory committee in order that the study could be completed and the final report presented to the State Legislature.

The CNA staff continues to support the suggestion that a multidisciplinary meeting be convened by the Governor in order to provide the momentum for initiating and following through in the development of a statewide plan for nursing education.

In the Fall of 1971, the California Joint Practice Commission (CJPC) was established through the efforts of the California Nurses' Association, the California Medical Association, and Dr. Virginia Barham, regional associate of the NCSNNE. Six nurses and six physicians were appointed initially and later the membership was increased to ten members each from medicine and nursing.

Initial topics of discussion included: the scope of nursing practice; various levels of education for nursing personnel; the role of physician assistants; expanded roles of the nurse; necessary legislation for the practice of nursing; and the expectations of nurses and physicians toward each other. To assist with these complicated issues, a steering committee was formed to delineate the key concerns and problems relevant to each area. In addition, the steering committee asked the Commission members to submit their thoughts regarding specific goals, directions and tasks that they felt the CJPC should undertake prior to the meeting of the steering committee in April, 1972. In order to facilitate its objectives, the steering committee recommended to the Commission that the group focus on areas of agreement rather than ones of disagreement.

One of the major activities of the CJPC to date has been the formulation of statements on the expanding role of the registered nurse in primary, acute, and long-term care. Each statement includes: a definition of terms used; conditions of practice with emphasis on academic and clinical preparation; continuing education and working relationships; scope and evaluation of practice; and public protection. The Committee's recommended statements have been forwarded to the CNA and CMA boards for their review and approval. The three statements also have been referred to legal counsel for examination. Recently, a resolution has been introduced in the State Assembly to utilize ensuing joint practice statements as the basis for determining and defining health care practice in California.

The joint practice committee plans for the future include: continued sponsorship by the CNA and CMA; holding four Commission meetings each year; and promoting increased communication between the two professional groups as well as eventual work with other health professional organizations.

GEORGIA

SMPC: Operational *SJPC: Operational*

The Georgia Educational Improvement Council (GEIC) conducted a detailed study of nursing education needs and resources in the state and published its report and recommendations in 1969. In the fall of 1970, the Georgia Commission on Nursing, a fifty-five-member multidisciplinary group, was appointed to examine methods for implementing the Georgia and National Commission reports.

This Commission on Nursing subsequently became the statewide master planning committee for nursing and nursing education in Georgia. In January, 1971, however, when the Governor's term expired, the Commission on Nursing was disbanded. Then on June 15, 1972, by an Executive Order of Governor Carter, the Georgia Commission was reactivated and relocated in the Georgia Educational Improvement Council. Organizational and structural changes were soon after made in Georgia's state government, one of which involved the transfer of GEIC to the legislative branch of government; therefore, the SMPC was reassigned to the Office of Comprehensive Health Planning under the executive branch.

The Executive Order identified thirty-nine members (most of whom had been on the original Georgia Commission), appointed to serve on the reactivated SMPC. This multidisciplinary committee includes educators, consumers, registered nurses, licensed practical nurses, and physicians. These members also represent the following organizations: the Georgia Hospital Association, the Regional Medical Program, the Practical Nursing Examining Board, the State Board of Nursing, the Georgia State Nurses' Association, the State Nursing Home Association, the Student Nurses' Association, the Georgia State League for Nursing, the State Department of Human Resources, and the Department of Education. In addition, all levels of nursing education in the state are represented on the committee. Recently, a project director was appointed to spearhead and coordinate the state's planning and education efforts.

The master planning committee has structured two subcommittees–Nursing Practice and Nursing Education–for the purpose of examining goals, establishing priorities, suggesting specific recommendations, and identifying specific methods for implementation. In addition, the committee plans to establish special committees within the Nursing Education subcommittee to deal with continuing education and legislation.

The SMPC published a brochure, entitled "National Commission for the Study of Nursing and Nursing Education and You," to be distributed for informational purposes throughout Georgia. This pamphlet has had wide distribution, to date, and continues to be issued to various groups in the state.

Since its official establishment, the SMPC has made several recommendations to Governor Carter, proposing that: nurses, along with various health professionals, be included in organizing, planning, and implementing health services; there be support of nurse practitioners in primary health care services within the Department of Human Resources; training programs be established to prepare qualified registered professional nurses in primary health care; support of personnel be increased to provide more and better comprehensive health services for school children; counseling and referral services be instituted for applicants who have been rejected from nursing schools; and the joint practice committee be recognized and supported. These recommendations were presented and discussed with the newly formed Board of Human Resources by the project director, director of Comprehensive Health Planning, and the committee chairman. The Governor's continued interest in nursing was evidenced when he immediately appointed nurse representatives to serve on the Governor's Advisory Council on Mental Health, Maternal and Child Health and Family Planning.

In mid-1972, Georgia officially established its State Joint Practice Committee, formerly a medical-nursing liaison committee. Fourteen persons each, representing Georgia State Nurses' Association and the Medical Association of Georgia, comprise this twenty-eight-member group. Since its inception, the committee has identified the need for involvement of individuals at the local level. Thus, one of their priorities is the creation of counterpart JPCs in regional and local areas of Georgia.

Topics for discussion by the committee presently focus on the current Nurse Practice Act, nursing practice patterns, and the congruent roles of the nurse and physician. As a result of these dialogues, the committee anticipates sponsoring, in the near future, joint statements on primary health care.

ILLINOIS

SMPC: Operational *SJPC: Operational*

The Illinois Nurses' Association and the Illinois League for Nursing (INA-ILN) Coordinating Council, appointed in 1965, functions as the designated committee to coordinate implementation efforts in the state. This Coordinating Council is made up of the executive committees of the two organizations: the INA Executive Committee consists of the five officers who are nurses, while the ILN Executive Committee members include one management consultant, one administrator, and three nurses. In 1966, the Coordinating Council was successful in obtaining funds for the support of the Illinois Study Commission on Nursing (ISCON).

In 1968, having completed their study, ISCON published a report of its findings on nursing needs and resources in Illinois which were quite compatible with those of the NCSNNE. Thereafter, summaries of the current status of the recommendations in the 1968 ISCON report were prepared in 1971, and updated in late 1972, in order to reassess its measurements of progress and to assist in delineating the scope of practice for future activities. Meanwhile, a comprehensive proposal, entitled "To Systematize Nursing Education in Illinois," was developed as a three-year project. This proposal, sponsored by the Coordinating Council, identified a design for implementing recommendations derived from the state and national studies. Submitted to the Division of Nursing, Bureau of Health Manpower Services, HEW, in January, 1972, the proposal was approved in July, 1972; however, it has not yet been funded. The materials developed for the proposal, in the meantime, have been widely used in the establishment of the Commission on Implementation.

The Illinois Implementation Commission on Nursing (IICON) was officially appointed in November, 1972, by the INA-ILN Coordinating Council to intensify implementation efforts in the state. In January, 1973, IICON accepted its charge to systematize nursing education in Illinois consonant with developing current trends for nursing manpower. IICON, an independent, multidisciplinary group, is composed of thirty-eight members. The appointing body, in selecting membership on this commission, sought individuals and leaders who represented: various types of nursing programs; educational, hospital and health planning groups; community health agencies; various fields of nursing and medical practice; and professional associations.

IICON has created standing committees to accomplish its work. The Committee on Nursing Education has been quite active in the planning and programming of nursing education so as to improve the quality of health services in Illinois. A Committee on Evaluation has been appointed. In addition, a Committee on Continuing Education was originally planned for IICON; however, INA has recently established a Council on Continuing Education and is giving it high priority in support and staffing. Therefore, the IICON Executive Committee has recommended that the INA Council on Continuing Education be IICON's arm for continuing education rather than set up its own standing committee, thereby duplicating efforts. This plan, acceptable to both the Council and ILN Board, will go to IICON for approval at its April, 1973 meeting. A fourth committee, on Medical/Nursing Joint Practice, has already been activated and is jointly responsible to the INA and ISMS. It will provide a formal structure for medicine and nursing to examine, discuss, and reformulate complementary practice roles in health services.

IICON has recently prepared a brochure on the "National Commission for the Study of Nursing and Nursing Education and You" for distribution in Illinois. This brochure briefly describes the NCSNNE and the past, present, and future activities of IICON.

In addition to the activities of IICON, a joint project between INA and the Health Education Commission of the Illinois Board of Higher Education has focused on promoting, facilitating, and coordinating institutional, regional, and statewide planning for nursing education. This twenty-month project was initiated in September, 1971, to accelerate the movement of registered nurses through baccalaureate and master's programs in nursing. Supported by a grant to INA from the Illinois Regional Medical Program, the project hopes to identify barriers for registered nurses who desire to further their education in nursing and plans to propose specific actions for overcoming those obstacles. Their findings should provide IICON with valuable information to use in their further planning for nursing education in the state.

The Illinois Joint Practice Committee, established in August, 1972, through the efforts of the two sponsoring organizations—the Illinois State Medical Society and the Illinois Nurses' Association—is part of the organizational network of IICON. The membership of the committee is composed of four nurse practitioners who are appointed by INA, and four physicians who are appointed by ISMS.

Recently, the committee reviewed programs that prepare nurse practitioners for expanded roles and reviewed the licensing laws for health workers in Illinois. Subsequently, they prepared a statement and proposed two recommendations suggesting that no changes be made in the nursing and medical practice acts that relate to the scope of practice; and furthermore, that the existing moratorium on licensure for new categories of health workers, who provide care, be continued at least through 1974. These two recommendations have been referred to the boards of directors of the two parent organizations for their approval. Currently, the committee is in the process of identifying its objectives and developing a plan and timetable to accomplish them.

KANSAS

SMPC: Operational *SJPC: Operational*

In Kansas, master planning is the product of interorganizational agreement. The umbrella group is the Master Planning Committee for the Study of Nursing and Nursing Education.

The administrative committee of this group, well established and operational, is composed of the executives of the six sponsoring agencies, namely: Kansas Medical Society (KMS), Kansas League for Nursing (KLN), Kansas Nursing Home Association (KNHA), Kansas State Nurses' Association (KSNA), Kansas State Board of Nursing (KSBN), and Kansas Hospital Association (KHA). The Kansas State Nurses' Association serves as the coordinating agency and chairs the meetings of the administrative committee which was created as an implementation mechanism for coordinating progress in statewide master planning and state joint practice, both areas of which are dealt with by specific task forces. Members have been involved with providing inter- and intra-agency communication; providing endorsement, support, and encouragement to the master planning committee; selecting a project director; and proposing and administering the budget.

The Master Planning Committee for the Study of Nursing and Nursing Education, officially established in May, 1972, is an eighteen-member interdisciplinary group organized in November, 1971, following a multidisciplinary meeting on statewide planning for nursing education. Since its formation, the master planning committee has accomplished several activities. The first achievement has been the identification of objectives which are: to develop a plan to provide adequate educational opportunities to meet identified needs; to provide opportunities for communication and cooperation among nurse and allied health practitioners, educators, recipients and employers of health care; to conduct a study to determine the health care needs and resources in Kansas; to cooperate with all groups who have similar objectives to those of the master planning committee; to improve the articulation of curricula among the various types of educational programs in nursing in order to enhance career advancement; to develop and implement a statewide program of continuing education in order to maintain and improve the competence of nurse practitioners; and to define various levels of nursing practice and seek such legislation as may be needed for the protection of the various publics.

During 1972, four task forces were organized: Continuing Education, Articulation of Curricula, Nursing Service Needs and Levels of Nursing Practice, and Joint Practice. The Task Force on Continuing Education has developed "Guidelines for Nursing Programs for Nurses in Kansas" which embody the Continuing Education Unit concept. These guidelines have been endorsed by the Kansas State Nurses' Association Committee on Credentials. Based on the utilization of the guidelines, 130 continuing education programs have been approved throughout the state of Kansas. The Continuing Education Unit Program has stimulated increased interest and attention to the problems of maintaining nursing excellence and has served to provide more opportunities for nurses to maintain their competence.

The Articulation of Curricula Task Force has been identifying and exploring possibilities for implementing essential concepts in career ladder curriculum. The Nursing Service Needs and Levels of Nursing Practice Task Force is concerned with various levels of nursing practice, including the registered nurse, nurse educator, nurse administrator, nurse researcher, licensed practical nurse, nurse aide, and their implications for change in nursing education. Several other groups that are concerned with these problems have expressed a desire to become involved and assist with the work of master planning.

A fourth task force is the Joint Practice Committee; which has been organized since March, 1972. This twelve-member group (six nurses and six physicians) was appointed by the Kansas State Nurses' Association and the Kansas Medical Society. During the initial phase of organization, the Joint Practice Committee reviewed the objectives of the National Joint Practice Commission; as a result of that examination, a subcommittee has been formed to develop objectives for the state Joint Practice Committee.

The master planning committee has distributed, throughout the state, numerous copies of the pamphlet, "National Commission for the Study of Nursing and Nursing Education and You," designed for Kansas. The brochure describes highlights of the Commission and the involvement of Kansas in implementing its recommendations. Currently, the master planning committee is in the process of developing a funding proposal for the continuing implementation phase and setting timetables for reaching its objectives.

MAINE

SMPC: In Process *SJPC: Operational*

Presently, Maine has no designated or existing group to deal with coordinating progress in statewide master planning and state joint practice. However, plans are underway for the development of such a group to be created sometime in 1973. Meanwhile, the Board of Directors of the Maine State Nurses' Association is assuming responsibility for coordinating implementation efforts of the NCSNNE report and recommendations.

A study, "Statewide Planning for Nursing Education in Maine," submitted by the MSNA to the Division of Nursing, Public Health Service (HEW) in September, 1970, was funded and has just recently been completed.

During the study, two groups—the Statewide Advisory Committee and the Technical Advisory Committee—served the project in an advisory capacity. The Statewide Advisory Committee, with an approximate thirty-member multidisciplinary membership, represented a cross-section of Maine's health care providers and consumers. The smaller group, the Technical Advisory Committee, included nurses from various nursing education programs and practice settings. Both advisory groups, having completed their function, were dissolved in May, 1972.

A preliminary report of the study findings and recommendations was discussed by the project director with nurses who attended the MSNA Annual Meeting in October, 1972. The final report of the study was then issued in December, 1972, and has been widely circulated to allied health agencies, health professional organizations, legislators, Maine's congressional delegation, and to the ANA and the NLN.

As a follow-up to the issuance of the final report, the MSNA feels strongly that interpretation of the study to others is essential toward increasing understanding within the profession so that progress can be made toward future planning. Therefore, meetings have been held throughout the state with local school nurse groups, the district nurse associations, and other organizations, to discuss the study, its findings and recommendations, and possible implementation efforts. Meanwhile, within the MSNA, the Commission on Nursing Education has been charged with examining the recommendations and making suggestions for implementation.

At present, an Ad Hoc Committee on Continuing Education, appointed several years ago by the members of the MSNA and MLN, and the MSNA Commission on Education assume responsibility for planning of nursing education, resources, and related concerns in the state.

The MSNA Board of Directors has been involved in initiating plans toward the development, sponsorship and establishment of a multidisciplinary SMPC in Maine. The board has plans underway to hold a meeting with representatives of the various health agencies, the university system and private colleges, governmental agencies, and the health professions. Hopefully, the overall outcome of this meeting will produce recommendations and suggestions for the sponsorship and establishment of a SMPC in Maine. A few considerations toward this goal include: inviting the Governor to create the committee; asking an existing agency such as Comprehensive Health Planning to sponsor the committee; or requesting the Maine State Legislature to establish the committee.

To progress with the implementation of the study's recommendations, financial assistance is sorely needed. A request to the Division of Nursing, Public Health Service, for funding was not approved. Therefore, additional funding sources are currently being identified by the MSNA Board of Directors.

Maine has had a liaison committee between medicine and nursing since June, 1972. This group, originally composed of five members each from nursing and medicine, increased its number of members in order to have more practitioners involved. Initially, the nurse representatives rather than being practitioners, had held administrative positions in nursing service and education. With the additional members, the nurse representatives now contain practitioners, including a pediatric nurse associate, a family nurse associate, a nurse-midwife, and a nurse clinician. To date, the MSNA-MMA liaison committee has developed and approved joint statements of policy on the practice of nurse midwifery and the practice of the pediatric nurse associate.

NORTH CAROLINA

SMPC: Operational *SJPC: Operational*

In September, 1971, the North Carolina Steering Committee for NCSNNE Implementation was established. This group, originally composed of eight members from the nursing profession, later became multidisciplinary and increased its membership to twenty. The objectives for the steering committee are: to make nurses and others in the state aware of the NCSNNE report and the progress toward implementing their recommendations; and to coordinate the implementation efforts.

To assist with these activities, five subcommittees were formed to deal with the following specific areas: the development of a proposal for a demonstration project involving cooperative planning for nurse inservice education in isolated areas; the design of an information "flyer" to be distributed throughout the state; the planning and organization of a retreat session for the steering committee; the development of a program packet, including a tape talk to familiarize people with developments in the state; and the planning of a program presentation for the State Nurses' Association (NCSNA) clinical sessions to take place in September, 1972.

The informational materials have been completed through the assistance of the NCSNA. The program packets, circulated throughout the state to interested groups, include information about the NCSNNE report and North Carolina's role as a target state. The retreat, a two-day conference held in February, 1973, was devoted to assessing the implementation progress to date and to establishing immediate and long-range goals in relation to NCSNNE recommendations. At the conference, a number of activities were identified as having been accomplished. These were: the beginning of interinstitutional planning; the formation of the joint practice committee along with the development of guidelines for task forces; the development of guidelines for nursing education programs; and the initiation of actions necessary for seeking continuing education funds. In addition, serious health problems were identified from group discussions, priorities were established for meeting short-term and long-term needs, and suggestions for accomplishing those priorities were identified.

The steering committee, too, has studied the recently published preliminary report (partially funded by HEW), of a survey of RNs in North Carolina in 1971, describing relevant findings pertinent to the nursing needs and resources in North Carolina. In addition, the committee had studied draft legislation resulting from the work of the Legislative Research Commission to Study the Lawful Role of the Nurse.

In North Carolina, the Joint Committee on Nursing Education of the State Board of Education and the State Board of Higher Education has been designated the state's Master Planning Committee for Nursing Education. This committee, existing since 1965, has developed "Guidelines and Criteria" for assessing nursing education programs in North Carolina to insure availability of nursing personnel with various kinds of preparation to meet nursing needs of the state and to insure an uninterrupted flow of nurses into the communities. These guidelines have been approved by the two parent state boards and have been widely distributed throughout the state. To date, the master planning committee has assisted in: seeking funds for continuing education; helping form the joint practice committee between medicine and nursing; and in beginning interinstitutional planning.

The master planning committee has formed two subcommittees—an Educational Programs Review Committee and a subcommittee to study geographical distribution of nursing education programs and resources in the state. Recently, a report was prepared by the Advisory Committee on Continuing Education (this committee is advisory to three state organizations dealing with health issues, including the master planning committee), proposing a statewide program of continuing education which would be: accessible to nurses where they live and work; funded by a state appropriation; coordinated through a central state office; and implemented through the State's System of Higher Education. This proposal was presented to the Legislative Research Commission's Committee to Study the Lawful Role of the Nurse, and hopefully, through this group, it will be directed to the Advisory Budget Commission for inclusion in the state's 1973-75 budget.

In October, 1971, with the approval of the boards of the North Carolina State Nurses' Association (NCSNA), and the North Carolina Medical Society (NCMS), the North Carolina Joint Practice Committee (NCJPC) was established. The NCJPC membership consists of eight nurses, eight physicians, one nursing student, one medical student, and the presidents of the two parent organizations who serve as ex-officio members. The majority of the members are practitioners who represent a variety of practice settings and specialties.

The NCJPC, to date, has pursued the following activities: 1) agreement on developing joint policy statements on medical and nursing practice as legal interpretations of the law for approval by NCSNA and NCMS as well as gathering information about current nursing practice in North Carolina for testimony to the Legislative Research Commission; 2) exploration of the need for, and areas of, possible joint statements by the two professions; 3) exploration of role modifications as related to the physician's assistant, the family nurse practitioner, the nurse midwife, and other "specialized" areas of nursing practice; 4) implications of the legal aspects of role changes for nursing education and liability insurance coverage; 5) meeting with representatives of the North Carolina Pharmaceutical Association and the North Carolina Board of Pharmacy to discuss recommendations of the Legislative Research Commission's Committee in relation to proposed changes in the Pharmacy Act; 6) discussion of the possibility for registering family nurse practitioners under Exemption 13 of the Medical Practice Act, under rules and regulations developed jointly by the two professions' licensing Boards, as recommended by NCMS's Committee on Legislation; and 7) development and adoption of "Guidelines for Task Forces" to explore role relationships of physicians and nurses in: school health services, emergency care services, nurse-manned clinics, occupational health services, long-term care services, and maternity and family planning services (including midwifery).

The task forces are currently being appointed and will most likely be composed of medical and nursing practitioners as well as representatives from other disciplines. The charge for each task force will be to develop guidelines for the practice of selected expanded nursing roles and then to determine the related educational requirements for that particular practice. Currently, legislative bills, which provide legal protection for the nurse functioning in the expanded role, have been introduced in the General Assembly. This legislation necessitates changes in the Nurse Practice Act, the Medical Practice Act, insurance laws, and possibly, the Pharmacy Practice Act.

PENNSYLVANIA

SMPC: Operational *SJPC: Operational*

Initially, an Interdisciplinary Planning Committee of Pennsylvania, representing the Pennsylvania League for Nursing (PLN), Pennsylvania Medical Society

(PMS), Pennsylvania Nurses' Association (PNA), and the Hospital Association of Pennsylvania (HAP), met to spearhead the establishment of two commissions—the Commission on Joint Practice and the Master Planning Commission for Nursing Education. Shortly thereafter, the planning group formalized its efforts by holding a joint organizational and orientation meeting for the two commissions in March, 1972. Following this session, the designated commissions met separately to appoint their officers and identify their roles.

The planning committee decided not to seek, at this time, official state recognition and appointment of the commissioners but to continue the close relationship with the four sponsoring organizations. Therefore, a plan was devised for the creation of a coordinating committee to serve as the official group to coordinate progress in master planning and joint practice within Pennsylvania. The membership of the coordinating committee numbers nine including the committee project director and four members each from the two commissions. Each commission appoints its chairman, vice-chairman, secretary, and one member-at-large to serve on the coordinating committee; the project director acts as the primary liaison person between the two commissions.

One of the first actions of the coordinating council was to publish a brochure, entitled "National Commission for the Study of Nursing and Nursing Education and You," designed specifically for use in Pennsylvania. These pamphlets, which describe the highlights of the Commission and Pennsylvania's involvement as a target state, have been widely distributed to various groups throughout the state.

The purpose of the Master Planning Commission for Nursing Education in Pennsylvania is to discuss and make recommendations for the restructuring of nursing education in the state. This forty-two-member group represents health planners, government agencies, administrators of health care, nursing education programs, and professional organizations. Because of the large membership of this commission, a steering committee of eighteen members was formed to function as the nucleus working group to explore and develop relevant materials and recommendations for review by the total commission. To provide continuity between these two groups, the chairman of the Commission for Nursing Education also serves as the chairman of the steering committee. Since the fall of 1972, the Master Planning Commission for Nursing Education has met approximately every three months, and its steering committee every six weeks.

The goals of the Commission for Nursing Education were determined by asking the steering committee to establish priority rankings for the NCSNNE recommendations. Those recommendations receiving the highest rankings became the goals for the commission, and they are: restructuring nursing education within the general system of education in Pennsylvania; supporting collaboration between general education and nursing education in planning and implementing innovative educational programs and policies; enlarging activities and efforts directed toward the recruitment and retention of minority groups in nursing; ensuring the availability of graduate education in nursing for the potential student population throughout the Commonwealth; and extending and expanding learning opportunities for nurses through planned and organized continuing education programs. To date, other accomplished activities of the commission and/or its steering committee include: establishing a timetable for the existence of the commission; identifying the need for hard data on nursing manpower supply and demand; reviewing data on schools of nursing in Pennsylvania; reviewing possible curriculum models; and selecting two models to function as model demonstrations during the project period.

Recently, the steering committee completed a draft of recommendations and evaluation of activities for review by the Commission on Nursing. This document also includes the development of hypotheses regarding the future of nursing education in Pennsylvania. Hopefully, available data as well as other information which support the hypotheses will form the base for the final recommendations. The present timetable indicates that: approval of the final recommendations and reports is tentatively planned for November, 1973; the publication of the report is scheduled in 1974; and a final meeting is planned for March, 1974, at which time the Commission on Nursing will dissolve.

The Pennsylvania Commission on Joint Practice has been established since March, 1972, to discuss and make recommendations for the effective use and expansion of health manpower in the Commonwealth of Pennsylvania. The specific objectives of this commission are to formulate and distribute a joint position statement on the congruent roles of the nurse and physician; and to ensure a position statement on advanced clinical practice and specialization as nursing assumes more responsibility and accountability for individual practice in all kinds of health services.

This thirty-six-member group includes representatives from: various health associations; health licensing boards including pharmacy, nursing, medicine, and osteopathy; nurse and physician practitioners; comprehensive community health programs, regional medical programs, insurance companies for the health professionals, third party payers; and consumers. Like the SMPC, the Commission on Joint Practice has a large membership. Therefore, a seventeen-member steering committee was created to act as the working core for the commission. This committee has been meeting every six weeks and the larger Commission on Joint Practice, every three months since October, 1972.

A few activities of the Commission on Joint Practice and/or its steering committee to date include: appointing a task force to study the role of the physician's assistant (associate); accepting the recommendation that Directors of Nursing of all hospitals be members of their hospital's governing board; reviewing current statements on nursing roles and functions as well as the current issues in health delivery and manpower; and accepting a definition of nursing as contained in the current Pennsylvania licensure legislation. (A new State Nurse Practice Act, recently introduced in the House and Senate Licensure Committees, provides for the expanded role of the nurse.) Also, an initial draft of recommendations and evaluation of activities has been prepared for consideration by the total commission. The timetable indicates that the final approval of the report and recommendations is scheduled by the commission for January, 1974. The completed, published report is expected in March, 1974, at which time the Commission on Joint Practice, as presently established, will be terminated.

TEXAS

SMPC: Operational *SJPC: Operational*

The Commission on Nursing in Texas is an independent, multidisciplinary group formed and chartered in 1971 for the purposes of: assuming the leadership role in the state for implementing the NCSNNE recommendations; and improving health care in Texas through the effective education and utilization of nursing personnel on the health care team.

The commission objectives, and a plan of action for carrying them out, were adopted in July, 1972. These objectives focused on: informing health professionals and community leaders in Texas of the essence of their program; implementing recommendations dealing with nursing roles and functions, nursing education, nursing career mobility and nursing research; and developing financial sources to support the activities necessary in implementing the recommendations.

The twenty-one-member commission involves a cross-section of Texas health care providers—physician and nurse practitioners, hospital administrators and a member from Comprehensive Health Planning; nurse educators and educators from other disciplines; and members from the public-at-large. The commission feels a strong commitment to remaining interdisciplinary in order to deal objectively with all issues and concerns which relate to all health professional roles in Texas. Currently, the Commission on Nursing is in the process of becoming incorporated in order to receive funds from available sources; final actions for incorporation are expected to be completed by May, 1973.

The Commission on Nursing has created three committees to help accomplish its work. The first is a committee to implement the pilot project involving nurse practitioners, which has been designed to demonstrate the possible use of nurse practitioners as deliverers of primary health care in a medically deprived area of the state. To date, two such possible sites have been proposed. In both areas, community leaders have indicated much interest, and physicians have offered support for having the commission sponsor a program involving the expanded role of the nurse. Currently, funds are being sought by the commission to support this program.

The Committee on Publicity was appointed to: outline a public information program using printed materials, tapes, film-strips, and speakers; and to promote dissemination of information about the Commission on Nursing in professional health journals and the general media. One method of informing the public has been the newly prepared pamphlet entitled "National Commission for the Study of Nursing and Nursing Education and You," which describes the NCSNNE and the implementation activities in Texas. These brochures have been mailed directly to health professionals and distributed at professional conventions and meetings. In addition, several articles have been published in professional journals, newsletters, and bulletins. The newly organized Speaker's Bureau also provides information about the Commission on Nursing. This group comprises the members of the Commission for Nursing in Texas and, perhaps at a later date, will include other health leaders.

Initially, the Coordinating Board Nursing Project (CBNP) received a federal grant from the Division of Nursing (HEW) to conduct a three-year study of nursing education needs and resources in Texas. Shortly thereafter, the Commission for Nursing identified the CBNP, which is under the auspices of the Coordinating Board of the Texas College University System, as the state Master Planning Committee for Nursing Education, until August 31, 1974. The Commissioner of Higher Education in Texas then approved the CBNP as the state master planning committee. CBNP includes members who represent nursing education, nursing service, medicine, allied health, hospital administration, state funding agencies, and the public-at-large. Their study is currently at midpoint and areas similar to those identified by the National Commission are being investigated.

To help carry out the CBNP's objectives, three task forces have been created to study certain problem areas of nursing education. The Task Force on Education will analyze curricula of the various levels of professional nursing programs in order to determine common curricular areas. This information will be gathered by conducting a survey on the behavioral objectives of each participating nursing program. The purpose of the Task Force on Utilization is to determine if the graduates of the various registered nurse programs are utilized on the basis of their educational preparation. The data will be collected from a survey which will include approximately sixty-five hospitals. The Task Force on Continuing Education, as the name suggests, will develop a statewide continuing education plan for nurses. This will be accomplished by participating in continuing education planning of major nursing programs and surveying all continuing education courses and processes now in use.

Membership on these task forces includes persons from hospital councils, nursing program faculty, educational institutions, state agencies and others who can make worthwhile contributions to the study. The three surveys have been initiated and the final task force reports will be available in July, 1974.

In mid-1972, the Texas Joint Practice Commission, previously the TNA-TMA Liaison Committee (in existence since 1964), was officially established to study the congruent roles between medicine and nursing. The membership of the commission includes nine physician practitioners, seven nurse practitioners (as well as two alternate persons from each profession), and the presidents of the two parent organizations who serve as ex-officio members. The criterion used by TMA and TNA in appointing the commission members was that the nurses and physicians, in addition to having an interest in serving on the committee, must spend at least fifty percent of their time in clinical practice.

Statewide conferences for nurses and physicians across the state of Texas have been held both prior to and after the establishment of the TJPC. Most of the conference participants have been nurses; very little representation was evident from other professions or from rural communities. Therefore, a decision was made to discontinue the statewide conferences and, in turn, to create a Speaker's Bureau so that members could help explain the SJPC goals to an increasing number of individuals in local communities.

Although it is a relatively young group, the commission has, thus far, been able to formulate its objectives, after intensive discussions on problems in medicine and nursing within their state. Plans are currently being made to implement those objectives. In addition, the TJPC is in the process of informing districts and medical societies about their existence and requesting assistance from local groups.

WYOMING

SMPC: Operational *SJPC: Operational*

In May, 1970, the Wyoming Commission for Nursing and Nursing Education (WCNNE) was formed through the cooperative efforts of the Wyoming League for Nursing, the Wyoming State Board of Nursing, and the Wyoming Nurses' Association. An autonomous body, the WCNNE is neither attached to nor sponsored by any organization. Their purpose is to bring together the people most concerned with future nursing needs in Wyoming so that discussion, planning, and implementation may take place.

WCNNE includes approximately forty members with representatives from some seventeen organizations, including: various nursing organizations; the State Hospital Association; the State Medical Society; the State Health Department; the Regional Medical Program; the State Nursing Home Association; and all levels of nursing education in the state.

The commission is in the process of becoming incorporated in order to receive funds from any available source so that implementation of its recommendations can be accomplished.

WCNNE has created several committees to carry out its work. The Executive Committee, which handles administrative duties, originally was composed of the three elected officers and two additional members. However, it was later found necessary to increase the membership to nine persons. The Committee for Consumer Representation, appointed by the commission's chairman, exists to recommend to the commission the names of individuals and/or consumer organizations to serve on the WCNNE. The Committee for Mobility in Nursing was appointed in September, 1971, to: encourage the concepts of career and educational mobility; become familiar with the objectives of the various nursing programs; establish a framework for communications among the various levels of nursing education offered in Wyoming; and to establish a mechanism for working with, and sharing information among, various institutions. The Publicity Committee has been involved with publication of the information brochure entitled "National Commission for the Study of Nursing and Nursing Education and You," which was designed specifically for Wyoming. This pamphlet briefly describes the National Commission and Wyoming's efforts to implement some of the NCSNNE recommendations. These pamphlets have been widely distributed to various groups throughout the state.

Because the concerns of WCNNE are quite broad, covering areas wider in scope than most state master planning committees, they are considering enlarging their task force committee and charging it specifically with SMPC functions so that the commission will have the freedom to work on, and assist with, all areas of implementation.

In 1970, a committee (later to become the task force committee), was appointed to determine whether there was a need for establishing several new practical nursing programs in the state. This committee gathered much information and concluded that a detailed study of nursing needs and resources must be conducted in Wyoming. The original committee then expanded to become a task force to identify possible funding sources for the survey. The Regional Medical Programs (Colorado-Wyoming and Mountain States) provided assistance and, by the end of 1972, the study on nursing needs and resources in Wyoming was completed.

The study was designed to be updated annually and used as a basis to determine Wyoming's needs for all types of nursing personnel. A preliminary report will be available later in 1973. It is this task force which will likely become responsible for planning for nursing education in the state by examining nursing educational patterns, needs and resources, career patterns, and by proposing a plan for change.

Wyoming officially established its joint practice committee in mid-1972, to discuss and make recommendations concerning the congruent roles of the nurse and physician in providing quality health care, with attention to the use of skills in other professions long assumed to be the sole concern of the physician and/or the nurse.

The joint practice committee evolved from another committee established in January, 1971, to study Manpower and Better Utilization. The SJPC membership now includes four physicians, eight registered nurses, two licensed practical nurses, and one hospital administrator.

To date, the joint practice committee has created five subcommittees to: explore funding sources; formulate a statement on Emergency Room Care; formulate a statement on Home Health Care; explore the possibility of compiling a list of non-nursing functions; examine the idea of increasing their membership to broaden representation. This committee has also, in collaboration with other health related groups, prepared a bill for "Medical Support Personnel" which is presently being introduced in the Wyoming State Legislature. In addition, the SJPC has drafted a joint position statement on the role of the registered nurse in the hospital emergency room. Currently, the group has begun work on developing guidelines for home health care, reviewing non-nursing functions being performed by nursing personnel, and studying the roles of the physician assistant and the nurse practitioner.

Section II Non-Target States and the District of Columbia

ALABAMA

SMPC: In Process *SJPC: Unorganized*

The members of the Alabama Commission on Nursing, appointed by the Alabama State Nurses' Association, represent the various state nursing organizations and the five levels of nursing education programs in the state. By broadening its membership, it could become a SMPC according to the guidelines proposed by the NCSNNE and adopted by most other states.

There is no SJPC in the state. The Alabama Hospital-Medical Council deals with concerns between medicine and nursing in Alabama.

ALASKA

SMPC: Unorganized *SJPC: Operational*

The Alaska State Nurses' Association indicates no knowledge of any committee responsible for the planning of nursing education, resources, and related concerns in the state. However, nursing education in the state is extremely limited.

There are three nursing programs in Alaska, all located in Anchorage: one LPN, one Associate Degree, and one Baccalaureate program. The directors of the three programs and Dr. Virginia Barham, a NCSNNE regional associate, conceived the idea of holding a multidisciplinary statewide conference, in the Fall of 1972, to examine the potential for extending the contribution of nursing in the delivery of health care, and begin to improve the status and utilization of nurses in the health care system.

The Anchorage Higher Education Consortium (an agreement between Alaska Methodist University and the state schools in the area) has been involved with planning for interdisciplinary continuing education in the health professions. This consortium might be the logical beginning step in the organization of a state master planning committee in Alaska.

A joint practice commission between the ASNA and the AMS has been formed.

ARIZONA

SMPC: Operational *SJPC: Operational*

In late 1970, the Arizona Board of Nursing and the Arizona State Nurses' Association began discussing implementation of the NCSNNE report. At that time, a multidisciplinary steering committee was appointed with persons representing the state department of public health, varying levels and types of education, medicine, osteopathy, nursing, hospital administration and consumers. In October, 1971, the steering committee submitted to HEW a project proposal for "Establishing and Implementing a Master Plan for Nursing in Arizona" and, at about the same time, became incorporated as the "Council for Nursing in Arizona." This council is officially recognized by the Arizona Health Planning Authority as the organization to provide necessary information concerning nursing for the development of the Arizona Plan for Health Services. It is considered the state master planning committee for nursing in Arizona.

The proposal previously submitted to HEW has not been funded; the council is presently studying the document for the purpose of rewriting and resubmission. In addition, the group is examining alternative approaches to funding.

Arizona has had an operational state joint practice committee since October, 1972. Three persons each, representing the Arizona Medical Association, the Arizona Nurses' Association, and the Arizona Osteopathic Physicians Association, comprise the nine-member group. Topics for discussion by the committee thus far have been the Arizona Plan for Health Care, the new definition of professional nursing passed by the 1972 legislature, and anticipated legislation affecting health and health workers in the state.

ARKANSAS

SMPC: Operational *SJPC: In Process*

Arkansas has recently completed a study of the state's nursing needs and resources, supported by a Division of Nursing study grant. The final report has been written and will soon be ready for distribution, while a brief listing of the recommendations has already had wide circulation.

A twenty-eight-member multidisciplinary committee has been formed to implement the recommendations of the recently completed study in Arkansas. This committee, spearheaded by the state league and nurses' association, drew some members from an interdisciplinary advisory committee originally appointed to review the study results and plan for implementation. Members include consumers, health administrators, higher education specialists, nurse practitioners and educators, and physicians.

Arkansas has a liaison committee between medicine and nursing. The formation of a SJPC will be brought before the House of Delegates of the AMS for a vote in April, 1973.

COLORADO

SMPC: In Process *SJPC: Operational*

A Colorado Planning Committee for Nursing Education, in existence since 1967, has eleven members—all of whom are nurses, to the best of our knowledge.

That committee advises the state's Commission on Higher Education on matters concerning the opening of new nursing education programs. This committee has also implemented a certification program, appointed a Career Ladder Advisory Committee, and its continuing education subcommittee is working with the Commission on Higher Education to develop statewide continuing education activities for nurses.

A twelve-member joint practice committee between medicine and nursing exists with eight members representing nursing and four representing medicine.

CONNECTICUT

SMPC: Operational *SJPC: Operational*

In 1971, an ad hoc committee, representing the various professional disciplines in Connecticut, requested that the Governor establish a task force to plan for nursing in Connecticut. Subsequently, that ad hoc committee was broadened to include a truly multidisciplinary representation. It has received official sanction to act as a task force to the state's Commission on Higher Education for the purpose of *advising* that commission in their planning for nursing education in Connecticut. The task force has prepared a statement of policy on nursing education for Connecticut which, when approved, will go to the Commission on Higher Education for action.

Connecticut has had an operational joint practice committee since the fall of 1972. It is made up of the six nurse and eight physician members who sit on the liaison committee for medicine, nursing, and allied health groups. The group has encountered problems in communications and organization. Its continuation depends largely on whether or not the physician representation on the committee wishes to take up substantive matters on joint practice. The SJPC is operational, but it hasn't accomplished anything of note. The CNA remains enthusiastic about the committee, but the CSMS appears to have some real reservations.

DELAWARE

SMPC: Operational *SJPC: In Process*

The Delaware Comprehensive Health Planning Council has recently spent 1-1/2 years studying the resources and needs of the health disciplines and has published a two-volume report which includes a model for health care delivery in the state; priorities and programs have been determined for the next three years. The first volume was sent to the Governor in 1972; the second will be transmitted later in 1973. Nursing has been an active component in the study, and an eighty-member nursing task force helped determine the proposed state plans.

There is no JPC in Delaware. The DSNA proposed the establishment of such a committee to the DSMS, but the latter declined to participate. The medical society prefers to continue the liaison committee arrangement with nursing which already exists. The DSNA is, however, continuing to seek a joint committee conforming to the NJPC guidelines and they have received indications that a number of physicians are now interested in fostering such a group.

DISTRICT OF COLUMBIA

SMPC: Unorganized *SJPC: Unorganized*

There is no designated or existing group, at present, to deal with concerns for nursing education and resources in the District of Columbia. A Council on Education (provisional) is to be appointed shortly, and it is hoped that this can lead to a permanent planning body. Vigorous development of policy and program in continuing education has taken place, however.

The medical and nurse associations had a liaison committee at one time, but it no longer exists. When discussion must take place between the two organizations, an ad hoc committee is established for the specific purpose at hand. The immediate past president of the DCNA is a nurse representative on the medical society's Committee on Allied Health. The nurse association plans to pursue the establishment of a District of Columbia Joint Practice Commission.

FLORIDA

SMPC: In Process *SJPC: Operational*

In June, 1971, a statewide informational meeting on the NCSNNE report and recommendations was held, sponsored by the State Board of Nursing, the Florida Nurses' Association, and the State League for Nursing. Other health professionals were in attendance and legislators, educators, consumers, and allied health personnel were invited. Thereafter, the nursing organization expected the Governor to appoint a SMPC but no action has yet been taken on that request. At present, a subcommittee of the State Comprehensive Health Planning Council is working with FNA and State Board of Nursing representatives to locate funds to conduct a study of nursing education in Florida. They hope that action will begin by the summer.

In late 1972, the Committee on Nursing of the Florida Medical Association and the Medical Liaison Committee of the FNA held a joint meeting, decided to become a SJPC, and formed an ad hoc group to draft a list of objectives. At their February, 1973 meeting, the Joint Practice Committee of Medicine and Nursing met and heard the ad hoc group's proposed objectives. At this point, the committee has identified their objectives and is considering criteria for Joint Position Statements on Practice.

HAWAII

SMPC: In Process *SJPC: Operational*

An ad hoc committee to establish and coordinate progress in state master planning and state joint practice did exist but has disbanded since it completed its work. The University of Hawaii Council on Nursing Education, established in late 1971, is responsible for the continued planning of nursing education, resources, and related concerns in the state.

A state joint practice committee has been established between medicine and nursing with four nurse members and three physician members being initially designated to serve.

IDAHO

SMPC: Operational *SJPC: Operational*

Idaho's forty-member interdisciplinary Commission on Nursing and Nursing Education has completed and submitted to the Idaho Board of Education, a master plan for nursing education which includes both findings and recommendations. One recommendation was that a consortium of schools of nursing be organized and functional by September, 1973. That consortium is now active and the master plan has been approved by the Board of Education.

A joint practice committee between medicine and nursing has been reactivated. Idaho also possesses an extremely active liaison committee comprised of the executive boards of the state hospital, medical, and nurse associations. Their cooperative efforts have influenced legislation, arranged for joint continuing education efforts, and the projection of future activities.

INDIANA

SMPC: In Process *SJPC: Operational*

Indiana has no multidisciplinary state master planning committee; however, a task force of the state nurse association's Council on Education submits recommendations on nursing education to the Health Careers Education Advisory Subcommittee of the state's Commission on Higher Education, for inclusion in statewide planning for all post secondary education. If representation is broadened, this task force could constitute an ideal state master planning committee.

In November, 1970, a broad-based committee composed of representatives from the state organizations of medicine, dentistry, hospitals, practical nursing, and registered nursing was established to deal with examining roles and functions of medicine and nursing and identifying health care needs in Indiana. A lack of adequate staffing (and possibly the structural size of the committee) has delayed progress, but plans are underway to review the organization and objectives to determine how it might function more effectively.

IOWA

SMPC: In Process *SJPC: In Process*

In 1971, the combined nursing education committees of the state nurse association and citizens league met to discuss a state planning commission. Late in that year, the Iowa Board of Nursing submitted a proposal to the Governor that would establish a multidisciplinary state commission to study nursing in Iowa, funded by the Board of Nursing. In 1972, the Governor approved establishment of such a commission, to include fifteen members who would be charged with studying, projecting, and making recommendations for the direction of nursing practice, education and continuing education.

For many years, the state's medical and nursing associations have maintained liaison through various committees and joint efforts on the Iowa Health Council. In June, 1972, a special committee of the Medical Society (Committee on Delegation of Authority) met with representatives of the INA and Board of Nursing to discuss the broad subject of delegation of authority by physicians to nurses and others, as well as other matters of mutual interest and concern. This group has continued to meet on a regular basis.

KENTUCKY

SMPC: Unorganized *SJPC: Unorganized*

There is no single coordinated group dealing with concerns about state master planning and joint practice in Kentucky; there are, however, a number of diverse groups grappling with such concerns. The Kentucky Hospital Association has an active multidisciplinary committee charged with making recommendations to its board of trustees for implementing *An Abstract for Action.* That association has worked with nurses at the state and district levels to address mutual concerns. The Nursing Education Committee of the Kentucky Nurses' Association also has been involved in related activities. That association, along with the State Board of Nursing, co-sponsored a multidisciplinary meeting to discuss the implementation of *An Abstract for Action* for Kentucky in 1971.

A liaison committee between the executive committees of the state nurses' association and the state medical society does exist in Kentucky.

LOUISIANA

SMPC: In Process *SJPC: In Process*

There is an active ad hoc committee in Louisiana seeking to establish a task force on nursing to coordinate progress in state master planning and joint practice. In 1971, that organization began efforts to organize a meeting of interested organizations and agencies to mobilize support for the concept of multidisciplinary statewide planning. An Executive Order creating a Committee on Statewide Planning for Nursing has been in the Governor's office since December, 1972. The LSNA is not encouraged about the prospect for it being signed.

Louisiana has a liaison committee between medicine and nursing which is not very practice-oriented. The nurses would like to see the committee change direction or be replaced by a SJPC but the physicians have thus far not agreed to their suggestions.

MARYLAND

SMPC: In Process *SJPC: Operational*

The Maryland Commission for Nursing, a thirty-eight-member, multidisciplinary group, has held one meeting and plans to continue as a preliminary planning group if the grant proposal for statewide planning, submitted in October 1, 1972, to HEW, is not funded. If and when the project is funded, this group would make an assessment as to the composition that would be required. They might continue as they are presently constituted or assist in designating a new committee.

Maryland has a twelve-member committee on joint practice between medicine and nursing. The president of the Maryland LPNA is also a member of this committee.

MASSACHUSETTS

SMPC: In Process *SJPC: Operational*

At present, there is an eight-member ad hoc nursing group attempting to get master planning off the ground in Massachusetts. The group, which is limited to MNA members, is planning to broaden representation by including nurse members from the state board of nursing, the LPN association, and the Weston Assembly, an active group of deans, department heads and chairmen of LPN and all basic nursing programs in the state.

The Massachusetts Board of Higher Education has developed a proposal and will most likely function as the planning agency for the public (and eventually the private) sector of education, including nursing and health education in general. They have established a nursing steering committee to the Board of Health Educational Advisory Committee in Health Affairs Education. The chairman of the ad hoc nursing group is the only nonpublicly employed nurse on that committee. Hopefully, a multidisciplinary group will evolve which will be designated to plan for all nursing education in the state.

A sixteen-member JPC exists in Massachusetts with eight representatives each from medicine and nursing.

MICHIGAN

SMPC: In Process *SJPC: Operational*

A steering committee, including representation from the state nurses' association, state league for nursing, state board of nursing, and state association of LPNs, is seeking to establish and coordinate progress in state master planning in Michigan.

A State Plan for Nursing Education was developed under the aegis of the CHPC of the State Board of Education but has not been acted upon, as yet, by either group. The steering committee is concerned with this lack of action and, along with evaluating the plan and changes which have occurred since its development (1969-1970), the committee is evaluating the effect of federal budget reduction for nursing education, utilization of revenue sharing funds for health and health education, and other movements which affect planning for nursing education today. They will then again contact the State Board of Education to see what their intentions are concerning the master plan.

Michigan's eighteen-member JPC is composed of representatives from medicine, nursing, osteopathy, and pharmacy. They have been meeting bimonthly and are presently: defining objectives and examples of joint practice; and discussing problems of joint decision making related to practice. Efforts are being directed at enhancing interdisciplinary educational opportunities, particularly at the preparatory level of medicine and nursing.

MINNESOTA

SMPC: Operational *SJPC: In Process*

The Minnesota Higher Education Coordinating Commission (MHECC) began, in late 1972, a study to develop a comprehensive statewide plan for nursing education in their state. The commission was appointed by the governor and the establishment of this study is a major development for nursing education in Minnesota. The state nursing organizations had been trying for a number of years to establish such a formal link with the state agency responsible for the coordination of higher education. MHECC has appointed an advisory committee composed of nurse educators, employers, practitioners, students, and representatives from medicine. Staff members from government agencies and professional organizations also serve as consultants to the advisory committee.

A steering committee of MNA (Council on Nursing Practice) and MSMA (Committee on Nursing) members is being established to develop guidelines for a SJPC. Presently, concerns between the two professions are being dealt with by the MSMA committee which has nurse representatives.

MISSISSIPPI

SMPC: Operational *SJPC: Operational*

The Board of Trustees of Institutions of Higher Learning in Mississippi has a Nursing Education *Advisory* Committee which is multidisciplinary, fulfilling the function of a SMPC in Mississippi.

Mississippi has an eleven-member JPC (six nurses and five physicians) between medicine and nursing designated as such in January, 1972.

MISSOURI

SMPC: In Process *SJPC: Unorganized*

A statewide informational meeting on nursing and nursing education was held in September, 1972. The multidisciplinary steering committee which planned the meeting was charged to select from its membership the nucleus of a committee that would undertake planning for nursing education in Missouri. This group was subsequently formed with representation from the major state nursing organizations (including LPNs and students), the state hospital and osteopathic associations, and the three types of basic nursing education programs. Twelve persons comprise this committee which is named the Missouri State Committee on Nursing and Nursing Education. Their first meeting was held in January, 1973 and their purpose, objectives, and functions will soon be formalized, at which time they will seek endorsement of health organizations throughout the state and then seek authority as a master planning committee. Committee representation will have to be broadened to include representatives from across the state and from other disciplines.

One of the major objectives of the Missouri Commission on Nursing and Nursing Education will be to push for the development of a SJPC. At present, liaison between the state medical and nursing associations in Missouri consists of an advisory committee to the medical society's Ad Hoc Committee on Health Manpower and Nursing is only one group represented on that body.

MONTANA

SMPC: Operational *SJPC: In Process*

The Montana State Commission on Nursing and Nursing Education, a twenty-three-member multidisciplinary group, has as one of its purposes to carry out studies of needs and resources and then to formulate definite plans for nursing and nursing education in their state. They plan to use the HEW statement on the expanded role of the nurse to identify, assess, and analyze the utility of these roles for planning continuing education programs for nurse practitioners to meet their needs. They have established five subcommittees and hope to develop and submit a grant to a private foundation for funding; the greatest need is for full-time assistance to continue their work.

A liaison committee exists between the state medical and nursing associations but it has been relatively ineffective. The nurses' association feels that it has had little or no support from the medical association and has been unable to persuade medicine that some joint planning between the professions is needed for improved health care in their state. The nurses' association, however, plans to continue its efforts. In addition, the MSCNNE has decided to work for the establishment of a SJPC through the medical and nursing associations to assist in preparing nurses for expanded roles.

NEBRASKA

SMPC: Operational *SJPC: Unorganized*

The State Comprehensive Health Planning Agency in Nebraska has identified nursing needs and resources in their state and formulated a number of recommendations regarding nursing and nursing education. The group is necessarily a multidisciplinary one.

A JPC in Nebraska is nonexistent. When there is a need for discussion between the state medical and nursing associations, the NNA Council on Practice and the NSMA Allied Health Committee establish an ad hoc group for that purpose. We have no indication that any effort is being made to establish a standing group for interdisciplinary planning.

NEVADA

SMPC: In Process *SJPC: In Process*

The NNA currently has plans underway to establish a SMPC in Nevada. In August, 1972, a conference was held and selected nurses from the state attended.

At that time, NCSNNE recommendations were reviewed, their implications for Nevada discussed, and attention given to where nursing is in Nevada now and where it should be going.

At present, three physicians have been appointed to work with the NNA Committee on Practice. In addition, an ad hoc group from NNA is studying the possibility of establishing a SJPC. They have initiated contact with the NSMA for that purpose.

NEW HAMPSHIRE

SMPC: In Process *SJPC: In Process*

In April, 1971, the NHNA submitted a tentative guideline for planning nursing education in their state to Governor Peterson and requested him to appoint an interdisciplinary SMPC for nursing education. Thereafter, the Governor directed the Office of Comprehensive Health Planning and the NHNA to work together to develop a SMPC for nursing education. In October, 1972, a statewide informational meeting was held at which time the consensus was to establish a SMPC, under the aegis of the CHP office. Steps are now being taken to constitute such a group from the membership of the multidisciplinary steering committee that planned the conference.

There has existed a liaison committee between the NHNA, NHHA and NHMS for some time, but we are told that it is a committee in name only. Representatives from the NHNA and the NHMS are meeting in the spring and the nurses' association is hopeful that this meeting will provide a beginning for joint practice in the state.

NEW JERSEY

SMPC: Operational *SJPC: Operational*

The State of New Jersey Department of Higher Education's Office of Health Professions Education has a nineteen-member multidisciplinary advisory council that is charged with providing an effective advisory mechanism for coordinating policy, program approvals, and evaluation in the health professions.

The final revised draft of the *Health Professions Education Master Plan* was released in December, 1972. This plan is part of the New Jersey Master Plan for Higher Education and includes nursing as one of its major components.

New Jersey's thirteen-member SJPC organized by the state medical and nursing associations meets on a monthly basis. Their attention to date has been focused on: the general objectives as set down by the NJPC; the need for changing the state's nurse practice act; taking a stand regarding institutional licensure; and the expanded role of the nurse, as well as other topics regarding practice.

NEW MEXICO

SMPC: In Process *SJPC: In Process*

There is presently no multidisciplinary group to deal with concerns of nursing education and resources in New Mexico, but plans for such a group are being discussed by several organizations. A study of nursing needs in New Mexico has been completed and published; one of the recommendations is that an overall committee be established to deal with statewide planning for nursing education. The Career Ladder Project has been funded until August, 1973, to create a statewide plan for career mobility in nursing. In addition, there is an Interagency Council on Education which includes universities as members and all the technical schools in the state as associates. Consideration is being given to the possibility of involving this group in state master planning for nursing education.

A liaison commitee exists between the NMMS, the NMNA, and voluntary health agencies in the state. The concept of a SJPC has been approved by the state medical society House of Delegates and the SMA Board of Directors. The NMNA has appointed the six nurse members and the NMMS is now in the process of selecting their representatives.

NEW YORK

SMPC: Operational *SJPC: Unorganized*

In New York, the State Board of Regents is legally responsible for preparing, every four years, a statewide plan for all higher and professional education.

In 1972, the State Education Department, the administrative arm of the Regents, submitted a proposal to the Division of Nursing (NIH) entitled "Developing a Statewide System for Continuous Regional Planning for Nursing Education." The project, now being reviewed by the division, focuses on the problem: How can NYS plan for the orderly development of nursing education, with respect to quantity and quality to ensure that the nursing needs in the state can be met through 1985? The purpose of the project is to develop for NYS, a statewide, long-range, regionally based plan for the development of nursing education. Hopefully, the resultant plan will be incorporated into the Regents statewide plan, and represent ongoing planning activity.

In each of the eight designated regions, a multidisciplinary community planning group will assume the initiative for regional planning. These plans will be integrated into a statewide plan, after having been reviewed by a Statewide Advisory Council and a Health Professions Advisory Panel.

The NYSNA and MSSNY (state nurses' and medical associations) have two avenues of communication: 1) at the executive level, the organization presidents, chief executive officers and other designees, meet; 2) NYSNA's Committee on Medicine and Para-Medical Personnel and MSSNY's Committee on Nursing and Allied Health provide a liaison between the two professional organizations.

There is no state joint practice committee organized in New York. However, there is a joint practice committee organized on the regional level and at least two other local areas are considering establishing such committees.

NORTH DAKOTA

SMPC: Operational *SJPC: In Process*

The twenty-seven-member multidisciplinary Joint Committee on Needs and Resources acts in an advisory capacity to the state's Board of Higher Education. This committee, initiated in 1967, completed a report on the status of nursing education in North Dakota with the assistance of the Upper Midwest Study.

There does exist a sixteen-member Joint Committee on Professional Nursing Practice between the state nurse, medical, and hospital associations. The Board of Directors of the North Dakota State Nurses' Association, in early 1973, called for an investigation of the possibilities of expanding the purposes of the joint committee to meet the requirements of the NJPC. They hope to meet with the joint committee in the Spring of 1973.

OHIO

SMPC: Operational *SJPC: Unorganized*

The Ohio Committee for Nursing and Nursing Education was organized in late 1970 to plan for the implementation effort in Ohio. Consisting of a broad representation of the state's nurses, the group's function is to initiate and provide for the ongoing coordination and evaluation of the National Commission's recommendations and to provide for the continued coordination and evaluation of implementation.

The Governor's office has recommended the appointment of a Nursing Task Force, under the aegis of the Ohio Department of Health and its Office of Comprehensive Health Planning, to carry out a study of nursing needs and resources in the state. This Nursing Task Force will include representatives from voluntary health organizations, private industry, professional organizations, and consumers of health services. Part of this study group's objectives is to develop a master plan for nursing education in Ohio for a ten-year period. The task force members are to be appointed in the Spring of 1973.

Ohio's liaison committee between medicine and nursing is presently inactive.

OKLAHOMA

SMPC: In Process *SJPC: Unorganized*

Some time ago, the very active Oklahoma Board of Nursing requested the Governor to consider establishing a SMPC for nursing and nursing education. Consideration was given by the Governor and his staff members to the development of a nursing commission under the aegis of Comprehensive Health Planning, but representatives of the Regents for Higher Education indicated that their single concern is with the area of education and do not wish to become involved with practice and the delivery of health care.

On December 7, 1972, the State Health Planning Council adopted a State Plan for Nursing Education, identified by the Board of Nurse Registration and Nurse Education and submitted to the State Health Planning Council for adoption. The Board of Nursing has called for an organized planning effort and recognizes this state plan as the focus for statewide planning for nursing in Oklahoma.

There does exist a liaison committee between medicine and nursing in Oklahoma, but it has been rather inactive over the past few years.

OREGON

SMPC: In Process *SJPC: Operational*

The Oregon Commission on Nursing, a multidisciplinary group, was established through the initiative of the Oregon League for Nursing. To our knowledge, that commission has been neither very active nor successful, making little headway in evaluating and planning for nursing education in the state. The Oregon Nurses' Association through their Committee on Nursing Education is planning to form a master planning committee but, at least initially, without representation from groups other than the ONA.

Oregon's JPC has six representatives each from the state medical and nurse associations. The purposes of the committee are to maintain liaison with the NJPC; to assure orderly, ongoing communication; to plan both current clinical practices and procedures and new methods of providing patient care; to discuss relationships with new categories of health care personnel; and to deal with other areas of mutual concern.

RHODE ISLAND

SMPC: Operational *SJPC: Operational*

Rhode Island's thirty-eight-member, multidisciplinary Committee on Nursing completed Phase I of their report in 1972. It has been submitted to the Board of Regents. The report reviews nurse manpower resources, current and projected needs, and the educational programs required to meet those needs. The committee is presently developing a plan for Phase II of the study. This will include the experimental study of nursing practice patterns in at least two hospitals in order to demonstrate and encourage altered approaches to nursing service.

The eighteen-member SJPC in Rhode Island evolved from the liaison committee between the state nurse and medical associations. The committee has increased its membership to include nurse as well as physician practitioners. The group meets monthly and plans to discuss the laws governing each of the two professions. In addition, they are planning to schedule a meeting of the membership of each profession with an NJPC member as speaker.

SOUTH CAROLINA

SMPC: Operational *SJPC: Operational*

South Carolina's nineteen-member SMPC is multidisciplinary with both student and consumer, as well as legislative, representation included along with that from the professions.

The SJPC between medicine and nursing has fourteen members, seven each from medicine and nursing. This group has endorsed nurse midwifery for South Carolina and is continuing to explore the congruent roles of nurses and physicians.

The members of the SMPC and the SJPC have met together one time for the purpose of exchanging information. South Carolina Nurses' Association has assisted in the coordination of the two planning groups.

SOUTH DAKOTA

SMPC: In Process *SJPC: Operational*

No single committee, at present, is responsible for the planning of nursing education, resources, and concerns in South Dakota, but there have been attempts to establish such a committee and there are now plans underway to do so again.

The Core Curriculum Project, charged by the State Health Department, RMP/CHP, to develop a core curriculum for the sixty-two health programs in the state has a subcommittee of practicing nurses and nurse educators. The director of the project plans to suggest to the members of the subcommittee that they consider spearheading the development of a multidisciplinary, independent, SMPC. CHP is presently updating the data on South Dakota's nursing needs and resources and the SMPC could begin working with that revised data to develop a nursing education plan for the state.

South Dakota has had a JPC between medicine and nursing since late 1972.

TENNESSEE

SMPC: Operational *SJPC: In Process*

The Tennessee Higher Education Commission has a legislative mandate to conduct statewide planning for all higher education, including the professions, in Tennessee. Their Nursing Advisory Committee has presented recommendations to the Tennessee Higher Education Commission in relation to the master plan for nursing education in the state. This advisory committee anticipates developing a more formal organization in the near future. Presently, the Tennessee Higher Education Commission staff is revising the 1969 nursing study and plans to continually update the data.

The state nurse and medical associations have a fourteen-member liaison committee. Discussion is presently underway between the two professional organizations regarding a joint statement on nursing practitioners (clinicians) and the establishment of a SJPC.

UTAH

SMPC: Operational *SJPC: In Process*

The Board of Higher Education in Utah is responsible for the overall education planning in the state. The Administrators' Conference Group, composed of nurses, acts in an advisory capacity to the Board of Higher Education. In late 1971, this advisory group submitted a master plan for nursing education to the Board of Higher Education Committee for their consideration.

There is a liaison committee between the state nurse and medical associations in Utah. The nurse members view the committee as a SJPC—their ten members are practitioners and represent the nursing areas of surgery, community health, obstetrics, pediatrics, medicine, geriatrics, emergency room care service and operating room service. The state medical association sees the committee as a traditional liaison group and has yet to accept fully the changing concept of joint practice.

VERMONT

SMPC: Unorganized *SJPC: In Process*

There is presently no designated or existing multidisciplinary group to deal with concerns of nursing education and resources in Vermont. The VSNA is attempting to coordinate activities in these areas and there is a movement within the state nurses' association to form a multidisciplinary council on continuing education.

The executive committee of the VSNA has met with the executive committee of the VMS in an attempt to establish a SJPC in Vermont. Two resolutions have been sent to the board of each organization: 1) to establish a task force which would be a SJPC between medicine and nursing; 2) to appoint a liaison from each organization to the other.

VIRGINIA

SMPC: In Process *SJPC: In Process*

The Committee on Education for Health Professions and Occupations of the State Council of Higher Education in Virginia is planning the development of health education programs throughout the state. The executive secretary of the State Board of Nursing is a member of the committee and chairs the Task Force on Nursing and Nursing Education which will act in an advisory capacity to the above named committee.

There is a liaison committee between the state nurse and medical associations in Virginia and efforts are being made to establish a SJPC. The medical society, however, tabled action on SJPC formation in 1972, and its board of directors took no further action in January, 1973. The Liaison Council to Organized Nursing of the Medical Society of Virginia is recommending to the Medical Society Council that the current liaison committee be dissolved and a SJPC formed in its place.

WASHINGTON

SMPC: In Process *SJPC: Operational*

There exists a very active Ad Hoc Committee for Statewide Master Planning in Nursing Education in this state. The committee is sponsored by the State Nurse Planning Council (a multidisciplinary committee), the State Board of Nursing, and the State Nurses' Association. They have considered expanding or altering the Nurse Planning Council to become a SMPC, funding for such a committee, and preparing a projected proposal to submit to HEW. Plans for integrating with the Council on Higher Education in early June, 1973, are being finalized.

Washington has a six-member SJPC, with three representatives each from medicine and nursing.

WEST VIRGINIA

SMPC: Operational *SJPC: Unorganized*

The West Virginia Planning Commission for Nursing has been organized since mid-1971 and is endeavoring to develop a statewide mechanism of planning for nursing. Funded by the state nurse associations and private donations, the commission is seeking long-term financing. A one-year federal planning grant was used to organize task forces in nursing service education and community nursing to develop the planning mechanism. The group is presently developing a proposal to submit to the Appalachian Regional Commission through the CHP group in West Virginia, for funding. The commission is expanding its membership and has already broadened the membership of the advisory committee to include representatives from CHP, the state student medical and nursing associations, the state nursing home, hospital and medical associations and the Appalachian Center Extension Services.

There is a liaison committee between medicine and nursing in West Virginia.

WISCONSIN

SMPC: Operational *SJPC: In Process*

The Commission on Statewide Planning for Nursing Education in Wisconsin published their needs and resources study in March, 1970, and submitted it to the State Board of Nursing. An advisory committee to the state board was appointed to implement that report. This twenty-four member committee is also multidisciplinary and plans to publish an updated report for nursing education in Wisconsin.

The Wisconsin Nurses' Association has appointed ten members as their representatives to a SJPC. However, the Wisconsin Medical Society designated one of their existing committees to meet with the nurse "ad hoc JPC." In essence, the nurses were then attending meetings of the state medical society's "Commission on Hospital Relations and Medical Education." At the meetings the physician contingent carried on their own commission business as well as the joint practice part of the agenda. The chairman of the physician committee agrees that the JPC shouldn't be part of another commission but the situation currently has not been corrected.

STATUS OF STATEWIDE COMMITTEE ORGANIZATION—APRIL 1, 1973

State	Master Planning Committee			Joint Practice Committee		
	Operational	In Process	Unorganized	Operational	In Process	Unorganized (none)
Alabama		X				X
Alaska			X	X		
Arizona	X			X		
Arkansas	X				X	
California		X		X		
Colorado		X		X		
Connecticut	X			X		
Delaware	X				X	
District of Columbia			X			X
Florida		X		X		
Georgia	X			X		
Hawaii		X		X		
Idaho	X			X		
Illinois	X			X		
Indiana		X		X		
Iowa		X			X	
Kansas	X			X		
Kentucky			X			X
Louisiana		X			X	
Maine		X		X		
Maryland		X		X		
Massachusetts		X		X		
Michigan		X		X		
Minnesota	X				X	
Mississippi	X			X		
Missouri		X				X
Montana	X				X	
Nebraska	X					X
Nevada		X			X	
New Hampshire		X			X	
New Jersey	X			X		
New Mexico		X			X	
New York	X					X

STATUS OF STATEWIDE COMMITTEE ORGANIZATION—APRIL 1, 1973 (*continued*)

State	Master Planning Committee			Joint Practice Committee		
	Opera-tional	In Process	Unorga-nized	Opera-tional	In Process	Unorga-nized (none)
North Carolina	X			X		
North Dakota	X				X	
Ohio	X					X
Oklahoma		X				X
Oregon		X		X		
Pennsylvania	X			X		
Rhode Island	X			X		
South Carolina	X			X		
South Dakota		X		X		
Tennessee	X				X	
Texas	X			X		
Utah	X				X	
Vermont			X		X	
Virginia		X			X	
Washington		X		X		
West Virginia	X					X
Wisconsin	X				X	
Wyoming	X			X		

Appendix D

A PLAN FOR THE LONGITUDINAL STUDY OF IMPACT ON HEALTH CARE EXERTED BY THE NATIONAL COMMISSION FOR THE STUDY OF NURSING AND NURSING EDUCATION

In its final report, *An Abstract for Action*, the National Commission for the Study of Nursing and Nursing Education proposed fifty-eight specific recommendations for the improvement of health care delivery through the reconstruction of American nursing—its roles and functions, educational patterns, and career enhancement. We are now in the third and final year of a planned implementation phase designed to initiate efforts toward the accomplishment of those recommendations. Recognizing that only a beginning can be expected within so short a time when society-wide change has been urged, the Commission is nevertheless committed to accomplishing as much as possible over the remaining months so that a foundation can be constructed and continuing building efforts assumed by significant others.

Because the concept of planned implementation is, in itself, somewhat unique, and because nursing has for a long time been grappling with many of the underlying problems identified in the Commission's report, it seems particularly appropriate that some measurements be taken over time of the impact of *An Abstract for Action.* To this end, at a meeting on October 6, 1972, the members of the Commission directed the staff to consider:

1. The reconvening of the Commission, together with its National Advisory Council composed of former commissioners at a suitable time three years after the conclusion of the implementation phase.

2. The development of hypotheses or standards of measurement for the assessment of long-term impact of the Commission's report and activities.

3. The separation, insofar as possible, of "outside" factors from the longitudinal analysis of Commission accomplishments.

The first item is, of course, the simplest. Because the Commission can anticipate some continuing royalties and income from its publications, ample funds should be afforded for the support of such a meeting. The director and former associate director have indicated their willingness to accept responsibility for planning that meeting and for contacting all present and past commissioners. The meeting would be scheduled for the fall of 1976 at a place and time of general convenience. Materials would be provided in advance, and the cooperation of such organizations as the American Nurses' Association and the National League for Nursing would be sought in the assemblage of relevant data and information.

The second and third considerations are closely intertwined. We fully recognize that a large number of our recommendations are based on general societal trends and felt needs. Many of our proposals would likely have been enacted even if the Commission had not existed. (Parenthetically, we would observe that change well might *not* have taken place so fast or so neatly, if the Commission had not provided structure and impetus.) For example, it seems clear that public support of nursing education will continue and increase because of population growth, health care requirements, and, hopefully, the end of wartime demands for budget priority. While our Commission's urging may influence the rate of increase, this will be only one of several forces at work—and one that is almost impossible to isolate and assess.

To provide a valid measure of impact, then, it is necessary to select a subset of the recommendations urged by the Commission—ones that are more unique, less likely to have occurred by natural social evolution, and perhaps, more controversial in terms of initial acceptance. By examining a limited set of "change variables" we can more nearly isolate them from contaging factors, and more fairly generalize the probable impact of the Commission's influence on the total movement within the health care system.

Based on this reasoning, the staff has made a preliminary survey of Commission recommendations and has developed a profile of recommendations in each of the three general areas of the final report: nursing practice, nursing education, and nursing careers. Within each of these fields, seven critical proposals have been selected and corresponding statements of expectation (or hypotheses) generated. These have been selected for their capacity to demonstrate:

1. Concomitant variation, and
2. Temporal relationship

Briefly, we have attempted to determine important issues which have: (a) clearly observable and measurable results; and (b) some causal relationship through clear before-after sequences of events. If we let the selected Commission recommendations, the assumed causal or independent variable, be represented by X_n, and the assumed effects, or dependent variables, to be represented by Y_n, then we should be able to determine that there is a concomitant variation between the two factors and that X_n preceded Y_n in time. While there can never be, in nonexperimental research, conclusive evidence that other factors did not intrude and did not affect variations, we should by analysis be able to determine whether, in fact, there was some major relationship or correlation between the recommendations and changes in nursing.

In the sections below, we propose the "critical profiles" for longitudinal study. From their observed outcomes, we might generate probabilistic statements about the overall impact of the Commission, its report, and its implementation activities.

Nursing Roles and Functions

The National Commission recommended seventeen specific proposals in the area of roles and functions. Many of these are couched in terms of expanded public and private support for research and demonstration projects, while others are clearly in line with present trends toward distinguishing non-nursing functions and assigning them to appropriate personnel.

There are, however, seven recommendations which have specific possible outcomes that fall in the category of desired concomitant variability and temporal relationship. For analytic purposes, these would be represented as follows:

XR_1 Federal funds be supplied through the ERIC program, or through the Division of Nursing, as well as private and state funds, to the American Nurses' Foundation so that it might become a national clearinghouse for the collection and dissemination of information about research and innovations in nursing.

YR_1 There will be, in 1976, an operational Clearinghouse on Nursing Research, maintained by a variety of funding agencies, and operated under the auspices of the American Nurses' Foundation.

XR_2 . . . private funds [should] allocate increased monies for applied research and demonstration grants that would examine new methods, procedures, settings, and personnel relationships for improved nursing practice.

YR_2 There will be, in 1976, a statistically significant increase both in the number of foundations making grants in support of nursing research related to practice and in the amounts of money being provided for that purpose.

XR_3 A National Joint Practice Commission be established between medicine and nursing to discuss and make recommendations concerning the congruent roles of the physician and the nurse in providing quality health care.

YR_3 There will be, in 1976, an operational National Joint Practice Commission jointly sponsored by the American Medical Association and the American Nurses' Association, this Commission to be actively engaged in carrying out the activities proposed by the NCSNNE.

XR_4 Counterpart joint practice committees be established in each state between medicine and nursing to consider the congruent roles of physicians and nurses.

YR_4 There will be, in 1976, joint practice committees in each state, involved in improving the delivery of health care through better nurse-physician practice patterns.

XR_5 Two essentially related but differing career patterns be developed for nursing practice—episodic and distributive.

YR_5 There will be, in 1976, a statistically significant shift in the allocation of nursing manpower with a major increase in the numbers and percentage of nurse practitioners functioning in the area of distributive care.

XR_6 Nursing career patterns should be so organized that recognition, reward and increased responsibility for practice are based on increasing depth of knowledge and demonstrated competence to perform in complex clinical situations.

YR_6 There will be, in 1976, a statistically significant upward shift in the proportion of time spent by nurses in all health care facilities in direct client contact and a statistically significant downward shift in the utilization of nurses for supervisory and administrative functions within all health care facilities.

XR_7 Nursing leadership work actively to bring education and service together in joint planning and decision making.

YR_7 There will be, in 1976, a statistically significant upward shift in the number of institutions offering joint appointments in education and service, and in the number of individual faculty members who are actively engaged in the practice of nursing in addition to teaching.

For each of the antecedent variables, we have baseline data on the level of activity or penetration as of the issuance of the National Commission report in 1970, as well as change information over the period of the implementation phase. This will permit us to measure change through the fall of 1976 by means of direct observational or statistical comparison. We know, for example, that fewer than six of the 100 largest private foundations in 1971 provided grants to support research into nursing practice. This has been an area in which the Commission has been active, both in providing general information to foundations and in exercising direct follow-up to interested foundations and researchers. Likewise, we know that, in

1971, approximately 89 percent of our full-time nurse practitioners were engaged in essentially episodic care as compared with approximately 11 percent engaged in health maintenance and disease prevention activities associated with distributive care. In the case of all seven selected recommendations, there is relative freedom from "contagion" by other independent variables prior to the issuance of *An Abstract for Action.*

Nursing Education

In this area, the National Commission proffered twenty-two recommendations, many of them consistent with the urgings of past nursing studies, and several of them congruent with strong social forces. For example, while the Commission and staff have worked zealously to ease the transition from hospital school to collegiate campus as the locus for nursing education, Altman has argued that the change is inevitable on the basis of economic determination alone. So, we can hardly claim credit for the outcome, though we may derive satisfaction from our efforts to make the operation as rational and nonabrasive as possible.

To arrive at some configuration by which we might assess the Commission's impact on nursing in this area, we have selected seven recommendations that seem to lie within our defined parameters. These may be stated in study form as follows:

XE_1 Each state have a master planning committee that will take nursing education under its purview.

YE_1 There will be, in 1976, a designated, interdisciplinary planning committee in each state charged with general responsibility for coordination of nursing education.

XE_2 Hospital schools of nursing move systematically and with dispatch to effect interinstitutional arrangements with collegiate institutions.

YE_2 There will be, in 1976, a significant increase in joint planning between hospital schools and colleges prior to the termination of diploma programs.

XE_3 Junior and senior collegiate institutions cooperatively develop programs and curricula.

YE_3 There will be, in 1976, a significant increase in the articulation between two- and four-year institutions with a statistically significant increase in the number of baccalaureate institutions which offer upper division programs in anticipation of enrolling graduates of ADN programs.

XE_4 Small programs be terminated or consolidated into larger programs in order to reduce the per unit cost of education and in order to make better allocation of qualified faculty.

YE_4 There will be, in 1976, a significant increase in the number of area or regional consortia for nursing education with shared facility, faculty, and resources.

XE_5 No less than three regional or interinstitutional committees be funded for the study and development of the nursing curriculum to develop educational objectives, universals, alternatives, and sequences for instruction.

YE_5 There will be, in 1976, no less than three completed regional or area studies of the nursing curriculum with proposals for universals or core studies, alternatives or specializations, and sequential approaches to articulation.

XE_6 These regional or interinstitutional committees should seek to specify appropriate levels of general and specialized learning for the different types of educational institutions.

YE_6 There will be, in 1976, a significant increase in the number of programs at *both* the two- and four- year institutions which offer a concentration in episodic or distributive care.

XE_7 The state master planning committee for nursing education identify one or more institutions to be responsible for regional coverage of continuing education programs for nurses.

YE_7 There will be, in 1976, a significant increase in the number of states that have designated agencies and master plans for the offering of continuing education for nurses and a significant increase in the number and percentage of nurses participating in continuing education activities.

For each of the selected antecedent variables, there is again sufficient baseline data to permit direct observational and statistical comparison. There is, to our knowledge, only one consortium for nursing education presently operating in the United States. There are a number of others at the proposal or developmental stage—most of them with direct communication to the Commission staff. This provides a clear instance for determining over time whether change is induced and the concomitant relationship between recommendation and response. We are just beginning to see the installation of episodic and distributive curricula in two- and four-year institutions and we can readily determine the extent of penetration of this recommendation over the coming months. Again, these examples illustrate the prescriptive selection of measures that avoid the contagion of general tendencies in the society at large that will affect nursing education, its institutions, and its patterns.

Nursing Careers

One of the major contentions of the National Commission is that there is not a shortage of nurses in the conventional sense—rather there is an obvious lack of retention coupled with a high degree of turnover which causes most of the manpower problems experienced. This can only be solved when the demand side of the manpower equation is addressed along with supply. To enhance the long-term perspectives of careers in nursing, and to improve related concerns of licensure and certification, the National Commission proposed nineteen recommendations for enactment. As in the case of the other two general areas, several of these are likely to be carried out even without further influence from the Commission; a number of them, however, are dependent upon the success of implementation efforts.

The staff proposes a profile of seven recommendations with their concomitant variables as the analytic basis for assessing the impact of the Commission in this area. Stated in study terms, these would be:

XC_1 Nurses be appointed to, and hold full membership in, groups involved in health manpower planning at all governmental and regional levels.

YC_1 There will be, in 1976, a statistically significant increase in the number of nurses involved in comprehensive and regional health planning and a significant increase in the percentage of such bodies having nurse members.

XC_2 Health management administrators and clinical directors of nursing service build on current improvements in starting salaries to create a strong reward system for remaining in clinical practice.

YC_2 There will be, in 1976, a statistically significant alteration in the organizational apportionment of nursing salaries with significant increases being provided to clinical nurses and master nurse clinicians in comparison with supervisory nurses.

XC_3 The professional health organizations, including those in nursing, take responsibility individually and collectively for interpreting the characteristics of contemporary nursing to the public.

YC_3 There will be, in 1976, a Congress or other interorganizational group of nursing associations that will plan and act collectively to present nursing's goals and functions to the public and to other health organizations.

XC_4 Institutions for nursing education develop career enhancement programs for licensed practical nurses.

YC_4 There will be, in 1976, a significant increase in the number of programs offering a combined LPN/RN program and a significant increase in the number of RN programs that offer special programs to meet the needs of LPNs wishing to become RNs.

XC_5 Institutions for nursing education provide more preparatory programs for liberal arts and science graduates seeking a professional career in nursing.

YC_5 There will be, in 1976, a significant increase in the number of institutions offering programs designed for the arts and science graduates and there will be a significant increase in the variety of forms such programs will take.

XC_6 All state licensure laws for nursing be revised to require periodic review of the individual's qualifications for practice as a condition for license renewal.

YC_6 There will be, in 1976, a significant number of states requiring, as a condition for renewal of the nursing license, evidence of continued learning, maintenance of clinical skills, and/or related professional capacity.

XC_7 Advanced levels of nursing practice should be recognized through designation by approved bodies for such purposes, presumably the Academy of Nursing.

YC_7 There will be, in 1976, through professional and interprofessional planning, a systematic process for determining and certifying advanced levels of clinical skill among nurse practitioners.

Again, there is sufficient information available on each of the antecedent variables for us to assess, over time, the direction and amount of change anticipated in the dependent statements. Through the assistance of other data gathering groups, including the research and statistics sections of ANA and NLN, we should be able to determine the economic and legal changes. Other information can be gathered by institutional and state surveys.

Commentary

While there is general evidence that most of the Commission's report and recommendations have struck a responsive chord among nurses, other health professionals, and the general public, as attested both by the number of supporting resolutions adopted, and the lack of violent controversy, there is still a great need to see that there is positive action as well as approval. Based on the historic precedents in nursing, this Commission undertook the added burden and responsibility of a three year implementation phase—over and above the initial three years of study. Even at this point in time, it is obvious that many of the recommendations are well on the way to acceptance. All the more reason, then, to attempt the assessment of overall effectiveness in terms of longitudinal change processes.

In nonexperimental research, it is difficult to determine and assign causation. In many cases, this is true, in part, simply because there is no provision for implementation, let alone deferred evaluation. In the case of the National Commission, there is the opportunity for analysis and assessment over time. And this is such a rare opportunity in social research that it should not be ignored.

It is also true in nonexperimental research that we seldom can determine concomitant variability and temporal relationship simply because we have too many givens in terms of restrictions and time limits. In this particular case, we have baseline data, we have formulated a manageable set of postulates, each of which satisfies the required conditions, and we have the means at our disposal to make observational and statistical comparisons at a designated point in 1976.

Finally, there is the intrinsic need to know what we really accomplished. This would be reason enough to do the longitudinal survey if it were only for self-satisfaction. But the real value may lie in our ability to look over the selected profiles and determine relative success and failure—and thus provide better guidance for other researchers. Perhaps in our shortcomings and "misses" they may find the means to avoid our errors and capitalize on our experience. This, in the end, may be the Commission's most enduring contribution.

Note: At their February 2, 1973 meeting, the Commission unanimously agreed to undertake the proposed follow-up study and directed the staff to plan the necessary arrangements.

Appendix E

THE NATIONAL COMMISSION AND THE LICENSED PRACTICAL/VOCATIONAL NURSE

At the early organizational meetings of the National Commission, it was agreed that the NCSNNE study of nursing should examine the generic problems of nursing. In view of the very real limitations on time and resources, however, the investigation was directed to focus its energy within definite parameters. The commissioners then agreed that the primary inquiry should be aimed at registered nurses (RNs), but, at the same time, recognized that recommendations coming out of this study would be intimately involved with the present practice and future course of licensed practical/vocational nursing.

At the advent of the investigatory phase, the staff and its advisory panels became fully aware that one could not wholly—or practicably—separate licensed practical nursing from registered nursing in any of the three dimensions being examined: practice, education, and career perspectives.

There are today more than 345,000 licensed practical nurses (LPNs), of whom almost 75 percent are actively employed in nursing at any given time.[1] The magnitude of contribution to the health care system provided by these nurses can be seen when we compare their numbers with the 440,000 RNs currently employed full-time. By extrapolation, LPNs occupy roughly 40 percent of the practitioner positions in nursing service across the nation.

In the course of more than 100 site visits to practice settings and educational institutions, the NCSNNE staff also discovered that the problems of the two nurse groups are closely related, similar in nature, and differing most frequently in detail rather than kind. For example, the educational curriculum of the LPN nominally prepares her to practice under the supervision of an RN. Increasingly, however, we find instances of LPNs being designated to serve as charge nurses, supervisors, and even directors of service.

The growing emphasis on distributive health care, also, has increased the opportunities for practical nurses to find challenging employment outside the hospital setting, and there is every reason to assume that, in both episodic and distributive care, LPNs are involved in sophisticated systems requiring decisions and judgmental acts that should be based upon deeper knowledge of health sciences than they may now be provided by their educational programs.

While, at this point, there is little systematic data on the enlarged role of practice for the LPN, a reexamination of the earlier analyses indicates that, for a long time, there has been, in many situations, a considerable overlapping in the functional nursing areas between the LPN and the RN. As revealed in *Sickness and Society*,[2] this has frequently resulted in such a blurring of personnel that distinct roles are difficult to define. It is vital that we give serious consideration to the determination of congruent roles and to the development of rational approaches to utilization.

The educational patterns for LPNs, like those for the RN, are characterized by a variety of institutional forms and curricula. LPN programs may be found in hospitals, community colleges, vocational educational programs, high schools, and a variety of OEO and Health Manpower centers. Preliminary examination again indicates a wide variety of content variation, sharp differences in course length, and, most likely, a wide range in learner outcomes. Certainly, the ability of the student to pass the licensure examination may be a minimal guarantee of knowledge, but by no means an accurate measure of the differences that individuals exhibit because of the imposed internal ceiling effect.

Finally, in terms of career perspectives, we find LPNs facing difficulties in both horizontal and vertical mobility—just as do RNs. These problems are heightened by the variety of institutions and curricular patterns for preparation which make it almost impossible to generalize about what an LPN is or what she/he should be able to do. The need for a general reassessment of our system of rewards and career inducements is quite evident.

In view of these several concerns, the National Commission strongly recommended that an invitational meeting between the NCSNNE, their staff and selected licensed practical/vocational spokesmen, practitioners, and educators be planned to explore further the problem areas. Out of this meeting, it was hoped that mutual understandings would evolve and that suggestions for further activities aimed at tackling the prevailing problems would be identified.

1972 INVITATIONAL CONFERENCE

As an initial step in planning an invitational conference, the NCSNNE staff contacted the major organizations representing licensed practical/vocational nursing—namely, the National Association for Practical Nurse Education and Service (NAPNES), the National Federation of Licensed Practical Nurses (NFLPN), and the National League for Nursing Council of Licensed Practical Nurse Programs. These organizations expressed their support for such a meeting as well as a willingness to participate. Shortly thereafter, the NCSNNE staff again contacted the officials of these organizations and members of the Commission's advisory panels requesting that they submit the names of individuals who are experienced in working on the concerns and problems of licensed practical/vocational nursing. Approximately sixty persons representing a wide variety of experience and knowledge were nominated to assist the Commission. From this initial list, some twenty-eight individuals, including licensed practical/vocational nurses, administrators, employers, consumers, officers, and executives of national organizations, were selected for participation in the planned meeting. The number of invitees was limited so that maximum opportunity for discussion and comment, during the two-day meeting, would be available. At the same time, these individuals seemed representative of all the varied points of view in the field.

The Invitational Conference on Issues in Licensed Practical/Vocational Nursing was held on October 24-25, 1972, in Rochester, New York. Of those invited, twenty-four persons attended. The participants included:

Edith Ankers, Director, Columbia Presbyterian School of Practical Nursing, New York, New York.

Ola Caldwell, Director, Postgraduate Practical Nurse Vocational Program, Dallas, Texas.

Evelyn Chamberlin, Member, Board of Vocational Nurse Examiners, Sacramento, California.

Elizabeth V. Cunningham, former Editor, NAPNES publications, Mastic, New York.

Jerald S. DeWeerd, Director, Nursing Education, Pine Rest Christian Hospital, School of Practical Nursing, Grand Rapids, Michigan.

Sallie Draney, Educational Coordinator, Licensed Practical Nurses of New York, Inc., New York, New York.

Ruth Edelson, Chairman, Council of Practical Nursing Programs, National League for Nursing, New York, New York.

Grace Estes, Licensed Practical Nurse Practitioner, Midwest City, Oklahoma.

Helen Feeney, Coordinator, Continuing Education and Community Services, Queensboro Community College of the City of New York, Bayside, New York.

Ethel P. Franklin, Director, Dodge City Community College, Department of Practical Nursing Education, Dodge City, Kansas.

Shirley Mannion, State Supervisor, Health Occupations Education, State Department Vocational Education, Phoenix, Arizona.

Rose Martin, Executive Director, National Association for Practical Nurse Education and Service, New York, New York.

Ruth Morrison, Assistant Director, Professional Examinations Division, The Psychological Corporation, New York, New York.

Ronald Nichols, Director, Shepard-Gill School of Practical Nursing, Massachusetts General Hospital, Boston, Massachusetts.

Jean Poulos, Licensed Vocational Nurse Practitioner, Santa Cruz, California.

Pearl Rasin, President, Licensed Practical Nurses of New York, Inc., New York, New York.

Sandra Rasmussen, Research Associate, Department of Behavioral Sciences, Harvard School of Public Health, Boston, Massachusetts.

Mary Rhode, Licensed Practical Nurse Practitioner, Bismarck, North Dakota.

Mary Runnels, President, National Federation of Licensed Practical Nurses, Inc., New York, New York.

Etta Schmidt, Executive Director, National Federation of Licensed Practical Nurses, Inc., New York, New York.

Mildred Smith, President, National Association for Practical Nurse Education and Service, New York, New York.

Sister Mary J. Walsh, Director, Department of Practical Nursing, National League for Nursing, New York, New York.

Pauline Wright, Executive Director, Tennessee Licensed Practical Nurses Association, Nashville, Tennessee.

Lillian Zeffaro, Administrator, Van Dyk Manor Nursing Home, Montclair, New Jersey.

Prior to the invitational conference, background materials including general information about the major concerns of LPNs, a profile of one state's specific problems relating to licensed practical nursing, and a preliminary agenda were mailed to each attendee so that she/he could review them before the meeting.

The primary purpose of the invitational conference was to provide an opportunity for the exploration and discussion of key issues affecting the present and future of licensed practical/vocational nurses, particularly: roles and functions, including the changing demands placed upon LPNs; educational patterns, especially the problems of upward mobility and articulation; and career perspectives, particularly as future health care trends are projected.

The two-day program included general sessions which were moderated by: Ms. Joan Guy and Mr. Stuart Marylander, members of the NCSNNE, and Robert Hoekelman, MD, Chairman, National Joint Practice Commission; NCSNNE staff members also participated. The moderators introduced the topic for discussion and identified the primary objectives and related problems relevant to that topic. During the general sessions, the conference participants shared much information on a variety of subjects which pertained to the three designated, general areas of concern. Briefly, the major topics discussed were:

1. definition of the role of beginning practitioners and the expanding practice of the LPN.
2. action by RNs toward understanding and accepting the educational role, stated functions, and job descriptions of the LPN so that both might practice nursing efficiently and effectively as integral members of the nursing team.
3. identification of curricular objectives for basic practical nursing programs and establishment of goals for continuing education programs.
4. preparation of educators who can and will develop a core foundation for nursing within an overall pattern of preparatory and continuing education.
5. identification of occupational competencies for each level of nursing.
6. articulation among existing nursing education programs to facilitate lateral and vertical mobility as desired by the individual student and practitioner.
7. recognition of previous learning experiences and provision of a variety of career opportunities for the LPN.
8. continuing education system to develop or maintain occupational competencies and provide advanced credit standing for the individual practitioner and student.

During the third general session, which was primarily devoted to problems related to career perspectives, the draft of a study proposal for licensed practical/vocational nursing was introduced, and a copy given to each conference participant. The inability of the NCSNNE to undertake such a study, due to lack of funds and limited staff, was discussed. During the dialogue, several participants commented that the proposal would be useful and suggested that NAPNES, NFLPN, and the NLN jointly support such a study.

The final session of the meeting was devoted to focusing on suggestions for solutions to particular problems discussed in the previous sessions. Using a group conference technique—the Delbecq System[3]—participants were then divided into three groups. Each person within the group was directed to identify, list, and rank order, in each area of concern (practice, education, and career), three major problems, proposed actions or solutions to those problems, and suggested agencies which could assist with the specified actions. These issues were then discussed among the members within each of the groups and, afterwards, given to the staff for recording.

Prior to the adjournment of the conference, the President of the NFLPN submitted to the total conference group the following resolution:

> Be it resolved that this Conference request that the NCSNNE include practical nursing in its final report as an integral part of nursing; and Be it further resolved that the NCSNNE request that the representation on the NJPC and its state components be expanded to include the licensed practical/vocational nurse.

This resolution was agreed to unanimously by the participants with a single abstention recorded.

As a follow-up to the last session of the invitational conference, the NCSNNE staff prepared a composite of the priorities and concerns which evolved from each group during the final session. This information was then mailed to the conference participants shortly after the meeting.

To gain feedback from the meeting participants, the NCSNNE staff requested the attendees to submit their reactions and comments regarding the conference as a whole, the follow-up summary of priorities, and the proposed study for licensed practical/vocational nursing. Of all the participants, only nine persons (38 percent) responded. In general, the respondents expressed favorable comments regarding the meeting. They found the conference to be stimulating, worthwhile, and helpful as well as providing an opportunity to exchange viewpoints and learn from each other. In addition, most of the respondents strongly recommended that an independent study to explore, in greater depth, the three areas of expressed concern related to licensed practical/vocational nursing be pursued further. It was felt that such an investigation is essential and would be of significance in identifying the past, present, and future trends in licensed practical/vocational nursing.

In summary, the invitational conference achieved its purpose of providing the NCSNNE a forum to share the many facets of problems and concerns related to licensed practical/vocational nursing with individuals possessing a diversity of viewpoints and backgrounds in this field.

PRIORITIES ESTABLISHED BY CONFERENCE PARTICIPANTS

In determining those activities that should be taken up with regard to licensed practical nursing and its relationship to registered nursing and the health care delivery system as a whole, the conference participants, through a series of structured discussions and acting as small group task forces in each of three areas, developed a forced-choice listing of objectives and priorities. To some extent, these mirror the concerns and the prepotency of feelings held by many LPNs (and RNs as well). For its possible utility in shaping further study, these items are listed as arranged by the participants' task forces. Numbers in brackets refer to the relative weight assigned by the members of the related discussion group and are only significant for comparison within the single area—not across areas.

Area: Practice, Roles and Functions

A. Definition, identification, and examination of roles and functions in licensed practical nursing. (40)
   1. Define roles and functions of LPNs.
   2. Determine the roles of LPNs in interaction with RNs and other health practitioners.
   3. Standardize the roles and functions of LPNs across state and national levels.

4. Identify and examine the expanded role of the LPN in episodic and distributive health care.

B. Identification and examination of the utilization of the LPN. (35)
   1. Identify the proper utilization and responsibilities of the LPN in various settings.
   2. Formulate job descriptions for LPNs.
   3. Identify ways to improve quality of care provided by LPNs through joint efforts with RNs.

C. Improvement of communication among health team members. (30)
   1. Identify ways to gain acceptance of LPNs among health team members, particularly RNs and MDs.
   2. Recognize the contribution of LPNs to the health care delivery system by health team members.
   3. Determine ways to help health care members, particularly RNs, function with LPNs efficiently and effectively as integral members of the health team.

D. Identification and solution of the legal problems related to the practice of LPNs. (14)
   1. Identify legal limitations and restrictions imposed on the LPN by the state Nurse Practice Acts.
   2. Examine the possibilities of a national licensure for the LPN/LVN.
   3. Identify and propose remedies for legal problems that may evolve from role changes of the LPN.
   4. Suggest and provide ways to involve LPNs on boards of nursing, health professional groups, and other associations concerned with legal aspects of the LPN.

E. Identification and suggestions for how LPNs can enhance their practice. (2)
   1. Identify factors which facilitate or hinder acquisition of skills and knowledge relating to practice.
   2. Provide model in-service programs (continuing education) aimed at current developments which affect the role and functions of LPNs.

Area: Education

A. Identification and examination of problems, and proposed changes, in basic education for practical nursing. (73)
   1. Identify and examine the essentials in a basic nursing program (core curricula) for the LPN to reduce the wide variation in programs.
      a. Identify curricular objectives for an LPN program.
      b. Recommend an LPN program (curriculum) at the state and/or national level.
   2. Define and identify admission requirements.
   3. Identify criteria for selecting applicants into LPN programs.
   4. Recommend, at state and national levels, a standard for selecting applicants for the LPN programs.

5. Recognize that practical nursing education includes components of basic preparatory programs for all nursing.
6. Identify and develop occupational competencies for each level of nursing.
7. Examine restrictions imposed upon LPN programs because of legal and/or state board requirements.
8. Examine the possibilities of national accreditation for LPN programs.
9. Improve the public's view of the licensed practical nurse.

B. Identification and assessment of issues in continuing education programs. (18)
   1. Identify and determine the essentials in continuing education for LPNs.
   2. Identify and establish goals for continuing education programs.
   3. Explore and recommend means for increasing the availability of continuing education for relicensure.
   4. Assess and evaluate the validity of courses offered to fulfill legal requirements for continuing education for relicensure.
   5. Identify criteria for continuing education that will serve as a guide toward changing career goals.
   6. Develop refresher courses for the LPN returning to practice.

C. Identification and examination of articulation among the nursing programs. (24)
   1. Identify and provide ways to enhance understanding and articulation among the various nursing programs in order to facilitate vertical and horizontal mobility as desired by the individual practitioner.
   2. Suggest ways for improving articulation among existing preparatory and continuing education programs in nursing.
   3. Encourage LPNs toward upward mobility.
   4. Identify and assess qualifications of LPNs who desire to advance their education.

D. Identification, examination, and recommendations for recognition of experience and education of the LPN. (20)
   1. Recognize previous learning experiences through proficiency examination and equivalent college credit.
   2. Develop additional evaluation tools for articulation purposes.

E. Facilitation of communication and understanding of practical nursing among nurse educators. (11)
   1. Identify the perceptions of RNs toward LPN education as part of the overall pattern of nursing education.
   2. Suggest ways to facilitate and improve communication and understanding among all educators as well as with employers of LPNs.
   3. Prepare educators who can and will develop a core foundation for nursing within an overall pattern of preparatory and continuing education.
   4. Encourage team teaching among nursing educators and students.
   5. Encourage nursing educators to be innovative in regard to curricula.

F. Encouragement of organizational support to enhance the practice and education of LPNs. (4)
   1. Examine the need for strong organizational relationship among LPN educators.
   2. Encourage LPNs to assume responsibility in groups concerned with the delivery of health care and education of nurses.

Area: Career

A. Recognition and acceptance of licensed practical nursing. (30)
   1. Identify and recognize practical nursing as a career choice.
   2. Identify practical nursing as an integral part of nursing.
   3. Identify and recognize the LPN's potential for further growth and development in nursing practice.
   4. Identify the roles of other health care delivery personnel and their relationship with LPNs.
   5. Recognize, encourage, and provide opportunities for LPNs to become involved with various groups concerned with health planning at all levels—state, regional, and national.

B. Identification and assistance in the development of career mobility. (29)
   1. Examine the barriers which inhibit LPNs from further advancement.
   2. Study and identify the variety of career opportunities for LPNs.
   3. Identify the availability of opportunities for horizontal and vertical mobility for LPNs.
   4. Identify an understanding of and encourage a commitment to a career ladder on the part of nurse educators.
   5. Develop curricular designs/models to assist educators in planning for upward mobility.
   6. Establish a clearinghouse for obtaining and disseminating information related to mobility and articulation among the nursing programs.

C. Encouragement and assistance in career counseling. (4)
   1. Provide career counseling to high school students who are interested in entering a nursing program.
   2. Provide career counseling to LPNs who desire to further their education.

D. Identification and examination of health care provided by LPNs. (6)
   1. Examine whether practical nursing programs are producing products which are filling the health needs in the community.
   2. Examine the health care expectations that employers have of LPNs.
   3. Assess the system of rewards available to LPNs for providing health care.

LICENSED PRACTICAL NURSING STUDY PROPOSAL

In early 1971, pursuant to a request from the National Commission for a range of alternative actions related to licensed practical nursing, the NCSNNE staff developed a preliminary proposal for conducting a national study of licensed practical/vocational nursing that would be modeled after, and structured upon, the findings and data previously developed. To obtain some independent and expert criticism, the draft was transmitted to Dr. Ivan J. Fahs of Research Coordinators, Inc., and former director of the Upper Midwest Study of Nursing. After he made several suggestions for modification and addition, the revised copy of the draft was then presented to the commissioners for their consideration.

Upon reflection, the Commission agreed that such a study might assist in resolving some concerns regarding the role and future of the LPN, and that it would be most economical and logical to provide NCSNNE study data and materials for such an effort. At the same time, the Commission's implementation schedule and resources simply made it impossible for them or their staff to undertake the enlarged scope of such an activity. It was agreed, therefore, that the proposal and related background information would be supplied, if desired, to the appropriate LPN organizations for their use, either as the basis for an investigation, or as a preliminary document in the development of a new proposal.

The study proposal was provided for and discussed by the participants of the October, 1972 invitational conference held in Rochester, New York. Certain portions of the proposal, such as a suggested timetable, obviously were already in need of revision, but the primary concern was the objectives, methodology, and organizational support for such an investigation. Briefly noted, the general methodology and approaches suggested were those of a normative, descriptive study modeled on those described in the appendices to *An Abstract for Action.*[4] An extensive literature and data survey would be conducted, together with site visits to educational and service facilities. A national advisory council would be designated and liaison committees established between the study staff and the national organizations representing LPNs. The broad objectives of the inquiry would be to:

1. Determine current and emergent trends in licensed practical nursing practice, to relate these to the health care needs of the American public in both episodic and distributive settings, and to recommend changes in roles and functions of LPNs and other related workers that would enhance the quality and quantity of care provided.

2. Assess current patterns and curricula in education of licensed practical nursing, to measure these in terms of current and emerging practice patterns, and to recommend changes in patterns and content that would lead to better practice and to enhanced opportunities for the individual to continue formal education, if desired, beyond the preparatory stage.

3. Assess current patterns and levels of career perspectives for licensed practical nursing, including both upward and horizontal mobility opportunities; consider licensing and accreditation in terms of recommended changes in practice and education; and to propose alterations in career perspectives that could enhance the quality and quantity of health care while ensuring a satisfactory manpower base of competent practitioners.

As one portion of the follow-up to the conference, participants were asked to respond specifically to the study proposal and criticize any and all portions of it. The general reaction from all replies was favorable and no specific changes other than those related to the recasting of dates, timetables, and the like were proposed. The NCSNNE staff indicated its willingness to assist the LPN organizations in investigating possible support for this effort and in updating and strengthening the proposal. Further action must, however, be dependent upon initiatives taken by the LPN groups.

FOOTNOTES

1. *Facts About Nursing, 1970-71 Edition.* New York: American Nurses' Association, 1972. pp. 171-184.
2. Duff, R. S. and A. B. Hollingshead. *Sickness and Society.* New York: Harper and Row, 1968.
3. Delbecq, Andre L. and Andrew H. Van de Ven. "A Group Process Model For Problem Identification and Program Planning." Madison, Wisconsin: The University of Wisconsin Graduate School of Business. *mimeo,* undated.
4. The National Commission for the Study of Nursing and Nursing Education. *An Abstract for Action: Appendices.* Jerome P. Lysaught, Director. New York: McGraw-Hill Book Company., 1971. "Appendix A. Methodology of the Study." pp. 1-22.